HIV/AIDS Related Communication, Hearing, and Swallowing Disorders

WITHDRAWN

HIV/AIDS Related Communication, Hearing, and Swallowing Disorders

WITHDRAWN

De Wet Swanepoel, Ph.D.
Brenda Louw, Ph.D.

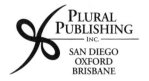

PLURAL
PUBLISHING
INC.
SAN DIEGO
OXFORD
BRISBANE

9194

kH

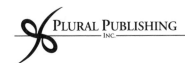

PLURAL PUBLISHING
INC.

5521 Ruffin Road
San Diego, CA 92123

e-mail: info@pluralpublishing.com
Web site: http://www.pluralpublishing.com

49 Bath Street
Abingdon, Oxfordshire OX14 1EA
United Kingdom

FSC

Mixed Sources
Product group from well-managed
forests and other controlled sources

Cert no. SW-COC-002283
www.fsc.org
© 1996 Forest Stewardship Council

Typeset in 11/13 Garamond book by Flanagan's Publishing Services, Inc.
Printed in the United States of America by McNaughton & Gunn

Library of Congress Cataloging-in-Publication Data

HIV/AIDS related communication, hearing and swallowing disorders / [edited by] De Wet Swanepoel and Brenda Louw.
     p. ; cm.
   Includes bibliographical references and index.
   ISBN-13: 978-1-59756-262-1 (alk. paper)
   ISBN-10: 1-59756-262-9 (alk. paper)
    1. Communicative disorders. 2. Ear—Diseases. 3. Hearing disorders.
4. Deglutition disorders. 5. AIDS (Disease)—Complications. 6. Neurologic manifestations of general diseases. I. Swanepoel, De Wet. II. Louw, Brenda.
   [DNLM: 1. HIV Infections—complications. 2. Acquired Immunodeficiency Syndrome—complications. 3. Communication Disorders—etiology. 4. Deglutition Disorders—etiology. 5. Hearing Disorders—etiology. WC 503.5 H6753 2009]
   RC423.H58 2009
   362.196'9792—dc22
                                                              2009030699

10/13/19

Contents

Preface   vii

Contributors   ix

SECTION I. BACKGROUND

Chapter 1.   Global Perspective on HIV/AIDS and   1
               Associated Communication, Hearing, and
               Swallowing Disorders
               De Wet Swanepoel and Brenda Louw

Chapter 2.   Pathogenesis of HIV Infection and Disease   11
               Progression
               Lynne M. Webber

Chapter 3.   Diagnosis and Management of HIV/AIDS   31
               Linda-Gail Bekker

Chapter 4.   Infection Control for Communication,   63
               Hearing, and Swallowing Disorders
               A. U. Bankaitis

Chapter 5.   Psychosocial Impact of HIV/AIDS in   97
               Communication Disorders
               Irma Eloff

Chapter 6.   Ethical Challenges in HIV Research and   115
               Clinical Care
               Ann Bartley Williams

SECTION II. COMMUNICATION DISORDERS

Chapter 7.   Communication Disorders in Children with   135
HIV/AIDS
Thomas L. Layton and Jianping (Grace) Hao

Chapter 8.   Communication Disorders in Adults with   173
HIV/AIDS
Lemmietta McNeilly

SECTION III. AUDITORY AND BALANCE DISORDERS

Chapter 9.   External and Middle Ear Disorders Associated   195
with HIV/AIDS
*Ivan Dieb Miziara, Ali Mahmoud, Raimar
Weber, Fernanda Alves Sanjar, and Bárbara
Elvina Ulisses Parente Queiroz*

Chapter 10.   Sensory and Neural Auditory Disorders   243
Associated with HIV/AIDS
Natalie Stearn and De Wet Swanepoel

Chapter 11.   Balance Disorders Associated with HIV/AIDS   289
Louis Hofmeyr and Malcolm Baker

SECTION IV. SWALLOWING AND FEEDING DISORDERS

Chapter 12.   Dysphagia and Related Assessment and   351
Management in Children with HIV/AIDS
Hilda Pressman

Chapter 13.   Dysphagia and Related Assessment and   385
Management in Adults with HIV/AIDS
Alexandra M. Stipinovich

Index   421

Preface

Disorders in communication, hearing, or swallowing are almost universally associated with HIV/AIDS. Unfortunately, these have largely been overlooked or masked by more acute and clinically obvious conditions. The fact that the majority of these disorders may not be life threatening does not, however, diminish their importance as foundational elements to quality of life and the ability to live as an integrated and active member of a community. In addition, the advent of highly active antiretroviral therapies has introduced an era in which HIV/AIDS can be managed as a chronic, rather than an acute, condition. Against this background, the imperative to provide persons living with HIV/AIDS with the necessary intervention for communication, hearing, balance, and swallowing disorders, becomes a pressing concern. This book is the first comprehensive text to address these neglected aspects of the HIV/AIDS epidemic across the life span. It is intended to serve as a complete resource for health care professionals, including speech-language pathologists, audiologists, otolaryngologists, primary care physicians, and nurses who provide services to persons living with HIV/AIDS.

Bringing together the accumulated experience and knowledge of a multidisciplinary group of internationally recognized clinicians and academics, this text applies current theoretical understanding and personal experience to clinical settings. Background chapters on the pathogenesis, medical diagnosis, and management of HIV/AIDS serve as a general orientation to the field. Novel aspects are also addressed in several chapters including HIV/AIDS associated balance disorders, the psychosocial impact of HIV/AIDS, ethical considerations, and infection control. Specific sections on the nature, diagnosis, and treatment of communication, auditory, and swallowing disorders across the life span, constitute the main focus of the text. Information is structured for easy access with concise updates on the theoretical underpinnings of communication, hearing, and swallowing disorders associated with HIV/AIDS, while including clinical strategies for identification, diagnosis, and intervention across all ages. The combination of communication, auditory, balance, and swallowing disorders associated with HIV/AIDS in a single text makes it the first comprehensive reference and clinical resource in the field.

It is our hope that the main beneficiaries of this text will be the persons living with HIV/AIDS through the dedicated efforts of the health care providers who serve them.

De Wet Swanepoel
Brenda Louw

Contributors

Malcolm Kevin Baker, M.D.
Professor and Consultant
  Neurologist
South African Military Health
  Services
University of Pretoria
Medical University of South Africa
Institute of Aviation Medicine,
  South Africa
Chapter 11

A. U. Bankaitis, Ph.D.
Vice President
Oaktree Products, Inc.
St. Louis, Missouri
Chapter 4

**Linda-Gail Bekker, MBChB,
DCH, DTM&H, FCP(SA), Ph.D.**
Associate Professor
Desmond Tutu HIV Foundation
University of Cape Town, Faculty
  of Health Sciences
Cape Town, South Africa
Chapter 3

Irma Eloff, Ph.D.
Professor and Dean
Faculty of Education
University of Pretoria
Pretoria, South Africa
Chapter 5

**Jianping Grace Hao, M.D.,
Ph.D.**
Associate Professor
Department of Communication
  Disorders
North Carolina Central
  University
Durham, North Carolina
Chapter 7

Louis Murray Hofmeyr, M.D.
Lt. Colonel
Chief ENT Surgeon of the South
  African National Defense
  Force(SANDF)
1 Military Hospital, Pretoria
Affiliated Extraordinary Lecturer
  at the Department of
  Otorhinolaryngology,
School of Medicine
University of Pretoria
Pretoria, South Africa
Chapter 11

Thomas L. Layton, Ph.D.
Professor and Chair
Department of Communication
  Disorders
North Carolina Central
  University
Durham, North Carolina
Chapter 7

Brenda Louw, Ph.D.
Professor Emeritus
Department of Communication
  Pathology
University of Pretoria
Pretoria, South Africa
Professor and Chair
Department of Communicative
  Disorders
East Tennessee State University
Johnson City, Tennessee
Chapter 1

Ali Mahmoud, M.D.
Division of Otolaryngology
Hospital das Clínicas
São Paulo University School of
  Medicine
São Paulo, Brazil
Chapter 9

**Lemmietta G. McNeilly, Ph.D.,
CCC-SLP, F-ASHA**
Chief Staff Officer, Speech-
  Language Pathology
American Speech-Language-
  Hearing Association
Rockville, Maryland
Chapter 8

Ivan D. Miziara, M.D., Ph.D.
Professor
Division of Otolaryngology
Hospital das Clínicas
São Paulo University School of
  Medicine
São Paulo, Brazil
Chapter 9

**Hilda Pressman, M.A., CCC-
SLP, BRS-S**
Principle Nutritional
  Management Associates LLC
West Orange, New Jersey
Chapter 12

Barbara E. U. P. Queiroz, M.D.
Division of Otolaryngology
Hospital das Clínicas
São Paulo University School of
  Medicine
São Paulo, Brazil
Chapter 9

**Natalie Anne Stearn,
M. CommPath**
Clinical Audiologist
Cape Town, South Africa
Chapter 10

Fernanda A. Sanjar, M.D.
Division of Otolaryngology
Hospital das Clínicas
São Paulo University School of
  Medicine
São Paulo, Brazil
Chapter 9

**Alexandra Maria Stipinovich
M. CommPath**
Speech-Language Pathologist
Department of Communication
  Pathology
University of Pretoria
Pretoria, South Africa
Chapter 13

De Wet Swanepoel, Ph.D.
Associate Professor
Department of Communication
  Pathology
University of Pretoria
Pretoria, South Africa
Adjunct Professor
Callier Center for
  Communication Disorders
School of Behavioral and Brain
  Sciences
University of Texas
Dallas, Texas
Chapters 1 and 10

Lynne M. Webber, M.D.
Head of Department
Department of Medical
  Virology
University of Pretoria

Pretoria, South Africa
Chapter 2

Raimar Weber, M.D.
Otolaryngology and Facial Plastic
  Surgery
Division of Otolaryngology—
  Hospital das Clínicas
São Paulo University School of
  Medicine
São Paulo, Brazil
Chapter 9

**Ann Bartley Williams, RN,
EdD**
Professor of Nursing and
  Medicine
Yale University
New Haven, Connecticut
Chapter 6

Dedicated to all children living with the direct or indirect consequences of HIV/AIDS and its associated sequelae.

These vulnerable victims demonstrate extraordinary courage.

CHAPTER 1

Global Perspective on HIV/AIDS and Associated Communication, Hearing, and Swallowing Disorders

De Wet Swanepoel and Brenda Louw

INTRODUCTION

Since the first reports describing the human immunodeficiency virus (HIV) as the primary cause of acquired immunodeficiency syndrome (AIDS) appeared in 1983, the HIV/AIDS pandemic has emerged as the top priority on current global health agenda (Barre-Sinoussi et al, 1983; Shiffman, 2006). The extent of its global reach and its pervasive and devastating nature has ensured that HIV/AIDS is the health care challenge of our time. Its effects are far reaching and impact not only those infected, but also the wider family, community, and societal structures.

Unfortunately, those who are most vulnerable suffer worst under the scourge of the pandemic—the poor, women, and children, and those living with disabilities. The complex relationship of HIV/AIDS

1

and disability hinges on an increased risk of acquiring disabling conditions related to the infection and its propensity to affect the most vulnerable, that is, persons with disabilities prior to HIV infection. In the case of disabling disorders in communication, hearing, and swallowing, this dual effect is seen most clearly in the increased occurrence of disabilities associated with HIV/AIDS and those living with such disabling disorders prior to infection being more vulnerable to HIV/AIDS (Groce, 2003; World Bank, 2004). The global extent of the HIV/AIDS pandemic means these effects are becoming increasingly widespread with associated disabilities proliferating, and increasing numbers of disabled individuals being infected with the virus.

GLOBAL EPIDEMIOLOGY OF HIV/AIDS

The number of persons living with HIV worldwide, estimated by the joint United Nations program on HIV/AIDS in 2007, was 33.2 million but may be as high as 36.1 million (UNAIDS, 2008). This means that everyday more than 6,800 persons are infected with HIV and more than 5,700 persons die daily as a result of AIDS (UNAIDS, 2008).

Although the global prevalence of persons infected with HIV is now remaining the same, the number of persons living with HIV/AIDS is increasing because of longer survival times in the context of a growing general population (UNAIDS, 2008). There are large differences in the incidence and prevalence of HIV/AIDS across and within world regions. Table 1–1 provides an overview of the global HIV/AIDS epidemic across world regions. Sub-Saharan Africa clearly is most affected by the global pandemic with two-thirds of all persons infected with HIV. Many countries in the region, especially in southern Africa, indicate national prevalence rates exceeding 15%. In this region of the world, HIV/AIDS has moved beyond an epidemic concentrated among populations at risk (i.e., injecting drug users, sex workers and their partners, men who have sex with men) to become a generalized epidemic sustained in the general population of many Sub-Saharan African countries (UNAIDS, 2008). HIV/AIDS remains the leading cause of death in this region with more than three in every four global HIV/AIDS-related deaths in 2007 occurring there.

Other world regions (i.e., East Asia, South, and Southeast Asia) present with much lower prevalence rates that are concentrated

Table 1–1. Global HIV/AIDS Epidemic

	HIV-Infected Persons	*HIV Adult Prevalence (%)*	*New Infections (per day)*	*Deaths From AIDS (per day)*
Sub-Saharan Africa	22.5 million	5.0	4,700	4,400
South and Southeast Asia	4.0 million	0.3	900	740
Eastern Europe and Central Asia	1.6 million	0.9	410	210
Latin America	1.6 million	0.5	270	160
North America	1.3 million	0.1	130	60
East Asia	800,000	0.3	250	90
Western and Central Europe	760,000	0.6	80	30
North Africa and Middle East	380,000	1.0	100	70
Caribbean	23,000	0.3	50	30
Australia, New Zealand and Pacific Region	75,000	0.4	40	3
TOTAL	*33.2 million*	*0.8*	*6,900*	*5,800*

Source: Adapted from UNAIDS (2008).

primarily in at-risk populations. Low national prevalence rates may, however, conceal serious epidemics such as HIV/AIDS, which initially are concentrated in specific population groups or localities but may spread to larger population sectors to become a more generalized epidemic (Kamps & Hoffmann, 2007).

Women

The tendency for HIV/AIDS to affect vulnerable populations most severely has had devastating effects on women. Globally, the ratio of men and women living with HIV/AIDS has remained stable and evenly divided but in sub-Saharan Africa, where it is a generalized population epidemic, women are far worse off with almost 61% of adults living with HIV in 2007 being women (UNAIDS, 2008). In 2006 prevalence rates of HIV/AIDS among women (15–49 years of age) attending antenatal clinics varied between 1 in every 3 to 1 in every 4 women. The prevalence rate for women of childbearing age (15-49 years of age) in South Africa, for example, is 29% and it is as high as 39% in Swaziland. Other world regions report much lower prevalence rates among women, but these appear to be increasing. In 2007 the percentage of women living with HIV/AIDS compared to men varied between 26 to 43% in these regions (UNAIDS, 2008). Women also bear the brunt of stigmatization in developing countries, as well as the emotional burden of mother-to-child transmission of the virus.

Children

The HIV/AIDS epidemic is a continuing scourge on those most vulnerable—infants and children. In 2007 an estimated 2.5 million children were living with HIV/AIDS around the world of which almost 90% reside in Sub-Saharan Africa. The global childhood deaths attributable to HIV/AIDS in 2007 were estimated at 380,000. Unfortunately the vast majority of these deaths were preventable, either through treating opportunistic infections with antibiotics or through antiretroviral treatment (UNICEF, UNAIDS, & WHO, 2007). The overwhelming majority of children with HIV/AIDS acquired it through vertical transmission from mother to child (Bond Horvath, Harvey, Wiysonge, & Read, 2007). Globally, approximately 1 in every 3 children born to HIV-infected mothers, contract the virus through this easily preventable transmission route. In addition to the direct effects for those infected, other children may not be infected but are severely affected by the scourge of the HIV/AIDS pandemic. In 2006 at least 15.2 million children under the age of 18 had lost at least one parent to HIV/AIDS and many millions more were made vulnerable. The millions of children affected by HIV/AIDS in any of these ways greatly increase their risk for poverty, homelessness, poor education, loss of opportunities, and early death (UNICEF, UNAIDS, & WHO, 2007).

People with Disabilities

A growing body of literature indicates that persons with physical, sensory (deafness, blindness), or intellectual disabilities are at a significantly increased risk of HIV infection (Groce, 2003; World Bank, 2004). The estimated 600 million persons living with a disability, 80% of whom reside in the developing world, are among the most vulnerable populations, often destined to be most stigmatized and poorest and least educated (Groce, 2003; Groce & Trasi, 2004; WHA, 2005). The risk factors for HIV/AIDS and for people with disabilities are very closely linked. For example, people with disabilities are more likely to be the poorest of the poor, to be poorly educated about sex, to be more vulnerable to sexual abuse, and to be at higher risk for substance abuse. All these factors are risks for a higher prevalence of HIV infection (World Bank, 2004). Initial reports from an international survey have confirmed that in all countries persons with disabilities were at a significant risk of becoming HIV infected (World Bank, 2004). Those with communication disorders such as hearing loss, are especially at risk because most of the information campaigns to educate and empower people with knowledge regarding HIV/AIDS may be inaccessible or inappropriate to individuals with such disabilities. The educational barriers for deaf and hard-of-hearing persons often lead to poor educational outcomes, which may furthermore inhibit their ability to obtain and process information (World Bank, 2004). Unfortunately, HIV/AIDS in people with disabilities has been a marginalized issue and much work remains to be done to accurately ascertain the extent, and closely related nature, of HIV/AIDS and disability, toward developing effective interventions.

LIVING WITH HIV/AIDS

Although no cure has yet been found for the HIV/AIDS epidemic, the advent of effective treatment regimens in the form of antiretroviral (ARV) therapies have changed the nature of HIV/AIDS from a terminal illness to a manageable, chronic condition for those with access to these therapies (Gifford & Groesel, 2002; Russel et al., 2007). At present the majority of individuals living with HIV/AIDS do not have access to ARV therapies with an estimated 31% of the 9 million people in need of treatment, as reported in December 2007, actually receiving it (WHO, 2008). However, there have, been significant improvements in access to treatment as evidenced by a 60% increase from 2005 to 2006 in HIV-positive pregnant women who received ARV prophylaxis to reduce mother-to-child transmission and a 70% increase in HIV-positive children who benefited from treatment in 2006 compared to 2005 (UNICEF, UNAIDS, & WHO, 2008). United global efforts to provide access to ARV therapies are reaching an ever increasing number of people with the goal of universal access to treatment set for 2010 (WHO, 2008).

The changing face of HIV/AIDS from a fatal to a chronic disease is resulting in a shift of emphasis to conditions associated with HIV/AIDS that may not necessarily be life threatening, but may impact the quality of life for individuals. Living with HIV/AIDS as a chronic condition still has a significant impact on the quality of life for affected individuals due to the pervasive effect of HIV/AIDS on the human body. There is a significant increase in disabilities secondary to HIV/AIDS, which may restrict societal participation, limit educational and vocational opportunities, exacerbate stigmatization, and severely diminish quality of life. Even though the effects may not be life threatening, their significance should not be underestimated. Health, after all, is not only the absence of disease but the total well-being of an individual, and HIV/AIDS managed as a chronic condition is a still a severe threat to the well-being of a person and his or her quality of life (Russel et al., 2007). As such, these associated conditions require serious consideration in addressing the total effect of HIV/AIDS on persons' health. This book addresses the disorders associated with HIV/AIDS in communication, hearing, balance, and swallowing as well as related aspects such as the psychosocial impact, ethics, and background information on disease pathogenesis, progression, treatment, and infection control.

Communication and Hearing Disorders

Communication and hearing disorders associated with HIV/AIDS are not life threatening but have a major, and underestimated, impact on quality of life. The occurrence of these disorders secondary to HIV/AIDS is much higher than in the general population and has been estimated to be as high as 75% in adults living with HIV/AIDS (Zuniga, 1999). This may be even more pronounced in children infected with HIV as they are more vulnerable to common opportunistic infections and to the direct effects of the virus on the central nervous system as well as associated developmental delays and disorders. Disorders that affect communication are very important as they may rob individuals of their means of accessing the world in which they live. Effective communication is at the heart of being human and allows us to connect and engage with each other. Any disruption in effective communication, whether in the faculty of language, speech, or hearing, therefore strikes at the heart of what constitutes quality of life and well-being for individuals. The complex interrelationship between communication, hearing, and the compromised immune system of persons living with HIV/AIDS requires a better understanding through continued investigations. It is imperative, however, that these conditions be recognized as important sequelae of HIV/AIDS that require appropriate and timely intervention to ensure optimal quality of life outcomes.

Balance Disorders

Despite a dearth of detailed population-based studies on HIV/AIDS associated balance disorders, and the fact that vertigo probably has been underreported due to the presence of more life-threatening and therefore more obvious symptoms, current evidence points toward frequent disturbances in balance functioning as a result of HIV/AIDS (Davis, Rarey, &Mclaren, 1995; Lalwani & Sooy, 1992; Marra et al., 1997; Teggi, Giardino, Pistprio, & Bisso., 2006). A disturbance in adequate maintenance of balance is a significant risk for fall accidents especially in elderly patients and also is an important consideration for ensuring quality of life.

Swallowing and Feeding Disorders

Disorders in swallowing not only are potentially life threatening but also are a severe threat to quality of life. It is the natural means by which food and liquids are taken to provide the necessary sustenance for daily functioning and ultimately for survival. For most people, the complex process of swallowing, which relies on highly coordinated neuromuscular interactions, is taken entirely for granted. In stark contrast, individuals living with HIV/AIDS often encounter significant difficulties with swallowing and feeding, which, if not life threatening, may have devastating effects on a person's quality of life (Bladon & Ross, 2007). The impact of a swallowing and feeding disorder is insidious and may be far reaching especially when invasive nonoral feeding methods are the only option.

SUMMARY

In just over 25 years since its first description, HIV/AIDS has turned into a worldwide epidemic, often described as a pandemic in Sub-Saharan Africa, and is at the top of global health priorities. As universal access to ARV therapies is being sought globally, the services for individuals living with HIV/AIDS require a change in perspective to reflect the chronic nature of the condition when managed with current treatments. Previously, the major emphasis related to the quantity of life associated with the HIV/AIDS pandemic. A growing emphasis, however, should now be placed on issues relating to the quality of life for persons who are living with HIV/AIDS. The increasing global population living with HIV/AIDS represents millions of people of all ages who require effective services to address the unique quality of life issues that accompany the condition. Associated disorders of communication, hearing, balance, swallowing, and feeding are central threats that undermine the well-being and effective functioning of individuals. It is imperative, therefore, that these aspects are raised and addressed as important concerns in the ongoing battle against HIV/AIDS.

REFERENCES

Barre-Sinoussi, F., Chermann, J. C., Rey, F., Nugeyre, M. T., Chamaret, S., Gruest, J., . . . Montagnier, L.. (1983). Isolation of a T-lymphotropic retrovirus from a patient at risk for AIDS. *Science, 220*, 868–871.

Bladon, K. L., & Ross, E. (2007). Swallowing difficulties reported by adults infected with HIV/AIDS attending a hospital outpatient clinic in Gauteng, South Africa. *Folia Phoniatrica et Logopaedica, 59*(1) 39-52.

Bond, K., Horvath, T., Harvey, K., Shey Wiysonge, C., & Read, S. (2007). The Cochran Library and mother-to-child transmission of HIV: an umbrella review. *Evidence Based Child Health, 2*, 4-24.

Davis, L. E., Rarey, K. E., & McLaren, L. C. (1995). Clinical viral infections and temporal bone histologic studies of patients with AIDS. *Otolaryngology-Head and Neck Surgery, 113*, 695-701.

Gifford, A. L., & Groessl, E. J. (2002). Chronic disease self-management and adherence to HIV medications. *Journal of Acquired Immune Deficiency Syndromes, 31*, S163-S166.

Groce, N. E. (2003). HIV/AIDS and people with disability. *Lancet, 361*, 1401-1402.

Groce, N. E., & Trasi, R. (2004). Rape of individuals with disability: AIDS and the folk belief of virgin cleansing. *Lancet, 363*, 1663-1664.

Kamps, B. S., & Hoffmann, C. (2007). Introduction. In C. Hoffman, J. K. Rockstroh, & B. S. Kamps (Eds.), *HIV medicine* (pp. 23-32). Paris: Flying Publisher.

Lalwani, A. K., & Sooy, C. D. (1992). Otologic and neurotologic manifestations of Aquired Immunodeficiency Syndrome. In T. A. Tami (Ed.), *Otolaryngologic Clinics of North America* (pp. 1183-1197). Philadelphia: Saunders.

Marra, C. M., Wechhin, H. A., Longstreth, W. T., Rees, T. S., Syapin, C. L., & Gates, G. A. (1997). Hearing loss and antiretroviral therapy in patients infected by with HIV-1. *Archives of Neurology, 54*, 407-410.

Russel, S., Seeley, J., Ezati, E., Wamai, N., Were, W., & Bunnell, R. (2007). Coming back from the dead: Living with HIV as a chronic condition in rural Africa. *Health Policy and Planning, 22*, 344-347.

Shiffman, J. (2006). HIV/AIDS and the rest of the global health agenda. *Bulletin of the World Health Organization, 84*(12), 923.

Teggi, R., Giardano, L., Pistorio, V., & Bussi, M. (2006). Vestibular function in HIV patients., *Acta Otorhinolaryngologica Italica, 26*(3), 140-146.

UNAIDS. (2008). *Report on the Global AIDS epidemic.* Joint United Nations Programme on HIV/AIDS (UNAIDS) and World Health Organization (WHO), Geneva, Switzerland: Author.

UNICEF, UNAIDS, & WHO. (2007). *Children and AIDS: A stocktaking report.* New York: UNICEF.

UNICEF, UNAIDS, & WHO. (2008). *Children and AIDS: A second stocktaking report.* New York: UNICEF.

World Bank. (2004). *HIV/AIDS and disability: Capturing hidden voices, report of the World Bank Yale University Global Survey on HIV/AIDS and Disability.* Washington, DC: World Bank.

World Health Assembly. (2005). *Disability, including prevention, management and rehabilitation.* Geneva, Switzerland: World Health Organization; May 25, 2005. WHA Resolution 58.23. Retrieved September 29, 2008, from http://www.who.int/disabilities/WHA5823_resolution _en.pdf

World Health Organization. (2008). *Towards universal access: Scaling up priority HIV/AIDS interventions in the health sector.* Progress Report 2008. Geneva. Retrieved September 29, 2008, from, http://www.who .int/hiv/pub/towards_universal_access_report_2008.pdf

Zuniga J. (1999). Communication disorders and HIV disease. *Journal of the International Association of Physicians in AIDS Care, 5*(4), 16–23.

CHAPTER 2

Pathogenesis of HIV Infection and Disease Progression

Lynne M. Webber

INTRODUCTION

It is now accepted that human immunodeficiency virus (HIV) is a descendant of simian immunodeficiency virus (SIV) as strains of SIV have a very close resemblance to HIV. HIV is officially described as a zoonotic disease and is classified as two different subtypes, namely, HIV subtype one (HIV-1) and HIV subtype two (HIV-2) (Wolfe et al., 2004). HIV-2 corresponds to SIVsm, a strain of SIV found in sootey mangabey primates indigenous to western Africa and the more virulent and successful pandemic subtype HIV-1 has its closest counterpart in SIVcpz found in forest dwelling chimpanzees of central Africa (Wolfe et al., 2004).

HIV remains within its host and gradually destroys the immune defense mechanisms over many years. The infection develops into HIV disease and advanced disease leads to the terminal phase called AIDS or acquired immunodeficiency syndrome. In the AIDS phase, the individual often suffers from opportunistic infections and events such as cancers that are due to a severely damaged and depleted immune system. In essence, HIV is a virologic infection but manifests as an immunological disease (WHO, 2006).

HIV belongs to the retroviridae family and displays the following important features:

- The virus reverses from an RNA core to a DNA provirus;
- It utilizes a unique and peculiar enzyme called reverse transcriptase;
- The viral DNA integrates into the host's DNA and becomes an integral feature of the host's physiology;
- The virus completes its life cycle by encircling its core structure with proteins; and
- The virus fuses with cellular receptors and coreceptors (Weiss, 1993).

Table 2–1 includes the common abbreviations used in the description of the mechanisms of HIV pathogenesis leading to disease progression. HIV-1 and HIV-2 differ at various junctions and, for treating clinicians, one of the crucial targets for some of the antiretroviral drugs, the reverse transcriptase enzyme, differ between the two subtypes (Rowland-Jones & Whittle, 2007). The differences between HIV-1 and HIV-2 can be summarized as follows:

- The structure of the reverse transcriptase enzyme is different between the subtypes, indicating that certain antiretroviral drugs effective against type 1 are not effective against type 2;
- HIV-2 appears to have a less virulent disease progression course than HIV-1 but both subtypes will result in an AIDS phase of disease and death;
- HIV-2 appears to be less prevalent than HIV-1 but the number of new cases is currently uncertain;
- HIV-2 appears to be geographically confined to certain western African regions of the globe but this pattern may be changing;
- Both HIV-1 and HIV-2 have the equal potential for mutational events and both have a constant mutation behaviour as part of their life cycle; and
- Most commercial tests currently testing for HIV nucleic acids only accommodate HIV-1 (Rowland-Jones & Whittle, 2007).

The characteristic feature of HIV is that the virus has the inherent potential to have RNA and DNA as part of its life cycle and this

Table 2–1. Common Abbreviations and Terms Used in HIV Pathogenesis

Abbreviation	Definition
HIV	human immunodeficiency virus
HIV-1	human immunodeficiency virus subtype one
HIV-2	human immunodeficiency virus subtype two
Viral DNA	viral nucleic acid found in the nucleus of the cell
Viral RNA	viral nucleic acid found in the cytoplasm of the cell
AIDS	acquired immunodeficiency syndrome
ARV	antiretroviral, drugs used to treat HIV
CD4+ T-cells	cluster designation T-cell infected by HIV
CD4 receptor	protein on the surface of the CD4 cell that binds HIV
CCR5 co-receptor	additional receptor/protein to which HIV binds
CXCR4 co-receptor	additional receptor/protein to which HIV binds
Viral tropism	viral expression or viral behavior
Reverse transcription	reversal of RNA molecules to DNA molecules
Antigen presenting cells	cells that present viral antigens/proteins to T-cells
Dendritic cells	antigen-presenting cells
NSI tropism	nonsyncytial inducing behavior
SI	syncytial inducing behavior

has important implications. Until quite recently, no antiretroviral (ARV) drugs were readily effective against the DNA component of HIV; thus, no cure seemed possible, although the new class of ARVs called integrase inhibitors are showing clinically promising results. HIV DNA becomes integrated into the host's DNA and this creates clinical complications such as the precipitation of autoimmune diseases, cancer formation, and metabolic disorders (Kamin & Grinspoon, 2005). HIV DNA also interferes with the proper functioning of the host's DNA telomeres and this leads to premature aging.

Finally, DNA reservoir ensures effective spread of the virus into "sanctuary sites" in the body, such as the eyes, testes, placenta, and brain, where the immune response is less effective than in other sites of the body (Graziosi et al. 1998).

This chapter on HIV pathogenesis discusses the natural course and disease progression of HIV-1 infection, the role of antigen-presenting cells, lymphatic tissue as the site for viral replication, and the practical concerns of the immunopathogenetic mechanisms of HIV infection. The last section considers some unanswered questions and future directions. Although considerable advances have been made in understanding the mechanisms of HIV-1 infection, many questions remain. A short argument on HIV vaccine development is addressed due to its dependence on understanding HIV-1 immunopathogenesis (Weiss, 2008).

NATURAL PROGRESSION OF INFECTION TO DISEASE

HIV transmission

HIV can be transmitted in a variety of ways, including:

- sexual contact (horizontally);
- contact with infected body substances and blood;
- blood transfusion;
- mother-to-child transmission (vertically);
- breast milk;
- occupational exposure;
- organ transplantation; and
- injection drug use.

HIV can still be transmitted by people on antiretroviral therapy (ARVs) and/or people with undetectable viral loads measured in their bloodstream. This emphasizes the need for everyone infected with HIV to exercise preventative measures at all times (Grazioisi et al., 1998). HIV-1 and HIV-2 are transmitted in the same ways but there is evidence than HIV-1 is more easily transmissible by the sexual and mother-to-child routes.

Staging System for Adolescents and Adults

The World Health Organization staging system (WHO, 2006) allows stratification of HIV-infected individuals into four prognostic stages on the basis of clinical criteria and immunologic markers in the form of four categories of cluster designation (CD) cell lymphocyte counts, as illustrated in Table 2-2. Another staging system in the form of the U.S. Centers for Disease Control, AIDS Surveillance Case Definition for Adolescents and Adults, is available. In this classification, HIV-infected individuals are assigned a stage according to a three-by-three matrix consisting of three CD4 cell count categories (1 to 3) and three clinical categories (A to C), as illustrated in Table 2-3. The WHO staging system for HIV infection and disease allows for stratification of individuals on clinical criteria to show HIV disease progression. The 1993 CDC case definition for AIDS includes all HIV-infected individuals with a CD4 cell count less than 200 cells/mm³ or a clinical AIDS indicator condition.

Acute HIV Infection

This phase of HIV disease also is called the primary infection or acute seroconversion phase. Here, some HIV-exposed and HIV-infected individuals present with a glandular-feverlike illness and tragically many individuals may not realize they are infected or even connect their symptoms to possible HIV-infection (Altfeld et al., 2001). The major pathogenetic mechanisms can be summarized with the following points, namely:

- The HIV-1 viral load or burden is very high and this enables the virus to spread effectively and thoroughly throughout the whole body;
- The virus attacks, infects and destroys the immune component called the CD4 T-cell, which is part of the cytotoxic T-cell immune response creating a clinical environment of severe immunosuppression;
- The host's body starts to produce HIV-specific antibodies but these only reach analytically detectable levels often within 3 to 6 weeks after exposure and this phenomenon is called the "window period"; and

Table 2–2. World Health Organization Clinical Staging System for HIV Infection and Disease

WHO Stage	Clinical Conditions	Performance Scale (CD4+ count)
1	acute retroviral infection asymptomatic persistent glands	Scale 1 CD4+ count = >500 cells/mm^3 asymptomatic normal activity
2	weight loss, <10% body weight minor mucocutaneous lesions herpes zoster recurrent urinary tract infection	Scale 2 CD4+ count = 350–499 cells/mm^3 Symptomatic normal activity
3	weight loss >10% body weight Unexplained diarrhea >1/12 Unexplained fever >1/12 Oral candida Oral hairy leukoplakia Pulmonary tuberculosis Severe bacterial infection	Scale 3 CD4+ count = 200–349 cells/mm^3 bedridden <50% of the day
4	HIV wasting syndrome Pneumocystis pneumonia Toxoplasma of the brain Cryptosporidiosis Cytomegalovirus Herpes simplex virus Progressive leukoencephalophathy Disseminated endemic mycosis Candida-esophageal, respiratory Atypical mycobacteriosis Nontyphoid salmonella septicemia Extrapulmonary tuberculosis Lymphoma Kaposi's sarcoma HIV encephalopathy	Scale 4 CD4+ count = <200 cells/mm^3

Source: WHO (2006).

Table 2–3. U.S. Centers for Disease Control, AIDS Surveillance, Case Definition for Adolescents and Adults

	Clinical Categories		
CD4+ count cells/mm3	A Asymptomatic Lymphadenopathy Acute retroviral syndrome	B Symptomatic Not defined in C	C Symptomatic AIDS events
>500	A1	B1	C1
200–499	A2	B2	C2
<200	A3	B3	C3

Source: CDC (1992).

■ These HIV-specific antibodies are not fully neutralizing and HIV-infection becomes a chronic and permanent disease for the host (Pantaleo, Graziosi, & Fauci, 1993).

Clinical Asymptomatic HIV Infection

In adults, there may be a lengthy, variable, and so-called historically "latent period" from HIV-infection to the onset of HIV-related disease events and the AIDS phase of the illness. An adult individual without any form of antiretroviral medication may be clinically well or obviously asymptomatic for longer than 10 years. In contrast, this period is shortened in HIV-infected children. For practical purposes, it must be noted that a clinician experienced in HIV medicine will notice subtle clinical changes in these so-called "asymptomatic individuals" and this depends on an extensive clinical history and a thorough medical examination (Gazzard & Murphy, 2003).

Persistent Generalized Lymphadenopathy

This phase is defined as enlarged lymph nodes clinically noted at two different anatomic sites other than the inguinal or groin-associated nodes. This description also explains part of the pathogenesis of HIV-associated disease whereby the virus migrates to the lymph glands and causes "immune-mischief" in the form of immunomanipulative behavior and immunodestructive strategies. The lymph tissue actually provides a reservoir for the virus and serves as an important anatomical site for the survival and perpetuation of the virus over many years. For clinical management of the patient, it should be noted that the presence of enlarged glands has little significance on disease progression, clinical prognosis, and viral replication strategies (Gazzard, & Murphy, 2003).

Progression to HIV-Specific Related Disease and Acquired Immunodeficiency Syndrome (AIDS)

Almost all, if not all, infected HIV-infected individuals will develop HIV-related disease events and problems and will progress to the terminal phase of AIDS. AIDS is a clinical WHO stage 4 disease and refers to individuals who are bedridden for greater than 50% of the day over the last month period. Table 2–2 lists the clinical conditions that are expected in this phase of the disease. How quickly such progression takes place is dependent on a number of factors and this determines the uncertainty of pathogenetic prediction of HIV-infection, namely:

- The genetic characteristics of the host;
- The immune response mechanisms of the host;
- The subtype of HIV;
- The quasispecies evolution of the subtype of HIV; and
- The concomitant opportunistic infection or disease of that HIV-infected individual (Weiss, 1993).

Advancing Immunosuppression and Immunocollapse

In an untreated HIV-infected individual, more than 10 thousand million new viruses are created every 24 hours; in turn, the body counteracts this attack by creating a thousand million new CD4+ T-cells that kill the viruses directly or indirectly. So, as the HIV-infection progresses and the immune system is slowly and systematically destroyed, the patients become more and more susceptible to opportunistic infections, auto-immune disorders, endocrine malfunctioning, and neoplastic development (Arts & Quinones-Mateu, 2003; Weiss, 1993).

Table 2–4. Common Types of Opportunistic Infections in Adults

MYCOBACTERIA	Human herpes virus 8
Tuberculosis	Polyomaviruses
Disseminated nontuberculous mycobacterial infection	Hepatitis B virus
	Hepatitis C virus
FUNGI	**BACTERIA**
Pneumocystis jirovecii pneumonia	Bacterial pneumonia
Candidiasis	Nontyphoid salmonella bacteremia
Cryptococcosis	Nocardiosis
Endemic mycoses	**PROTOZOA**
VIRUSES	Toxoplasmosis
Cytomegalovirus infection	Cryptosporidiosis
Herpes simplex virus	Isosporiasis
Varicella zoster virus	Microsporidiosis
Epstein-Barr virus	

Table 2–4 summarizes the list of opportunistic infections encountered in adults and children infected with HIV. Of specific relevance to this text on HIV/AIDS associated communication, hearing, and swallowing disorders are the selected list of opportunistic infections in Table 2-5.

THE LIFE CYCLE OF THE VIRUS

HIV-1 is an RNA virus that must bind to the CD4 receptor on the surface of the target cell. These target cells are usually the T-helper lymphocytes, dendritic cells, or macrophage cells. The virus also binds to co-receptors found on the surface of cells. Two important chemokine co-receptors are called CCR5 co-receptor and CXCR4 co-receptor. The CCR5 co-receptor is found on the surfaces of macrophages and dendritic cells and viruses binding to these cells are termed R5 viruses. These R5 viruses appear in the acute phase of infection and are responsible for the transmission of most HIV-1 infections. T-lymphocytes carry the CXCR4 co-receptor and viruses

Table 2–5. HIV/AIDS Associated Opportunistic Infections Particularly Relevant to Communication, Hearing, and Swallowing Disorders

Mouth and esophageal regions   • HIV gingivitis and periodontitis   • Common pharyngitis and tonsillitis   • Oral hairy leukoplakia   • Oral warts   • Oral rash of HIV seroconversion syndrome   • Secondary syphilis   • Oropharyngeal candidiasis   • Oropharyngeal herpes simplex viral disease, to mention but a few   *Ear region*   • Most of the human herpes virus species infections, in particular herpes zoster of the auditory canal   • Neurosyphilis   • Disseminated tuberculosis, as the more common presenting disorders

binding to these cells are termed X4 viruses. X4 viruses gradually emerge over time and as the disease advances are associated with the late and terminal phases of the illness. As the AIDS phase presents many viral species can be dual tropic, namely, CCR5/CXCR4 tropic. Tropism refers to the way viruses express their behavior and is reflected by their interaction with receptors on the cell surface. CCR5 and CXCR4 are classified as co-receptors for HIV entry into the human cell (Weiss, 2008).

Progression of Clinical Symptoms

Clinical symptoms are related to or can be correlated with the phases of HIV infection and the tropism or expression of HIV. In actual practice, viral utilization of these co-receptors can define the clinical presentation of the patient. Primary HIV infection or seroconversion and early infection with a CCR5 tropic virus often clinically presents with mucosal and skin problems, such as multiple abscesses in children; seborrheic dermatitis, especially over the facial region; and herpes zoster (shingles), skin, and neural eruptions. As the virus changes to the CXCR4 tropic behavioral strategy, it starts to create clinical problems of the neurons, microglia, and eosinophils with clinical manifestations noted in the pulmonary regions, the brain, spinal cord, and nerves (Pope & Haase, 2003).

Treatment Applications to the HIV-1 Life Cycle

The ARV drugs target specific sites of the HIV life cycle, hence the categorization into different classes of ARV drugs. The site of action of the ARVs within the HIV life cycle also determines to an extent their expected clinical side effects and toxicity profiles.

The full life cycle of HIV is summarized in Table 2–6. The life cycle of HIV is pertinent to the understanding exactly where the

Table 2–6. HIV Pathogenesis: The Life cycle of HIV-1

1. Binding	HIV-1 encounters a cell expressing the CD4 receptor and binds to the cell membrane
2. Membrane fusion and entry	fusion of the host cell membrane with the viral envelope, called gp41.
3. Reverse transcription	the viral RNA is transcripted to viral DNA
4. Integration	proviral DNA is incorporated into the host-cell genome
5. Proviral transcription	proviral DNA is transcribed into mRNA by the cell machinery of the host
6. Cytoplasmic expression	provides new viral genomes and encodes essential viral proteins
7. Translation	the translation of viral mRNA into new HIV-1 particles
8. Assembly	new HIV-1 cores assemble at the surface of the host-cell
9. Budding and maturation	new HIV-1 particles form as the viral core buds through the host-cell membrane

ARV drugs work, and this enlightens the clinicians to side effect profiles, toxicity events, and the eventual occurrence of ARV drug resistance. Although the full viral life cycle has 9 steps, only 4 steps are highlighted in this chapter as these four steps are the actual events in the life cycle where the inhibiting antiretroviral agents work. These four steps include:

- Fusion with the CD4 receptor/co-receptor and the cell membrane (the drugs are called fusion inhibitors);
- Transformation of the viral RNA into viral DNA, so called reverse transcription (reverse transcriptase inhibitors);
- Penetration of the nucleus of the cell and integration of viral DNA into the host DNA (integrase inhibitors); and
- Translated viral protease and genomic viral RNA are processed, assembled, package and released as a new infectious virus (protease inhibitors) (Coffin, 1996).

Destruction of the Immune Response

Dendritic cells are the most important antigen presenting cells (APCs) in the body and they appear to be the only cell type that can efficiently activate naïve T-cell lymphocytes. They also are the first cells that HIV confronts after immediate exposure and infection (Pope & Haase, 2003). The activation of CD4+ helper T-lymphocytes requires two protein signals and the dendritic cells commence this activation by producing interleukin-12 that stimulates naïve T-cells into active T-cells, as well as potentiating the natural killer cells function. Thus, a single dendritic cell can activate up to 3,000 T-cells.

Although dendritic cells are critical for generating an HIV-specific cytotoxic T-cell response, the interaction between HIV and dendritic cells also can be detrimental (Kedzierska & Crowe, 2001). Early in the infection, the dendritic cell acts as a Trojan horse carrying the virus to the rest of the immune system; and as the amount and the length of exposure increases, these dendritic cells then become dysfunctional. The dendritic cells carry HIV to the rest of the immune system via two mechanisms:

1. Infection of the dendritic cell by HIV after the virus binds to the CD4 cell receptor or the CCR5 and/or CXCR4 co-receptors; and

2. Binding of HIV to other surface receptors without infecting the actual dendritic cell (Pope & Haase, 2003).

HIV interacts with the dendritic cells using multiple surface receptors and these interactions differ depending on the type of subset of dendritic cells present. As an example, tonsil and blood subsets interact almost exclusively with the CD4 receptors and immature skin and mucosal subsets interact with C-type lectin receptors. After long-standing interactions, the dendritic cells become dysfunctional and this combination paradoxically fails to initiate T-lymphocyte proliferation. Viral suppression becomes less and less effective, the immune response fails to keep the ever growing viral burden under control, and the host enters the terminal phase of the illness dying from an AIDS-related event (Kedzierska & Crowe, 2001).

Viral Replication of HIV

Even in the early stages of HIV-disease, viral replication within the lymphatic tissue is already extensive (Orenstein, 2008). During the initial phase of HIV-1 infection, there is a burst of viruses into the plasma, which is then followed by a relative decline in viremia (Pantaleo, Graziosi, & Fauci, 1993). During this period, a strong HIV-1 specific cytotoxic T-cell response is generated and this coincides with the early suppression of plasma viremia in most infected individuals. Virions get trapped by the follicular dendritic cell network within the lymphoid tissue. Permanent reservoirs mostly in macrophages and latently infected CD4+ T-lymphocytes are established in the early stage of infection and this is the major obstacle to successfully eradicate HIV from the body with antiretroviral drugs. During the whole course of infection, the lymphoid tissue is the principal site of HIV-1 replication. It must be noted that the frequency of cells containing HIV-1 proviral DNA is 5 to 10 times higher in lymphoid tissue than in the circulating cells in the bloodstream, and the difference in viral replication in lymphoid tissue exceeds that in the peripheral blood by up to 10 to 100 times (Orenstein, 2008). The micromilieu of the lymphoid tissue creates the optimal environment for viral replication and can be illustrated with the following examples:

■ the close cell-to-cell contact between CD4+ T-cells and antigen presenting cells;

- the presence of infectious virions on the surface of the follicular dendritic network; and
- an abundant production of pro-inflammatory cellular cytokines such as interleukin-1, interleukin-6 or tumor necrosis factor alpha promoting the induction of viral replication in infected cells.

The above facts also illustrate that, in every situation where the immune system is activated, enhanced viral replication also can occur. This is a fairly recent understanding of HIV immunopathogenesis (Forsman & Weiss, 2008).

Although patients undergoing antiretroviral therapy show a significant decrease in the number of productively infected CD4+ T-cells within the lymphoid tissue regions, a pool of latently infected quiescent T-cells persists (Altfeld et al., 2002). It is these latently infected cells that perpetuate HIV viral replication even when the patient is taking ARVs. Recent studies also have shown that progression of disease is reflected by the destruction of the lymphoid tissue architecture and decreased viral trapping (Gazzard & Murphy, 2003).

For practical purposes, chronic activation of the immune system is the hallmark of progressive HIV infection. This predicts disease outcome through a number of mechanisms such as autoimmune manifestations, premature aging, neoplastic changes, and subsequent apoptosis of many components of the entire immune system.

PRACTICAL IMPLICATIONS OF HIV IMMUNOPATHOGENESIS

Tropism of the virus also means the manner in which the virus expresses itself or equates to the way the virus behaves. HIV has developed two behavioral strategies, namely, it is nonsyncytial inducing (NSI) or it is syncytial inducing (SI). NSI behavior means that the virus does not cause syncytial formation of cells in the organs that it infects or so-called "clumping" or a "stickiness" of the cells. SI behavior means the virus does cause syncytial formation or it further attacks the body by causing the clumpiness of the cells.

Practically, the SI behavior of the virus is a dangerous strategy development for the host's survival and occurs in advanced HIV disease (Ho et al., 1995; Weiss, 2002).

There are some practical implications for the health care practitioner, namely:

- HIV spreads throughout the whole body and infects a large number and variety of cells which means pervasive effects on everyday functioning may be expected;
- HIV will behave differently in different individuals and it is not easy for the clinician to predict exactly how the virus is going to react within that host;
- The behavioral changes of the virus as the disease progresses may impact on the phenomenon of discordant couples, whereby one sexual partner remains negative after continuous exposure to an HIV-positive partner in spite of unprotected sexual practices (Saez-Cirion et al. 2007); and
- It is not always possible to predict which HIV-infected individual will become a rapid disease progressor or a long-term disease nonprogressor.

Clinical manifestations in HIV-infected adults and children differ as listed in Tables 2–4 and 2–7. Children in the early phase (first 2 years) are prone to oral candidiasis, pneumonia, diarrhea, protein-energy malnutrition, and developmental delay. At any age, children present with invasive bacterial disease that can infect a wide range of organs. Older children may then present with swelling of the parotid glands, digital clubbing of the fingers, bronchiectasis of the lungs, and a nonspecific arthritic picture.

UNANSWERED QUESTIONS AND THE DEVELOPMENT OF A VACCINE AGAINST HIV

Improved knowledge and understanding of the pathophysiologic mechanisms during the course of HIV-1 infection has grown steadily over the years. However, many unanswered questions remain and there are currently too many to address within the scope of this

Table 2–7. Common Opportunistic Infections and Clinical Conditions in Children with Confirmed HIV-Infection

Infectious diseases	Other clinical events
• Extensive wart virus infections	• Unexplained persistent parotid enlargement
• Extensive molluscum contagiosum	
• Fungal nail infections	• Unexplained persistent fever
• Pulmonary tuberculosis	• Unexplained anaemia
• Severe recurrent bacterial pneumonia	• Severe wasting or severe malnutrition
• Esophageal candidiasis	• Chronic thrombocytopenia
• Chronic infective diarrhea	• Developmental delays
• Extensive and recurrent otitis media and externa	• Digital clubbing of the fingers
• Chronic bacterial sinusitis	• Bronchiectasis of the lungs
• Oral candidiasis	• Nonspecific arthritis

chapter. The following short list highlights some questions that remain unanswered:

■ Why do some individuals present clinically as long-term nonprogressors and other HIV-infected individuals as rapid progressors?

■ What protective mechanisms do HIV-negative partners have that prevent their exposure to HIV within a sexual relationship with an HIV-positive partner over an extended period of unprotected sexual practices?

■ What role does the genetic makeup of the host play in determining HIV disease progression?

■ Why do the HIV-specific antibodies have no or little neutralizing effect on the viral infection, as observed in other viral infections?

■ What are the challenges for researchers attempting to design a preventative vaccine against HIV-1?

One of the most common questions raised refers to urgent need for a protective vaccine to interrupt the epidemic. This requires a better understanding of current HIV-1 immunopathogenesis. In addition, as discussed, chronic activation of the immune system is deleterious to the HIV-infected host. Virtually all HIV-infected individuals test positive for HIV-specific antibodies yet the antibodies appear to have no obvious protective effect on their own. Recent studies have resulted in the belief that both humoral and cellular mechanisms contribute to protection. There also is considerable discussion about how to best monitor the induction of protective immune responses. As a concluding statement, despite all efforts so far, finding an effective and universally applicable vaccine lies far ahead in the future.

SUMMARY

Although there are two distinct subtypes of HIV, HIV-1 is the most predominant and the most virulent subtype globally. HIV is classified as a retrovirus, which means it can reverse its RNA structure to DNA provirus. Its life cycle has three enzymes that are inhibited by the ARVs, namely:

- Reverse transcriptase (reverse transcriptase inhibitors);
- Integrase (integrase inhibitors); and
- The protease (protease inhibitors) enzymes.

The natural history of HIV infection and disease is an integral component of the description of HIV-1 immunopathogenesis as the virus can alter its behavior strategies as the disease progresses. The different stages of disease progression can assist the health care practitioner in determining the possible type of infection or others that the patient might develop but these remain man-made artificial stages (Calza et al., 2008) Thus, the practitioner needs to focus clearly on a thorough medical history and an extensive medical examination.

HIV commences its life cycle by binding to receptors on the surfaces of cells and different cells have different receptors that determine HIV tropism. R5 tropic viruses bind to CCR5 co-receptors mostly found on the surfaces of macrophages and dendritic cells and X4 tropic viruses bind to CXCR4 co-receptors mostly found on the surfaces of T-lymphocytes. The virus changes its tropism as the disease advances and this influences the prediction risk for opportunistic events. The predominant cellular target for HIV-1 is the CD4+ T-lymphocyte and during the initial viremia HIV needs to spread within the host environment so that contact with the T-cells is possible. This is where the role of the antigen-presenting cells is so important for HIV transmission within the host's body as one of the first cells HIV encounters is the APC dendritic cells. HIV interacts with the dendritic cells using multiple surface receptors and is then transported to the T-lymphocytes. But, HIV also captures the dendritic cell for its own purpose and the longer HIV replicates within the host the more likely it will render this cell dysfunctional.

The virus can express its behavior as NSI or SI and this enables the virus to change its behavior during the natural history of the infection. This has a negative clinical impact on the host making the individual more susceptible to opportunistic infections and/or events. Thus, from a virologic and pathologic position, the early stage of HIV infection has a different immunopathogenetic environment to late stage infection.

Finally, chronic activation of the immune system is the hallmark of progressive HIV-1 infection and predicts disease outcome.

REFERENCES

Altfeld, M., & Allen, T. M., Yu, X. G., Johnston, M. N., Agrawal, D., Korber, B. T., et al. (2002). HIV-1 superinfection despite broad CD+ T-cell responses containing replication of the primary virus. *Nature, 420,* 434–439.

Altfeld, M., Rosenberg, E. S., Shankarappa, R., Mukherjee, J. S., Hecht, F. M., Eldridge, R. L., et al. (2001). Cellular immune responses and viral diversity in individuals treated during acute and early HIV-1 infection. *Journal of Experimental Medicine, 193,* 169–180.

Arts, E. J., & Quinones-Mateu, M. E. (2003). Sorting out the complexities of HIV-1 fitness. *AIDS, 15*(5), 780–781.

Calza, L., Manfredi, R., Pocatera, D., & Chiodo F. (2008). Risk of premature atherosclerosis and ischemic heart disease associated with HIV infection and antiretroviral therapy. *Journal of Infection, 57,* 16–32.

Centers for Disease Control and Prevention (CDC). (1992). 1993 Revised classification system for HIV infection and expanded surveillance case definition for AIDS among adolescents and adults. *Morbidity and Mortality Weekly Report, 41,* 1–5.

Coffin, J. M. (1996). Viral kinetics. *AIDS, 10,* 75-84.

Forsman, A., & Weiss, R. A. (2008). Why is HIV a pathogen? *Trends in Microbiology, 16*(12), 555-560.

Gazzard, B., & Murphy, R. L. (2003). European guidelines for the management and treatment of HIV-infected adults in Europe. *AIDS, 17,* 1-26.

Graziosi, C., Soudeyns, H., Rizzardi, P., Bart, P-A, Ghapius, A., & Pantaleo, G. (1998). Immunopathogenesis of HIV infection. *AIDS Research and Human Retroviruses, 14*(2), 135-142.

Ho, D. D., Neuman, A. U., Perelson, A. S., Chen, W., Leonard, J. M., & Markowitz, M. (1995). Rapid turnover of plasma virions and CD4 lymphocytes in HIV-1 infection. *Nature, 373,* 123-126.

Kamin, D. S., & Grinspoon, S. K. (2005). Cardiovascular disease in HIV-positive patients. *AIDS, 19,* 641-652.

Kedzierska, K., & Crowe, S. M. (2001). Cytokines and HIV-1 interactions and clinical implications. *Antiviral Chemistry and Chemotherapy, 12,* 133-150.

Orenstein, J. M. (2008). Hyperplastic lymphoid tissue in HIV/AIDS: An electron microscopic study. *Ultrastructural Pathology, 32,* 161-169.

Pantaleo, G., Graziosi, C., & Fauci, A. S. (1993). The immunopathogenesis of Human Immunodeficiency Virus infection. *New England Journal of Medicine, 328,* 327-335.

Pope, M., & Haase, A. T. (2003). Transmission of acute HIV-1 infection and the quest for strategies to prevent infection. *Nature Medicine, 7,* 847-851.

Rowland-Jones, S. L., & Whittle, H. C. (2007). Out of Africa: What can we learn from HIV-2 about protective immunity to HIV-1? *Nature Immunology, 8,* 329-331.

Saez-Cirion, A., Pancino, G., Sinet, M., Venet, A., & Lambotte, O. (2001). For the ANRS EP36 HIV CONTROLLERS study group. HIV controllers: How do they tame the virus? *Trends in Immunology, 28*(12), 532-540.

Weiss, R. A. (1993). How does HIV cause AIDS? *Science, 260,* 1273-1279.

Weiss, R. A. (2002). Virulence and pathogenesis. *Trends in Microbiology, 10,* 314-317.

Weiss, R. A. (2008). Special anniversary review: Twenty-five years of human immunodeficiency virus research: success and challenges. *Clinical and Experimental Immunology, 152,* 201-210.

World Health Organization (WHO). (2006). *WHO case definitions of HIV for surveillance and revised clinical staging and immunological classification of HIV-related disease in adults and children.* Geneva: Author.

Wolfe, N. D., Switzer, W. M., Carr, J. K., Bhullar, V. B., Shanmugam, V., & Tamoufe, U. (2004). Naturally acquired simian retrovirus infections in Central African hunters. *Lancet, 363,* 932-934.

CHAPTER 3

Diagnosis and Management of HIV/AIDS

Linda-Gail Bekker

INTRODUCTION

The HIV pandemic has had an impact on societies that is without precedent. The human immunodeficiency virus infection is caused by a retrovirus that infects and replicates in human lymphocytes and macrophages, eroding the integrity of the human immune system over a number of years, and culminating in immune incompetence and a susceptibility to a series of opportunistic and other infections as well as the development of malignancies.

An estimated 33 million (30–36 million) people were living with HIV in 2007 worldwide with 22.5 million of these in Sub-Saharan Africa (UNAIDS, 2008). At the turn of the century, Africa contributed over 70% to the global burden of people living with the human immunodeficiency virus (HIV). The success of this virus is based on its intrinsic molecular biologic properties and the pathogenesis of infection, namely, the erosion of the very immunity by which HIV infection may be controlled and eradicated itself.

In the United States, the country in which cases of AIDS were first recognized in 1981, 49% of all newly diagnosed HIV infections in 2006 were among men who have sex with men (UNAIDS, 2007). In contrast, the Sub-Saharan epidemic is predominantly heterosexual, with women comprising 60% to 70% of those living with HIV. Globally, the HIV incidence rate is believed to have peaked in the late 1990s and to have stabilized subsequently, notwithstanding increasing incidence in a number of countries, particularly in southern Africa, Asia, and Eastern Europe.

Changes in incidence along with rising AIDS mortality have caused global HIV prevalence to level off. However, the number of people living with HIV has continued to rise due to population growth and, more recently, the life-prolonging effects of antiretroviral therapy. In Sub-Saharan Africa, the region with the largest burden of the AIDS epidemic, data also indicate that the HIV incidence rate has peaked and is starting to plateau in most countries. However, the epidemics in this region are highly diverse and especially severe in southern Africa, where some of the epidemics continue to expand.

This chapter covers an approach to diagnosis of HIV infection in adults and newborns and outlines the recommended management and treatment of an HIV-infected individual from the time of the first clinical assessment. The chapter gives some indication of the expected natural history of the HIV infection until the time that medical intervention is indicated.

DIAGNOSIS OF HIV INFECTION

The global epidemic is stabilizing but at an unacceptably high level. In one of the worst hit countries, an estimated 5.5 million HIV-infected people live in South Africa today. Due to the chronicity of the infection and relatively long period of clinical latency prior to onset of symptoms, most are, as yet, unaware of their status (UNAIDS, 2008; South African Department of Health [DOH], 2007). HIV testing is key to both effective primary and secondary preventive strategies and critical for implementation of a management plan for those who test positive. Testing reduces risk behavior in people testing positive (Richardson et al, 2004). Regular follow-up, clinical examination, and blood test monitoring after a positive test enable timely commencement of various prophylactic treatments to prevent opportunistic infections. In addition, testing prior to onset of advanced HIV enables adequate preparation for antiretroviral therapy (ART).

HIV testing is indicated when:

■ someone requests a test;
■ someone believes that they are at risk of infection through unprotected sexual activity, needle stick injury, or unsafe injection drug use;
■ a pregnant woman wishes to know her status to protect her unborn child;
■ mother-to-child transmission of infection is suspected;
■ someone has a condition that indicates possible HIV infection;
■ public health and infection control is at stake (e.g., blood product safety);
■ someone presents with an opportunistic infection or unusual malignancy;
■ someone presents with newly diagnosed tuberculosis;
■ someone presents with a sexually transmitted infection;
■ a child/adolescent who may have been infected vertically presents;
■ someone lives in a high prevalence area and is sexually active.

Testing should be considered:

■ in anyone who is sexually active;
■ in anyone who engages in intravenous drug use;
■ at any contact with the health sector.

Laboratory Tests

A variety of diagnostic and monitoring tests available for HIV infection are available today. These tests vary in their complexity, which, in turn, determines their accessibility: some are at the point of care while others require sophisticated centralized laboratories. They also vary in their cost, which has determined their availability particularly in resource-constrained settings. Table 3–1 describes the merits and limitations of each test.

Table 3–1. Laboratory Diagnosis and Monitoring of HIV

Assay	Purpose	Comments
Rapid (finger prick)	Diagnostic	Point of care, cheap, immediate. Antibody test
Rapid (saliva)	Diagnostic/ surveillance	Point of care, cheap, immediate, less infection control issues. Antibody test.
ELISA	Diagnostic	Relatively cheap, laboratory required, patient usually must return for result. Antibody test.
Western blot	Diagnostic	Expensive, laboratory expertise, patient must return for result, confirmatory. Antibody test.
P24	Diagnostic	Occurs in acute infection and in advanced disease. Diagnostic during the window period. Relatively expensive and requires laboratory. Viral proteins.
Viral PCR (qualitative)	Diagnostic	Viral nucleic acid test. Diagnostic from 2 weeks postinfection onward. Requires laboratory expertise. Expensive. Used for neonatal infection from 4 weeks onward.
ELISA (4th generation)	Diagnostic	Combines ELISA with P24 to reduce the window period.
CD4 T-cell count	Monitoring	Assessment of immunological well being. Increasingly available at point of care. Inexpensive.
Viral load (quantitative PCR)	Monitoring	Three main methods. Relatively expensive. Monitors blood level of viral RNA both before and during antiretroviral therapy.
Resistance testing	Monitoring	Viral genotype determines the presence of resistance mutations in circulating virus.

Diagnostic Tests

HIV ELISA

ELISA is an acronym for enzyme-linked immunosorbent assay. This is the most widely used serologic technique today, and is used to detect antibodies against antigen from many infectious agents including HIV. An ELISA for HIV antibody uses HIV antigen to capture HIV antibodies in a blood sample. HIV antigen is fixed to a "solid-phase," for example, a plastic well in a multiwell plate. A second step is required to detect any captured antibody. This step commonly utilizes an enzyme-substrate color reaction. The intensity (optical density) of the resulting color can be measured, and the antibody levels can be judged as low or high, relative to control sera.

Currently, the most established tests for detecting HIV infection rely on ELISA as an initial screening test. During or shortly after infection, Immunoglobulin (Ig)M antibodies to HIV first appear. This is followed weeks to months later by IgG antibodies to Gag and Env and then to viral enzymes and regulatory proteins. The time to first detectable IgG by ELISA takes a median of 3 to 4 weeks, with almost all newly infected individuals having detectable IgG levels by 6 months. During this time, an ELISA test may be falsely negative, a period known as the window period. Figure 3–1 illustrates the natural history of HIV infection and by which stage the ELISA and other tests become reliable.

Current later generation ELISA tests reduce the window period to about 2 to 4 weeks, thereby reducing the number of false-negative results, especially in areas where incident infections are common. In most contexts, antibody tests are sufficient to make an accurate diagnosis of HIV infection. The use of two different enzyme-linked immunosorbent assay (ELISA) tests or two different rapid tests (on site) to confirm HIV infection meets the World Health Organization (WHO) testing recommendations for regions where HIV prevalence exceeds 10%. At lower HIV prevalence, a three-test strategy is recommended. Almost all ELISA tests are designed to detect both HIV-1 and HIV-2 antibodies.

The ELISA is the preferred screening method in the developing world because it lends itself to high throughput, rapid testing, and automation. Despite high specificity, the use of ELISA in populations where the prevalence of disease is low will lead to a high

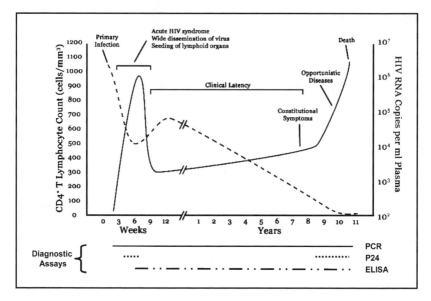

Figure 3–1. *Natural history of HIV and the role of diagnostic assays.*

proportion of positive results being false. Thus, in the developed world, the protocol is to confirm positive or indeterminate ELISA results with a second test, the Western blot. Western blots require significant time and resources and so are not suited to many high-prevalence areas.

The third-generation ELISA tests for HIV antibody have a sensitivity approaching 100% and a specificity greater than 99%. These tests have been in use since the early 1990s. Unlike earlier versions, the third generation ELISA tests detect both IgM and IgG antibody classes, and so detect HIV infection from an earlier stage.

Rapid Test Devices

A test that has worked well in resource-poor settings is the rapid test. Several have been endorsed by FDA and WHO. These tests have higher than 99% sensitivity and specificity when combined with a Western blot in the developed world and a second rapid test in the developing world. Because rapid tests are a "point of care" test and results are immediately available, rapid HIV testing can play an important role in expanding access to testing in both clinical and nonclinical settings and overcoming some of the barriers to early diagnosis. It is also thought that immediate disclosure of results may improve referral to care for infected persons. Rapid tests are primarily easy to perform, and require minimal equipment and user expertise. The majority of rapid tests are immunochromatographic, somewhat like an ELISA reaction in a simplified format. Others are latex agglutination tests. The better tests include a control to validate the result. Used correctly, the best rapid tests have an accuracy closely approaching that of ELISA tests. Only tested and approved tests should be used as many tests with varying degrees of quality are available.

Noninvasive HIV ELISA and Rapid Tests

Although immunoglobulin levels in saliva and urine are approximately 1000-fold lower than in plasma, technical advances are allowing increasingly accurate detection of HIV antibody in these body fluids. Saliva has higher concentrations of IgA and IgG and now both ELISA and rapid tests exist for saliva. At present, such noninvasive tests are largely used for surveillance. The results of epidemiologic research studies provide empirical insights into the occurrence of HIV in specific populations. This includes studies of both prevalence and incidence. They may involve large scale surveys or specific smaller communities or groups. This is known as surveillance data and often less invasive ways of determining HIV infection are preferred to simplify infection control, ethics, and logistics.

The Western Blot Test

The antibodies generated after HIV infection are not homogeneous, but are a population of antibodies to many of the protein components of the virus. A Western blot has the advantage of distinguishing these different antibodies, so that the patient's exact antibody profile can be visualized. The basis of the Western blot is a strip of cellulose membrane embedded with the different HIV proteins, arranged according to their molecular weights. A person's serum is incubated with the strip. A second phase reveals the "bands" where the antibodies have bound. Certain antibody bands have more diagnostic significance than others. Specific criteria exist for a positive or negative blot. Any other pattern of bands is regarded as an indeterminate result. Indeterminate results are common (up to 20% of uninfected persons). Western blot assays require a significant level of laboratory competency, are expensive, and not easily accessible in many parts of the developing world. With the advent of excellent ELISA tests, a Western blot is no longer regarded as essential for confirmation of HIV infection. However, HIV-2 infection may require a specific Western blot for reliable confirmation.

The p24 Antigen

The p24 protein is a core HIV protein. At times of high viral replication, p24 protein is directly detectable in the blood. This occurs during primary HIV infection and again in the late stages of acquired immune deficiency syndrome (AIDS). Notably, p24 is detectable in fewer than 10% of people in the asymptomatic phase of HIV infection. The p24 antigen test should, therefore, not be used instead of an antibody test, but only as a supplementary test to identify patients who are in early infection and in whom antibodies are not yet detectable by ELISA (i.e., the window period.)

Polymerase Chain Reaction (PCR)

Assays that detect the virus itself have been developed for two reasons:

- To detect incident infection earlier than would occur with antibody testing;
- more frequently, to monitor response to HAART.

To do this, tests that detect and measure viral nucleic acid in blood and other body fluids are available. Most commonly used is reverse-transcriptase PCR of viral RNA. There is an ultrasensitive version of this test that can reliably measure as low as 40 RNA copies per milliliter (ml) of plasma. In the polymerase chain reaction (PCR), "primers" target a specific DNA sequence, which is a portion of the HIV genome. Primers are short sequences of synthetic DNA that are complementary to one end of a gene sequence of interest. Primers prime a DNA polymerase enzyme to make copies of the DNA to which they are bound. Temperature shifts initiate different steps in the reaction. The final result is an exponential increase in copies of the targeted DNA fragment. This DNA then is readily detectable. The technique potentially can detect a single intact copy of HIV nucleic acid in a blood sample. Good laboratory technique is required to avoid cross-contamination of samples. Despite technical, logistical, and cost factors, this test is increasingly utilized and particularly blood transfusion services have moved towards this type of testing to improve safety.

Culture

HIV can be grown in cell culture, just like many other viruses. Fresh peripheral blood mononuclear cells from an uninfected donor are incubated with the sample for testing. The addition of the cytokine interleukin-2 is necessary to stimulate the cells. Growth of HIV is visible microscopically by cytopathic effect in the cells, and the detection of p24 antigen or reverse transcriptase activity in the culture. Culture is a research technology available in certain reference laboratories where safety and expertise permit.

Viral Load

HIV viral load is the concentration of free virus in the blood plasma. In its free form, HIV is an RNA virus and all the commercially available viral load tests measure HIV RNA. Note that commercial viral load assays are only available for HIV-1.

There are three main types of viral load tests: (1) Quantitative PCR; (2) Nucleic acid sequence-based amplification (NASBA) and; (3) Branch-chain DNA assays. All of these tests can measure free HIV in the range of 40 to more than 1,000,000 copies/ml. Although results obtained with different tests are comparable, it is best to remain with one type of test for ongoing monitoring of a particular patient.

The viral load should not be measured during an acute illness or within several weeks of a vaccination when, due to possible increased viral replication, the viral load may be transiently elevated. The viral load may help to assess whether treatment should be initiated. In developed countries, a baseline viral load followed by regular 3-month measurements (regardless of whether the patient is on therapy or not) is recommended (Department of Health and Human Services [DHHS], 2001). However, this is not common practice in resource-poor settings. The most important role of a viral load is in monitoring success of HAART (South African HIV Clinicians Society [SAHIVClinSoc], 2008).

The viral load is expressed as copies/ml or as a $\log_{10}$ value. The viral load fluctuates by a factor of 2 ($\log_{10}$ 0.3) in otherwise stable patients. Converting the viral load to the $\log_{10}$ value makes it easier to detect clinically meaningful changes over time: only viral load changes of greater than 0.5 $\log_{10}$, which represents a threefold change are significant. These changes are used when deciding to initiate therapy, and to monitor the response to therapy. Ideally, when monitoring the effect of highly active antiretroviral therapy (HAART), a patient's viral load should be less than 50 or less than 400 copies/ml (depending on the test) after 4 to 6 months of treatment—this is considered an "undetectable" viral load and the HIV infection is said to be fully suppressed in the patient on a particular therapy. If the viral load does not suppress by 6 months or it "rebounds" after an initial phase of suppression, the patient either is not taking the antiviral therapy or the therapy is no longer effective. This may be due to a number of reasons including drug reactions, acquisition of resistant mutations in an already established HIV infection, or acquisition of resistant virus de novo. Nonadherence is the most common cause for viral nonsuppression (Wilson et al., 2008).

CD4 Count

The cluster differentiation 4 (CD4) cell count indicates the health of the immune system and assists in the initial assessment and ongoing monitoring of the patient. This is the most important test to complete at entry into care as it establishes the patient's risk of developing HIV-associated complications and is an important means of deciding need for antiviral therapy.

All T-lymphocytes have T-cell receptors that are identified as CD3 molecules. CD4 is a molecule found on the surface of helper T-lymphocytes. CD8 is yet another molecule found on cytotoxic T-lymphocytes. CD4 and CD8 molecules play a subsidiary role in the binding of CD3 to MHC-II and MHC-I, respectively, during antigen presentation (Veazey et al., 1998).

CD4 is also the major receptor for HIV, and CD4+ T-lymphocytes are the main target of HIV infection. CD4+ T-lymphocytes are directly and indirectly destroyed by HIV. Although these cells initially are replaced as quickly as they are destroyed, over time the regenerative capacity of the immune system is exhausted, and the CD4+ cell numbers fall. As these cells play a central stimulatory role in the immune system, their falling numbers correlate with an increasing degree of immune suppression. CD4+ cells are detected using monoclonal antibodies to the CD4 molecule. A fluorescent-activated cell sorter (FACS) machine is commonly used to count them, but other options are available. Recently, innovative methods to quantify CD4 counts have driven the cost of the assay down and even point of care units are now available making the test far more freely available (MacLennan et al., 2007).

In uninfected healthy adults, an average CD4 count is 800 cells per microliter (μl), and the average drop in CD4 count in HIV-positive patients is 75 cells per μl per year (Wilson et al. 2008). Ideally, more than one CD4 count should be measured before treatment initiating decisions are made. People with a CD4 count of more than 500 cells per μl are usually asymptomatic. Many treatment guidelines around the world recommend a threshold of 350 cells/μl for the commencement of antiretroviral therapy (WHO, 2006a) Recent studies showing the extent of immune cell destruction early on in infection have reopened the debate about how soon after infection antiretroviral therapy should be reintroduced. Treatment is also now less toxic with less cumbersome pill burdens making the prospect of earlier and therefore longer therapy more feasible. Above 350 cells per μl, although HIV related symptoms and infections can occur, they are less common than under 350 cells per μl. By the time the CD4 count is 200 cells per μl or less, HIV infection is said to be advanced and the immune system is seriously damaged (Holmes et al., 2006). Patients with fewer than 200 CD4 cells per μl are at great risk for opportunistic infections and must be on appropriate prophylaxis. They should urgently be considered for antiretroviral therapy.

In children, normal CD4 counts are age dependent and vary widely. Therefore, CD4 counts often are expressed as a percentage of normal, rather than an absolute number. A CD4:CD8 ratio is sometimes reported. In a normal immune system, CD4 cells are in slight excess of CD8 cells so the ratio is slightly greater than 1. As CD4 cells are lost and some compensatory increase in CD8 cells occurs, the ratio falls to less than 1.

Drug Resistance Testing

The importance of drug resistance testing is growing as the prevalence of HIV strains resistant to ART grows and the transmission of drug-resistant HIV increases. Current estimates in the United States are that the frequency of new infection with a virus with at least one major resistance mutation is around 10 to 25% (Wainberg & Petrella, 2008). Genotypic testing is cheaper and easier than phenotypic testing and is more commonly performed at baseline in the United States due to increased transmission rates of genotype resistant virus in the United States. In patients receiving ART, an elevated viral load indicates possible drug failure or poor adherence. A confirmed viral load that remains elevated (1000–5000 copies/μl) after addressing adherence issues, is an indication for switching from first- to second-line therapy. For patients failing second-line therapy, who have further therapeutic options, drug sensitivity testing may help further management. The two main laboratory procedures used to assess susceptibility to antiretroviral drugs are the genotypic and phenotypic assays. As genotypic assays are most frequently used, we discuss only this methodology in more detail below.

Genotype Assays

Genotypic analysis identifies mutations of the HIV-*pol* gene sequences, encoding reverse transcriptase (*rt*) and protease enzymes (*pr*), which are associated with phenotypic resistance to ARVs. Following reverse transcription of the *pol* gene, DNA sequencing of the amplicons is compared with a consensus reference sequence. The genotype report is given in a "letter-number-letter" format. The initial letter indicates the amino acid of wild type consensus virus; the number, the codon of interest; and the final letter indicates the substituted amino acid at this codon. For example, "M184V" indicates that valine has been substituted for methionine at codon number 184 of the *rt* gene. Table 3–2 provides the amino acid letter code used in genotype reports.

Indications for genotype analyses include antiretroviral naïve patients if prevalence of resistant virus in the area or risk group exceeds 10% and for optimizing new regimens for those with viral failure on HAART.

Table 3–2. Amino Acid-Letter Code Used in Genotype Reports

A	Alanine	I	Isoleucine	R	Arginine
C	Cytosine	K	Lysine	S	Serine
D	Aspartic acid	L	Leucine	T	Threonine
E	Glutamic acid	M	Methionine	V	Valine
F	Phenylalanine	N	Asparagine	W	Tryptophan
G	Glycine	P	Proline	Y	Tyrosine
H	Histidine	Q	Glutamine		

Limitations of the genotypic assays include the following:

- they are expensive
- they can be performed only in relatively sophisticated laboratories;
- they can be performed only when viral load is high enough to be amplified (>1000 copies/μl);
- they only identify mutations present in more than 20% of circulating virions;
- they should be performed while patients are on a failing ARV regimen;
- they should be interpreted in conjunction with a knowledge of prior ARV usage.

Genotypic assays most reliably identify drugs that should be avoided and are less reliable for identifying drugs likely to be active.

Early Infection

Following HIV infection, there is a delay before HIV antibodies become detectable in the blood. This diagnostic "window" period: is approximately 4 weeks (see Figure 3-1). Tests that elicit viral antigen will reveal the infection earlier. The p24 antigen test is positive in the majority of patients a week before antibody ELISA tests become reactive. PCR testing, on the other hand, can detect HIV in the blood from approximately 2 weeks after infection.

Should a patient present with a suspected primary HIV illness and HIV-antibody tests are negative or indeterminate, a p24 antigen or a qualitative viral load test may confirm infection. Follow-up antibody testing can be performed 1 to 2 weeks later and repeated until detectable HIV antibodies are present and "seroconversion" is confirmed. Seroconversion describes the time after which the HIV-infected person begins to produce antibodies against the HIV antigens to a detectable level. Although there is variation in the timing, seroconversion, more than 3 months after infection is extremely unusual. Combined p24 and antibody ELISA tests are available, sometimes known as fourth-generation HIV tests, and these reduce the window period by a week or so.

The window period is particularly important in blood and organ donors and in these settings HIV screening using nucleic acid based tests that detect viral antigen are strongly advised. The p24 antigen test has been largely superseded by nucleic acid amplification technologies because it has approximately 75% sensitivity relative to PCR in identifying infectious persons in the window period.

Monitoring the Disease

The laboratory tests most commonly used to monitor a patient's progress both prior to and post commencement of antiretroviral therapy are the viral load and the CD4 count. The information that these tests give has been compared to that of a car traveling along a road that ends in a ditch: in this analogy, the viral load is indicative of the speed of the car, the CD4 count indicates the distance from the ditch, and the ditch indicates the onset of AIDS. In other words, viral load predicts the rate of disease progression (rate of loss of CD4 cells) and the CD4 count indicates the point of disease that the patient has already reached (Wilson et al., 2008).

HIV Diagnosis in Babies

Up to 30% of babies born to HIV-infected women will be infected either pre- or perinatally or during breast feeding. This can be significantly reduced with the use of antiretrovirals in the pregnant woman prior to birth, but there remains a risk that vertical transmission can occur (Conor et al., 1994). Recent studies have shown that survival in vertically infected babies is improved by commencing earlier antiretroviral therapy (WHO, 2006b). Vertical transmission of HIV presents a diagnostic challenge in the newborn in that placentally transferred maternal antibodies persist in the neonate. All babies newly born to HIV-positive women will test HIV-antibody-positive because of the transfer of maternal antibodies to the baby across the placenta. On average, most uninfected babies will become seronegative (no longer carry the maternal HIV antibodies) at 11 months of age but some may have detectable maternal antibody for up to 18 months. Infected babies will be persistently seropositive beyond 18 months of age (Stevens et al., 2008).

Therefore, to discriminate between infected and uninfected babies before the age of 18 months, it is necessary to utilize tests that detect the virus itself. Nucleic acid testing (usually PCR) has the highest sensitivity and specificity in this context. Standard p24 antigen testing is insensitive and will detect approximately 40% of infected babies. Therefore, a positive p24 antigen test indicates infection, but a negative result does not exclude infection. The recommended age for reliable HIV PCR testing in babies is after 4 weeks. If the mother is breastfeeding, there is ongoing risk of infection and the test may need to be repeated until after the child is weaned or is old enough to be tested with antibody tests (The Breast Feeding and HIV International Transmission Study Group, 2004).

The World Health Organization (WHO, 2006b) recently has posted new recommendations that consider recent pediatric studies and now recommends universal treatment of all HIV-infected babies less than 12 months of age. To benefit from early treatment and to reduce their risk of disease and death, infants need to be tested at the earliest opportunity.

For diagnosing infants the WHO (2006a) strongly recommends:

- Infants known to be HIV exposed, that is, born to mothers in prevention of mother to child transmission (PMTCT) programs, have a virologic test (HIV nucleic acid test) at 4 to 6 weeks of age.
- Any infant presenting at a health facility with signs or symptoms that may be an indication for HIV initially should be tested using an HIV antibody test with a positive test confirmed by virologic testing if possible.

■ All infants should have their HIV status established at their first contact with the health system, preferably before 6 weeks of age (in most cases this will be established by asking the mother and checking her history of HIV testing).

■ WHO also conditionally recommends that infants less than 6 weeks of age in settings of high antenatal HIV prevalence (i.e., >1%) should be offered maternal or infant HIV antibody testing.

Recommendations specify that infants are diagnosed using virologic tests (HIV DNA PCR, HIV RNA PCR, bDNa, NASBA, or ultrasensitive p24 antigen). The HIV DNA PCR is the only test that can be performed using dried blood spot (DBS) samples and is the most useful for early diagnosis in PMTCT follow-up (WHO, 2006b). Testing also is recommended around 4 to 6 weeks for PMTCT follow-up, and whenever an infant is sick or HIV is suspected in those known to be exposed. Testing at 4 weeks instead of at 6 weeks provides an additional 2 weeks at a time of great vulnerability to the infant.

If virologic testing is not available, presumptive diagnosis in accordance with nationally defined algorithms is recommended. Based on data from the CHER study, the WHO is refining an algorithm based on symptoms and signs of HIV at 6 weeks of age (WHO, 2008a). Although lacking sensitivity, suggestive signs include oral thrush, hepatomegaly, splenomegaly, lymphadenopathy diaper dermatitis, and clinical gastroesophageal disease (cough and/or vomiting during feeds).

Diagnosis of AIDS

The acquired immune deficiency syndrome (AIDS) occurs as a result of HIV infection, usually after approximately 6 to 9 years of infection and is a clinical diagnosis. It describes a constellation of clinical conditions, opportunistic infections and/or malignancies that may occur as a result of ongoing immune dysfunction and deterioration. After a thorough clinical examination during which the patient is clinically staged, a WHO stage 4 or CDC stage C would indicate AIDS. These staging systems for diagnosis were described in Chapter 2.

MANAGEMENT OF HIV/AIDS

Current research suggests that the host's initial response to HIV infection is critical and genetically determined. Less than 5% of patients show unusually slow or little immune damage for a long time (Beattie, Rowland-Jones, & Kaul, 2002). These nonprogressors are being carefully studied with the hope of developing immune-based therapies for HIV, and those that keep viral load undetectable despite no therapy are termed elite controllers (<1% of infections; Hatano et al., 2008).

HIV is a retrovirus that infects and replicates primarily in human CD4+ T cells and macrophages. The virus gains entry to the cells by attaching to the CD4 receptor and a coreceptor via its envelope glycoproteins. It is called a retrovirus because it encodes the enzyme reverse transcriptase, allowing a DNA copy to be made from viral RNA. The reverse transcriptase enzyme is inherently error-prone, resulting in a high rate of HIV mutation, which can rapidly lead to viral resistance in those on treatment.

HIV can be transmitted via blood, blood products, sexual fluids, other fluids containing blood, and breast milk. Most individuals are infected with HIV through sexual contact, vertically (before birth or during delivery, during breastfeeding), or when sharing contaminated needles and syringes (IV drug users). Sexual intercourse is the most common, albeit inefficient, mode of HIV transmission. The risk of transmission per exposure is low; estimates are on the order of 0.1% per contact for heterosexual transmission (Overbaugh, 2008).

Once integrated into the cellular DNA the provirus resides in the nucleus of infected cells and can remain quiescent for extended periods of time. Alternatively, it can become transcriptionally active (especially where immune activity is occurring) and can utilize the human host cell machinery to replicate itself. Viral RNA is then spliced singly or multiply to make a variety of structural and regulatory and accessory proteins. Viral proteases further process proteins and mature viral particles are formed when the virus buds through the host cell membrane. Within a few weeks of infection, there is a high level of viral replication in the blood that can exceed 10 million viral particles per μl of plasma. There is a concomitant decline in

CD4 T cells (Veasey et al., 1998). However, within a few weeks an immune response to HIV develops that curtails viral replication, resulting in a decrease in viral load and a return of CD4 T-cell numbers to near normal levels. The immune control is thought to be dependent on killer T cells and neutralizing antibodies. Depending on how effective this control is, the viral load will be known as the set point and this is thought to be prognostic of natural history outcomes for the infected person (Stekler & Collier, 2004) (see Figure 3–1).

Initial Assessment

Initial assessment of a person newly diagnosed with HIV should be thorough and include a comprehensive and focused medical history and clinical examination, as well as appropriate laboratory tests, in order to assess the stage of HIV disease in the individual. Baseline laboratory investigations will depend on available resources. All patients should have a CD4 count, hepatitis B and C screen, venereal disease research laboratory tests (VDRL), tuberculin skin test, and chest X-ray (CXR). HIV viral load should be performed at baseline in most developed countries. Drug resistance testing (genotype/phenotype) is recommended in settings—for example, the United States—where there are high levels of circulating resistant virus. At the end of the session, a comprehensive management plan for future care of this individual should be detailed, including a plan for "positive living" that incorporates any lifestyle modifications to accommodate the positive HIV status (DHHS, 2001; Kalichman, 2008; WHO, 2006a).

The patient may present at one of four stages:

- During the acute seroconversion illness
- Period of clinical latency
- Period of immune suppression before the development of AIDS
- With AIDS.

At the initial consultation with the medical practitioner, an infected patient may be at any stage of the natural history of this chronic infection, ranging from asymptomatic to severely ill. Diagnosis of HIV is the responsibility of all health care practitioners, and providers should also be sufficiently trained to manage the stage of positive living.

A person who feels he or she is at risk for being HIV positive should be offered a test. This should include determining risk factors for HIV acquisition or transmission and working out appropriate strategies to reduce risk. It may be prudent in cases where HIV is suspected to present the HIV test as an opt-out option among other diagnostics. Antibody tests, either ELISA or rapid tests, are the tests most frequently used to diagnose HIV. A positive result should be confirmed with a second specific confirmatory test: a Western blot or a second rapid test or ELISA.

The clinician should elicit a physical history of common symptoms likely to be related to HIV, paying particular attention to those symptoms that would assist in staging the HIV disease by CDC or WHO classifications (Center for Disease Control [CDC], 1992; WHO, 2005). Both the CDC staging and WHO clinical staging tables are included in Chapter 2. This includes fevers and night sweats, loss of weight, skin rashes, oral thrush or ulceration, diarrhea, headaches, and changes in mental status or neuropsychiatric function. All recent hospital admissions should be detailed as they may be related to HIV. Risk of TB should be assessed (symptoms and any known contact) and a vaccination history taken (particularly hepatitis A and B, pneumococcal, and tetanus). A note should be made of current medication and known allergies. All women should be asked about current and prior pregnancies and whether they have been pregnant since knowing their HIV status.

Attention should be paid to risk factors for contracting HIV, such as IV drug use and sexual history, including sexual orientation and risks of further HIV transmission, number of partners, whether partners are aware of HIV status, use of condoms, and previous sexually transmitted diseases (STDs) (including viral hepatitis). Social background and lifestyle issues should be discussed, including:

- Home environment—type of housing, how many people live there, water and electricity supply
- Children—ages and HIV status if known
- Disclosure of HIV status—to sexual partner, family, and/or friends

- Support structures—people who can provide emotional support for the patient
- Employment and other socioeconomic factors that may impede on adherence
- Smoking history
- Current and prior use of alcohol or other substance use.

In starting with the physician's general impression of the patient, it should be established if the patient is well or ill. The examination should be tailored to the extent of the patient's symptoms. Patients may appear very well despite quite extensive immune depletion (which may only be discovered once blood results are obtained) and represent potential for acute opportunistic infections. In these cases, prophylaxis should be considered and steps should be taken in preparing the patient for antiretroviral treatment. In other instances, the patient may be relatively early in infection but present with an acute infection (e.g., tuberculosis) and seem quite ill. Also, remember that patients may often have other sexually transmitted infections and are also still subject to other unrelated infectious and noninfectious illnesses.

Pregnancy testing should be done on all women of childbearing potential who are known to be HIV infected, and in high prevalence areas all pregnant women should be offered HIV testing. Hepatitis B, C, and syphilis serology should be performed to exclude these infections or detect them for treatment. Tuberculin skin test should be performed, if deemed clinically necessary. A reaction of more than 5 mm may require TB prophylaxis as long as active tuberculosis has been excluded. CXR should be requested if there are symptoms of TB or pneumonia. Once the initial assessment and CD4 count is completed, the patient should be staged according to either the CDC or the WHO classification systems as indicated in Chapter 2 (CDC, 1992; WHO, 2005). Continued management will depend on whether the patient is in early or late HIV disease.

The initial assessment is key for prognosis and formulation of medium- to long-term management plans. After clinical and laboratory staging, opportunistic infection such as TB and *Pneumocystis jiroveci* pneumonia prophylaxis as well as immunizations (pneumococcal, influenza, hepatitis B and A, and tetanus) should be discussed with the patient in the initial stages of evaluation. Decision on initiation of highly active antiretroviral therapy (HAART) will depend on the patient's clinical stage, CD4 count, medical comorbidities, and ability to adhere to chronic HIV treatment.

1. During the acute seroconversion illness:
   The acute retroviral syndrome occurs in up to 50% of patients following their infection with HIV (Lavreys et al., 2000). It is a symptom complex that ranges from mild, nonspecific influenzalike symptoms to a florid illness that may even require hospitalization. In the latter it may present with aseptic meningitis or meningoencephalitis, maculopapular rash, myalgia, arthralgia, fever, hepatosplenomegaly, and other neurologic findings such as peripheral neuropathy, Guillain-Barré syndrome, or facial palsies. Laboratory findings include lymphopenia, followed by lymphocytosis with atypical lymphocytes. In some cases, CD4 cell depletion may be severe, resulting in thrush or other infections such as *Pneumocystis jiroveci* pneumonia. These opportunistic infections and symptoms should be treated on their merit. During this time, serology may be negative or indeterminate, and diagnosis is most reliable by testing for viral RNA or DNA in plasma, although p24 antigen may also be positive at this time if the test is available. Whether to commence antiretroviral therapy at this stage is still an unanswered question. A number of clinical trials are ongoing at present exploring the merit of early treatment followed by withdrawal of treatment after varying periods of treatment. In some cases where clinically indicated, ART may be commenced as a life-saving intervention and the challenge in these patients often then is to know when to withdraw therapy, if at all (Kilby et al., 2008).

2. Period of clinical latency:
   Currently, most testing globally is done in individuals who are symptomatic and seeking health care. HIV testing is increasing in the sexually transmitted infection clinic, tuberculosis clinic, and in antenatal care. For this reason, asymptomatic individuals in the period of clinical latency are not seen that often. As testing is rolled out as a prevention strategy, more individuals will be living with a diagnosis of HIV infection prior to the onset of HIV-related illness. This asymptomatic period is of varying

duration for different individuals. It is a time when emphasis should be on lifestyle changes, the development of social support structures, preparation for treatment, and possibly disclosure to family, friends, and/or household. Medical encounters can be relatively infrequent and are important to monitor progress both clinically and with serial CD4 counts. If immunity is well preserved, CD4 counts may be performed initially 12 to 6 monthly, and with increasing frequency (3 monthly) as infection advances and the time to commence therapy draws near. Patients should pay attention to diet, smoking, and drinking habits at this time, with the goal of maintaining as healthy a lifestyle as possible. Importantly, positive prevention is critical at this time too with every effort made to reduce the risk of HIV transmission and to build a psychosocial environment conducive to the challenges that progressive HIV and lifelong therapy will present. Vaccination status should also be reviewed and updated at this stage.

3. Period of immune suppression before the development of AIDS: Ideally, patients should be offered treatment before the onset of AIDS. Recent reports confirm that HIV infection wreaks havoc on the immune system almost from the start of infection (Veazey et al., 1998). Clinical data indicate that the baseline CD4 is predictive of both morbidity and mortality and that patients with low CD4 counts are more at risk of opportunistic infections (Holmes et al., 2006) and complications in the early stages of treatment. In addition, patients with low CD4 counts have a much increased susceptibility to tuberculosis (Lawn, Myer, Bekker, & Wood, 2006). Guidelines of when to start treatment have taken this into consideration and many countries now have adopted an approach where treatment is recommended when the first indicators appear that immunity is beginning to fail (i.e., WHO stage 3 illness or a CD4 count less than 350). All of these patients should be screened for occult opportunistic infection, particularly tuberculosis; they should be offered prophylaxis to *pneumocystis jerovici* pneumonia (PJP) and TB and steps should be taken to ready them for treatment initiation (DHHS, 2008; SAHIVClinSoc, 2008; WHO, 2006a). Before patients commence HAART, the following tests should be done and monitored during the course of therapy:

- CD4 count
- Viral load
- Liver function tests
- Full blood count
- Serum creatinine and U/A for proteinuria
- Hepatitis B surface antigen
- VDRL

Also consider (depending on setting):

- Hepatitis C serology: most commonly seen in setting where intravenous drug use is occurring.
- Viral genotype: consider where high background rate of de novo viral resistance to antiretrovirals.

Practitioners should have a clear understanding of clinical staging for HIV. Two internationally recognized clinical staging systems currently exist: the World Health Organization, which describes four clinical stages (stages 1–4) from asymptomatic to AIDS and the CDC, which describes 3 (stage A to C) (CDC, 1992; WHO, 2005).

4. With AIDS:
   Patients who have reached the clinical stage described as AIDS are at high risk of morbidity and mortality. They should be quickly assessed for opportunistic infections and if clear should be offered antiretroviral therapy with urgency (Badri, Lawn, & Wood, 2006). Where suspected, concomitant opportunistic infections should be investigated aggressively in order to commence treatment for the opportunistic infections without delaying ART for too long. In most cases, ART can be commenced shortly after initiating opportunistic infection treatment. In some cases, where CD4 counts are particularly low, commencement of ART may result in unmasking or exacerbation of an opportunistic infection. This is known as immune restoration inflammatory syndrome or IRIS and reflects an immune response to ART (Lawn, Bekker, & Miller, 2005; Lawn et al., 2008). In most cases, if this is anticipated in patients with advanced HIV, it can be supportively managed without interrupting ART. It is rare that a patient will be considered too ill or too advanced to initiate ART. Patients need to understand that daily adherence and

lifelong therapy is indicated. If patients are very ill at the time of commencement, a family member may need to assist with pill taking until the patient recovers sufficiently to manage his or her own treatment.

Antiretroviral Therapy

HIV and its therapy, that of lifelong antiviral combination therapy with excellent adherence, has seen a paradigm shift in managing patients. Patients are encouraged to take responsibility for their treatment, become knowledgeable about the drugs and their side effects, to disclose where possible to friends and family, and adopt a self-help and independent attitude to their illness. In many settings, peers are becoming treatment supporters and mentors to others on treatment (Bekker et al., 2006). Some programs in countries where there are very large treatment programs, for example, South Africa, are showing that, despite the rapidity and scale of ART roll out in the public sector, high rates of adherence and good outcomes are being maintained so far (Keiser, Anastos, et al., 2008). The challenge will be to maintain these outcomes for as long as possible.

Data from developed countries show that, if patients are adherent, viral load can be chronically suppressed with ongoing immune restoration and return of good health and well-being for many years (Keiser, Orrell, et al., 2008). Conversely, the virus in patients who take their treatment poorly will develop drug resistance and that treatment eventually will no longer be efficacious for the patient. This will be indicated by a rise in viral load and falling CD4 count. After some time, health also will begin to fail. If the viral load is being monitored, it is advisable to intensify adherence counselling and measures such as reminders, pill boxes, and so forth, in the hope that improved adherence will lead to viral suppression even on the same drug regimen (Orrel et al., 2007). If, however, viral load continues to increase despite all efforts to improve adherence, the drug regimen is said to be failing and a change to another drug regimen is indicated. It is advisable to consider any prior therapy when choosing a new regimen as cross-resistance among antiretroviral agents does occur. Patients preferably should not be left too long on a failing regimen as additional resistance mutations will be incurred by the infecting virus in the presence of a suboptimal drug regimen. Most countries, and the World Health Organization, have both pediatric and adult treatment guidelines that consider new drugs, de novo resistance rates, and new data and are continually reviewed and revised (see DHHS Guidelines, 2001; South African Guidelines, 2008; WHO, 2008a, 2008b). By and large, highly active antiretroviral therapy consists of at least three potent agents and should include at least two classes of agents.

Adults

The first regimen that a patient is exposed to has the best chance of sustained success. Antiretroviral agents have a range of specific and well-described side effects (Murphy et al., 2007). Different patients will experience these side effects to varying degrees. Some are life threatening and it is up the practitioner to be aware and to both warn patients and monitor for them. Intolerance to side effects is another, less common cause for treatment changes. If a patient's viral load is undetectable, treatment can be swapped without breaks in therapy (Boulle et al., 2007). There may be other compelling reasons to select or avoid particular ARVs in particular patients.

Conventional combination antiretroviral therapy consists of two nucleoside reverse transcriptase inhibitors (NRTI) together with either a non-nucleoside reverse transcriptase inhibitor (NNRTI) or a protease inhibitor (PI). NNRTIs are at least as effective as PIs when combined with two NRTIs in clinical trials. NNRTIs are often cheaper, mostly have a lower pill burden, and offer no increased risk of cardiovascular disease although they generally have a lower genetic barrier making them a less popular choice for second-line therapy where mutations may have compromised NRTI performance. Efavirenz should be avoided in women of child bearing potential and in patients with uncontrolled depression or psychosis. Nevirapine should be avoided with coexisting liver disease and in patients with higher CD4 counts because of increased risk of rash-associated hepatitis. When selecting a second-line regimen, ideally two new NRTIs should be used, together with a third drug from a new class. A ritonavir boosted PI is recommended in second-line therapy. Ritonavir boosted PIs have a relatively high genetic barrier to resistance and the second-line regimen may be effective even if there are some mutations that limit the efficacy of the NRTIs. Table 3-3 provides a list of antiretroviral drugs commonly used in adults and their recommended dosages.

Table 3–3. List of Commonly Used Antiretroviral Agents and Their Recommended Doses for Adults

Drug Class	Generic name	Dosage
Nucleoside reverse transcriptase inhibitor	Zidovudine (AZT)	300 mg every 12 hrs
Nucleoside reverse transcriptase inhibitor	Didanosine (ddl)	400 mg daily (250 mg daily if <60 kg) (take on empty stomach)
Nucleoside reverse transcriptase inhibitor	Lamivudine (3TC)	150 mg every 12 hrs or 300 mg daily
Nucleoside reverse transcriptase inhibitor	Stavudine (d4T)	30 mg every 12 hrs (note higher doses for >60 kg no longer recommended due to toxicity
Nucleoside reverse transcriptase inhibitor	Abacavir (ABC)	300 mg every 12 hrs or 600 mg daily
Nucleotide reverse transcriptase inhibitor	Tenofovir (TDF)	300 mg daily
Nucleoside reverse transcriptase inhibitor	Emtricitabine (FTC)	200 mg daily (coformulated with TDF)
Non-nucleoside reverse transcriptase inhibitor	Nevirapine	200 mg daily for 14 days then 200 mg every 12 hrs (2 tabs daily)
Non-nucleoside reverse transcriptase inhibitor	Efavirenz	600 mg at night
Protease inhibitor	Nelfinavir	750 mg every 8 hrs or 1250 mg every 12 hrs
Protease inhibitor	Indinavir	800 mg every 8 hrs (on an empty stomach) or 800 mg every 12 hrs with 100 mg Ritonavir every 12 hrs (no food restrictions)
Protease inhibitor	Ritonavir	600 mg every 12 hrs
Protease inhibitor	Saquinavir	1000/100 bd or 2000/100 daily (only if PI naïve)

Table 3–3. *continued*

Drug Class	Generic name	Dosage
Protease inhibitor	Atazanavir	400 mg daily (only if PI naïve) or 300 mg with Ritonavir 100 mg daily
Protease inhibitor	Fosamprenavir	1400 mg every 12 hrs or 1400 mg with Ritonavir 200 mg daily
Protease inhibitor	Lopinavir/ Ritonavir	400/100 mg every 12 hrs or 800/200 mg daily (only if PI naïve)

Infants and Children

The revised pediatric guidelines from WHO (2008b) recommend ART regimens for pediatric patients should not be commenced on a nevirapine containing first-line regimen when there has been maternal or infant ARV exposure previously, non-nucleoside reverse transcriptase inhibitor ARV drug exposure or when there has been ARV exposure of unknown type. In these cases then, a protease inhibitor containing regimen should commenced to avoid possible early failure in the infant due to NNRTI resistance.

Pediatric formulations for children too young to swallow tablets traditionally have been liquids or syrups. These formulations are expensive and not easy to store or transport. Cost and logistical issues have prohibited their widespread use. This example has been given to illustrate the challenge this gives to the caregiver:

> *A 10-kg child being treated with standard doses of stavudine, lamivudine, and nevirapine, for whom a 3-month supply of drugs is dispensed at a clinic visit, would require 18 bottles of liquid weighing almost half as much as the child (4.3 kg). For a rural family who may have walked a long distance to reach the clinical centre, this is a significant issue.* (Clayden, 2008)

More recently, manufacturers have developed more convenient crushable minipills or dispersible formulations and fixed dose combinations (FDCs), which can be used by very young children (Clayden, 2008). Many programs now use these formulations and the WHO (2008b) recommends dosing according to their simplified weight band tables.

Prevention of mother to child transmission and postexposure prophylaxis guidelines should include at least two agents or more. This is to reduce the risk of viral resistance mutations occurring. In the developing countries, the WHO (2008a, 2008b) has recommended a public health approach to ART rollout. This entails the provision of antiretroviral therapies in a scheduled approach. Fewer drug options and drug costs have meant that individualized ART is practiced only in the private sector and the developed world. Significantly, this has resulted in far less frequent drug changes and much less frequent laboratory monitoring in most public sector programs (Keiser et al., 2008), making the cost of the management of an individual far less costly in the developing world. This is important as the unmet ART need and the scale of rollout in this sector of the world is far greater than in the developed world (Walensky et al., 2008).

Research has shown that the patients of practitioners who have some experience in ART management do better than those of inexperienced practitioners (Kitahata et al., 2003). Thus, in countries where HIV is prevalent, it is important that all health care workers develop some understanding of HIV pathogenesis, progression, and management.

SUMMARY

This chapter outlines the indications for HIV testing and recommended laboratory tests that should be employed in various settings. It also describes the variety of laboratory monitoring available once a patient tests HIV positive. From the time of infection, there is rapid viral replication and slow but inexorable loss of immune function. The natural history and variations in the rapidity with which this occurs in patients is described. Finally, an approach to the first assessment, ongoing care, and inevitable commencement of antiretroviral therapy is also discussed. Although there is not an exhaustive list of antiretroviral therapy at the disposal of the practitioner, a pragmatic approach to the initial commencement of adult and pediatric antiviral therapy is offered.

REFERENCES

Badri, M., Lawn, S. D., & Wood, R. (2006). Short-term risk of AIDS or death in people infected with HIV-1 before antiretroviral therapy in South Africa: A longitudinal study. *Lancet, 7,* 368(9543), 1254-1259.

Beattie, T., Rowland-Jones, S., & Kaul, R. (2002). HIV-1 and AIDS: What are protective immune responses? *Journal of HIV Therapy, 7*(2), 35-39.

Bekker, L. G., Myer, L., Orrell, C., Lawn, S., & Wood, R. (2006). Rapid scale-up of a community-based HIV treatment service: Programme performance over 3 consecutive years in Guguletu, South Africa. *South African Medical Journal, 96*(4), 315-320.

Boulle, A., Orrel, C., Kaplan, R. Van Cutsem, G., McNally, M., Hilderbrand, K., . . . Wood, R. (2007). Substitutions due to antiretroviral toxicity or contraindication in the first 3 years of antiretroviral therapy in a large South African cohort. *Antiviral Therapy, 12*(5), 753-760.

CDC. (1992). 1993 revised classification system for HIV infection and expanded surveillance case definition for AIDS among adolescents and adults. *MMWR.* Retrieved December 18, 1992, from http://www.cdc.gov/mmwr/preview/mmwrhtml/00018871.htm

Clayden, P. (2008). Starting infants on antiretroviral therapy. *Southern African Journal of HIV Medicine, 32,* 25-31.

Connor, E. M., Sperling, R. S., Gelber, R., Kiselev, P., Scott, G., O'Sullivan, M. J., . . . Jacobson, R. L. (1994). Reduction of maternal-infant transmission of human immunodeficiency virus type 1 with zidovudine treatment. *New England Journal of Medicine, 3312,* 1173-1180.

Department of Health. (2007). *HIV and AIDS and STI strategic plan for South Africa,* 2007-2011 DOH, SANAC. http://www.doh.gov.za/docs/misc/stratplan

DHHS Guidelines. (2001). *Guidelines for the use of antiretroviral agents in HIV-infected adults and adolescents.* Retrieved October 23, 2008, from http://www.aidsinfo.nih.gov/ContentFiles/AdultandAdolescent GL02052001009.pdf

Hatano, H., Delwart, E. L., Norris, P. J., Lee, T.H., Dunn-Williams, J., Hunt, P. W., . . . Deeks, S. G.. (2009). Evidence for persistent low-level viremia in individuals who control HIV in the absence of antiretroviral therapy. *Journal of Virology,* 83(1), 329-335.

Holmes, C. B., Wood, R., & Badri, M. (2006). CD4 decline and incidence of opportunistic infections in Cape Town, South Africa: Implications for prophylaxis and treatment. *Journal of Acquired Immune Deficiency Syndromes*, 42(4), 464–469.

Kalichman, S. C. (2008). Co-occurrence of treatment nonadherence and continued HIV transmission risk behaviors: Implications for positive prevention interventions. *Psychosomatic Medicine*, 70(5), 593–597.

Keiser, O., Anastos, K., Schechter, M., Balestre, E., Myer, L., Boulle, A., . . . Egger, M. (2008). ART-LINC Collaboration of International Databases to Evaluate AIDS (IeDEA), Antiretroviral therapy in resource-limited settings 1996 to 2006: Patient characteristics, treatment regimens and monitoring in Sub-Saharan Africa, Asia and Latin America. *Tropical Medicine and International Heath*, 13(7), 870–879.

Keiser, O., Orrell, C., Egger, M., Wood, R., Brinkhof, M. W., Furrer, H., . . . Boulle, A. (2008). HIV cohort study (SHCS) and the international epidemiologic databases to evaluate AIDS in Southern Africa (IeDEA-SA). Public-health and individual approaches to antiretroviral therapy: Township South Africa and Switzerland compared. *PLoS Medicine*, 5(7), e148.

Kilby, J. M., Lee, H. Y., Hazelwood, J. D., Bansal, A., Bucy, R. P., Saag, M. S., . . . UAB Acute Infection, Early Disease Research Program (AIEDRP) Group. (2008). Treatment response in acute/early infection versus advanced AIDS: Equivalent first and second phases of HIV RNA decline. *AIDS*, 22(8), 957–962.

Kitahata, M. M., Van Rompaey, S. E., Dillingham, P. W., Koepsell, T. D., Deyo, R. A., Dodge, W., . . . Wagner, E. H. (2003). Primary care delivery is associated with greater physician experience and improved survival among persons with AIDS. *Journal of General Internal Medicine*, 18(2), 95–103.

Lavreys, L., Thompson, M. L., Martin, H. L., Mandaliya, K., Ndinya-Achola, J. D., Bwayo, J. J., & Kreiss, J.. (2000). Primary immunodeficiency virus type 1 infection. Clinical manifestations among women in Mombasa, Kenta. *Clinical Infectious Diseases*, 30, 486–490.

Lawn, S. D., Bekker, L. G., & Miller, R. F. (2005). Immune reconstitution disease associated with mycobacterial infections in HIV-infected individuals receiving antiretrovirals. *Lancet Infectious Diseases*, 5(6), 361–373.

Lawn, S. D., Myer, L., Bekker, L. G., & Wood, R. (2006). Burden of tuberculosis in an antiretroviral treatment programme in Sub-Saharan Africa: Impact on treatment outcomes and implications for tuberculosis control. *AIDS*, 20(12), 1605–1612.

Lawn, S. D., Wilkinson, R. J., Lipman, M. C., & Wood, R. (2008). Immune reconstitution and "unmasking" of tuberculosis during antiretroviral therapy. *American Journal of Respiratory and Critical Care Medicine*, 177(7), 680–685.

MacLennan, C. A., Liu, M. K., & White, S. A. Diagnostic accuracy and clinical utility of a simplified low cost method of counting CD4 cells with flow cytometry in Malawi: Diagnostic accuracy study. *British Medical Journal, 335*(7612), 190.

Murphy, R. A., Sunpath, H., & Kuritzkes, D. R. (2007). Antiretroviral therapy-associated toxicities in the resource-poor world: The challenge of a limited formulary. *Journal of Infectious Diseases, 196*(Suppl. 3), S449–S456.

Orrell, C., Harling, G., Lawn, S. D., Kaplan, R., McNally, M., Bekker, L. G., & Wood, R. (2007). Conservation of first-line antiretroviral treatment regimen where therapeutic options are limited. *Antiviral Therapy, 12*(1), 83–88.

Overbaugh, J. (2008). Biology of HIV transmission. In P. A. Volberdling, M. A. Sande, J. Lange, W. C. Greene, & J. E. Gallant (Eds.), *Global HIV/AIDS medicine* (p. 75). Philadelphia: Saunders.

Richardson, J. L., Milam, J., Mc Cutchan, A., Stoyanoff, S., Bolan, R., Weiss, J., . . . Marks, G. (2004). Effect of brief safer sex counseling by medical providers to HIV-1 seropositive patients: A multicentre assessment. *AIDS, 18,* 1179–1186.

South African Guidelines. (2008). Southern African HIV Clinicians Society Guidelines for Antiretroviral Therapy in Adults. *SAJHIVMED, 29,* 18–33.

Stekler, J., & Collier, A. C. (2004). Primary HIV infection. *Current HIV/AIDS Report, 1*(2), 68–73.

Stevens, W., Sherman, G., Downing, R., Parsons, L. M., Ou, C. Y., Crowley, S., . . . Nkengasong, J. N. (2008). Role of the laboratory in ensuring global access to ARV treatment for HIV-infected children: Consensus statement on the performance of laboratory assays for early infant diagnosis. *Open AIDS Journal, 2,* 17–25.

The Breast Feeding and HIV International Transmission Study Group. Late postnatal transmission of HIV-1 in breastfed infants: An independent patient data meta-analysis. *Journal of Infectious Diseases, 189,* 2154–2166.

UNAIDS. (2007). *Annual Report: Knowing your epidemic.* Retrieved October 24, 2008, from http://data.unaids.org/pub/Report/2008/jc 1535_annual_report07_en.pdf

UNAIDS. (2008). *Report on the Global AIDS epidemic.* Joint United Nations Programme on HIV/AIDS (UNAIDS) and World Health Organization (WHO), Geneva.

Veazey, R. S., DeMaria, M., Chalifoux, L. V., Shvetz, D. E., Pauley, D. R., Knight, H. L., . . . Lackner, A. A. (1998). Gastrointestinal tract as a major site of CD4+ T cell depletion in gut lymphoid tissue in SIV infection. *Science, 280,* 427–431.

Wainberg, A., & Petrella, M. (2008). Development and transmission of HIV drug resistance. *Global HIV/AIDS medicine* (p. 154). Philadelphia: Saunders.

Walensky, R. P., Wood, R., Weinstein, M. C., Martinson, N. A., Losina, E., Fofana, M. O., . . . CEPAC-International Investigators. (2008). Scaling up antiretroviral therapy in South Africa: The impact of speed on survival. *Journal of Infectious Diseases, 197*(9), 1223–1225.

WHO. (2005). *Interim WHO clinical staging of HIV/AIDS and HIV/AIDS case definitions for surveillance: African region.* Retrieved August 17, 2009, from http://www.who.int/hiv/pub/guidelines/clinicalstaging.pdf

WHO. (2006a). *Antiretroviral therapy for HIV infection in adults and adolescents: Recommendations for a public health approach.* Retrieved October 23, 2008, from http://www.who.int/hiv/pub/guidelines/adult/en/index.html

WHO. (2006b). *Antiretroviral drugs for treating pregnant women and preventing HIV infection in infants: Towards universal access.* Retrieved October 23, 2008, from http://www.who.int/hiv/pub/mtct/pmtct/en/

WHO. (2008a). *Scale up of HIV-related prevention, diagnosis, care and treatment for infants and children: A programming framework.* Retrieved March 3, 2009, from http://www.who.int/hiv/paediatric/Paeds_programming_framework2008.pdf

WHO. (2008b). *WHO antiretroviral therapy for infants and children.* Retrieved March 3, 2009, from http://www.who.int/hiv/pub/paediatric/WHO_Paediatric_ART_guideline_rev_mreport_2008.pdf

Wilson, D., Cotton, M., Bekker, L. G., Meyers, T., Venter, F., & Maartens, G. (2008). *Handbook of HIV medicine.* South Africa: Oxford University Press.

CHAPTER 4

Infection Control for Communication, Hearing, and Swallowing Disorders

A. U. Bankaitis

INTRODUCTION

The emergence of acquired immunodeficiency syndrome (AIDS) during the early 1980s and subsequent discovery of the human immunodeficiency virus (HIV) moved infection control to the forefront throughout the medical and scientific communities. The concern for cross-contamination associated with HIV/AIDS led to the development of federally mandated infection control requirements, providing health care employers and workers with specific guidelines on how to reduce the risk of exposure to potentially infectious agents. The concept of applying infection control principles in the clinical environment is relatively straightforward; however, implementing an effective infection control program involves not only an appreciation of its importance, but also an understanding of general principles, appropriate organization and planning, and the consistent application and execution of such principles.

INFECTION CONTROL

Infection control refers to the conscious management of the environment for the purposes of minimizing or eliminating the potential spread of disease (Bankaitis & Kemp, 2003, 2005). The discovery of HIV impacted all areas of health care with regard to infection control, including speech-language pathology and audiology (Bankaitis, Kemp, Krival, & Bandaranayake, 2005). It is critical to recognize that infection control is not limited to minimizing the spread of HIV; quite frankly, the potential encounter with an HIV-infected individual should not serve as the determining factor as to whether or not infection control protocols should be followed. Rather, HIV simply served as the catalyst of change for infection control (Kemp & Roeser, 1998).

Infection control is driven by two foundational principles. First, the goal of infection control is to minimize or eliminate the spread of disease that potentially may be caused by any infectious agent, including but not limited to something as seemingly innocuous as *Staphylococcus*. Again, the concept of infection control is not dedicated to preventing exposure to HIV alone or to those pathogens perceived as more aggressive such as hepatitis B (Bankaitis & Kemp, 2007). Rather, infection control is intended to reduce or eliminate the probability of exposure to any potentially infectious microorganism regardless of how remote the possibility of cross-contamination is perceived by the clinician. Second, infection control is based on the foundational assumption that every patient, bodily fluid, substance, or agent is potentially infectious. As such, diagnostic and rehabilitative services, including those provided by speech-language pathologists, audiologists, and other health care professionals managing communication, hearing, and swallowing disorders, must be delivered in a manner consistent with infection control guideline requirements and applied uniformly across all patients.

RELEVANCE OF INFECTION CONTROL RELATED TO COMMUNICATION, HEARING, AND SWALLOWING DISORDERS

As primary health care providers for communication, hearing, and swallowing disorders, speech-language pathologists and audiologists have always been expected to practice routine hand washing and general housekeeping; however, infection control extends well beyond these two general practices. Prior to reviewing infection control guidelines in more detail and reviewing practical applications to the broad range of international professionals involved in the provision of diagnostic, rehabilitative, and/or habilitative services to individuals with communication, hearing, and swallowing disorders (e.g., speech-language pathologist, community speech-language and hearing workers, audiologists, hearing aid acousticians), it is important to appreciate its relevance to these fields.

Infection control is a relevant topic to clinicians managing patients with communication, hearing and swallowing disorders as follows.

Guidelines and Mandates Related to Infection Control

Infection control guidelines and mandates have been issued by a variety of governing bodies and/or agencies worldwide whereby adherence to established guidelines are expected and/or legally required. For example, the World Health Organization (WHO) recently issued infection control guidelines designed specifically to reduce or eliminate the incidence of nosocomial or hospital-acquired infections (WHO, 2002). In direct response to the emergence of severe acute respiratory syndrome (SARS) earlier this decade, it was recognized that many countries lacked the necessary infrastructure to minimize the spread of SARS. As a result, the regional WHO offices for Southeast Asia and the Western Pacific expanded the original WHO infection control guidelines, issuing updated information and revising current guidelines in hopes of strengthening infection control capacities throughout health care facilities in both developed and developing countries (WHO, 2004).

In a country like the United Sates, the Occupational Safety and Health Administration (OSHA) is the federal agency governed by the United States Department of Labor that is responsible for regulating the work place to ensure safety and healthful working environments. OSHA enforces established federal standards related to work-safety, which include infection control standards. In direct response to concerns related to HIV exposure in the workplace, OSHA developed guidelines based on the Universal (Standard) Precautions originally developed and issued by the Centers for Disease Control and Prevention (CDC), the federal epidemiologic agency governed by the U.S. Department of Health and Human Services. These guidelines were submitted in the form of a Federal Register in May 1989 with the final standard approved and published in 1991. With this standard in place, OSHA oversees and enforces infection control programs in health care settings throughout the United States to ensure compliance with current mandates and regulations. In other words, infection control is the law; failure of compliance results in citations and fines.

For territories outside the United States, OSHA standards are not legally binding as other territories most likely adhere to their own established standards. Putting aside jurisdictional issues, infection control guidelines issued by OSHA and separately issued by the WHO remain conceptually similar. Instead of delineating differences between infection control guidelines issued by two different agencies, this chapter focuses on general concepts that are universal in terms of infection control.

Nature of Professional Practice in Communication, Hearing, and Swallowing Disorders

The nature of clinically managing patients with communication, hearing, and swallowing disorders involves a notable degree of patient contact, including the use of various reusable objects that come in direct and indirect contact with multiple patients. Contact transmission, whether direct or indirect, represents the most common means of disease transmission in clinical environments where these types of services are provided (Bankaitis et al., 2005; Bankaitis & Kemp, 2003, 2005, 2007). Contact transmission involves the physical transfer of a microorganism from one location in the environment to a location within the vicinity of the human body. Touching a draining ear with a bare hand is an example of direct contact transmission. Indirect contract transmission occurs when patients and/or clinicians are exposed to or handle contaminated objects. For example, performing a listening check on a different patient's hearing instrument without first cleaning and then disinfecting the listening bell from the previous patient will cross-contaminate the current patient's hearing instrument.

Furthermore, speech-language pathologists, audiologists, and other professionals managing similar patient loads often manipulate body orifices including the nose, mouth, and ears, which serve as natural routes or portals of entry for microorganisms to access the human body. Microorganisms require both a mode (i.e., contact transmission) and route for potential disease transmission. Although a number of other things need to happen for disease to manifest, the nature of speech-language pathology and audiology creates an environment that is inherently susceptible to the occurrence of cross-contamination. From this perspective, speech-language pathologist and audiologists must be diligent in minimizing such risks with the application of appropriate infection control procedures.

Scope of Clinical Practice

The scope of clinical practice related to communication, hearing, and swallowing disorders dictates the need for infection control. The scope of practice for speech-language pathology is vast and diverse, involving many types of noninvasive and invasive patient contacts that potentially expose the clinician to saliva, mucus, blood, or other bodily fluids (Bankaitis et al., 2005). For example, some speech-language pathologists or community speech and hearing workers are involved in the selection, fitting, and management of adaptive and/or prosthetic devices for individuals with swallowing or other upper aerodigestive functions. These procedures involve insertion, handling, and manipulation of tracheoesophageal voice prostheses, one-way speaking valves (e.g., Passy-Muir Inc., Irvine, CA), pneumatic and electronic artificial larynges, palatal lift prostheses, and obturators. Other clinicians involved in nasoendoscopy, videostroboscopy, EMG, or nasometry (Kay Elemetrics Corp., Lincoln Park, NJ) studies manipulate instruments or materials placed in the nasal or oral cavities. Similarly, many audiologists are involved in procedures that potentially may result in exposure to blood or other bodily fluids (Bankaitis & Kemp, 2005). Worldwide, audiologists and other recognized health care professionals may be involved in intraoperative monitoring procedures that require interaction in an operating room (OR) environment. Many clinicians are involved in vestibular testing that, on occasion, can cause patients to become nauseous and physically sick. Given the importance of an unoccluded external auditory canal, the scope of practice in audiology has expanded to include cerumen management. As more and more of these types of procedures are performed by speech-language pathologists and audiologists, the incidence of exposure to blood and other bodily fluids and the subsequent risk of exposure to bloodborne pathogens substantially increase (Kemp & Bankaitis, 2000).

Types of Patient Populations Served

Communication, hearing, and swallowing services are sought by a wide range of patients who vary across several factors known to include, but not limited to, age, underlying disease (i.e., diabetes, cancer), nutritional status, socioeconomic status and exposure to past and current pharmacologic interventions (Bankaitis & Kemp, 2003, 2005). Each of these factors may directly influence the overall integrity of the immune system (Bankaitis & Schountz, 1998) and can create subtle degrees of immunocompromise that may be associated with an exponential susceptibility to ubiquitous microorganisms and subsequent development of opportunistic infections.

Opportunistic infections result from ubiquitous organisms residing in abundance throughout the environment (Bankaitis & Kemp, 2003, 2005). Microorganisms associated with opportunistic infections rarely cause disease or infection in healthy individuals; rather, these types of microbes take the opportunity to infect those exhibiting some degree of immunocompromise. Given the right conditions, in some cases, infections can be life threatening. For example, the bacterium *Staphylococcus* resides on skin surfaces. As such, it is not surprising that a study found physicians' stethoscopes were significantly contaminated with this bacterium because the instruments make contact with skin surfaces (Breathnach, Jenkins, & Pedler, 1992). Given the universal nature of the bacterium, the assumption by clinicians may be that *Staphylococcus* is an innocuous bacterium for which infection control procedures are not necessary. On the contrary, although this bacterium is ever present throughout the environment, it accounts for a high percentage of nosocomial or hospital-acquired infections (Murray, Kobayashi, Pfaller, & Rosenthal, 1994). As most hospital patients are sick and exhibit varying degrees of immunocompromise, despite the universal nature of *Staphyloccocus*, these patient populations remain extremely susceptible to such microorganisms. From this perspective, speech-language pathologists and audiologists must adhere to a proactive strategy to minimize the possibility of the inadvertent spread of disease in the clinical environment.

Cerumen Exposure

Worldwide, audiologists, hearing instrument specialists, hearing aid acousticians, and audioprosthologists come in contact with cerumen on a daily basis. Speech-language pathologists and community speech-language and hearing workers who perform hearing aid listening checks or participate in hearing screenings may also be exposed to cerumen. Cerumen is not an infectious agent unless it is contaminated with blood, dried blood, or mucus (Bankaitis & Kemp, 2002; Kemp, Roeser, Pearson, & Ballachanda, 1996). Given the color and viscosity of cerumen, it is difficult to determine through visual inspection with any degree of accuracy whether it is contaminated with blood or mucous by-products (Kemp & Roeser, 1998). Audiologists and speech-language pathologists are not in a position to predict with accuracy the composition of cerumen and should treat it as an infectious substance (Kemp et al., 1996).

Microbial Contamination of Medical Instruments, Hearing Instruments

Objects coming in direct or indirect contact with patients may be contaminated with potentially infectious microorganisms. Breathnach et al. (1992) documented the presence of *Staphylococcus aureus*, a bacterium that can cause serious infections in immunocompromised individuals, on the majority of physicians' stethoscopes swabbed in their study. A variety of microbes were also recovered from standard airline headsets including *Staphylococcus aureus* (12/20 headsets), *Staphylococcus epidermidis* (10/20), *Streptococcus* (8/20), and *Corynebacterium* (6/20) (Brooks, 1985). Most recently, Bankaitis (2002) documented the presence of light to heavy amounts of bacterial and/or fungal growth on the surface of hearing instruments removed from the ears of adult patients. The predominant organism recovered was *Staphylococcus*; however, each hearing aid was contaminated by a unique combination of bacterial and/or fungal microbial growth including *Acinetobacter lwoffi, Lactobacillus, Pseudomonas aeruginosa, Enterobacter, Aspergillus flavus,* and *Candida parapsilosis.* A follow-up study conducted by Sturgulewski, Bankaitis, Klodd, and Haberkamp (2006) revealed similar findings. Based on the findings of these researchers, particularly that of Bankaitis (2002) and Sturgulewski et al. (2006), it is plausible to assume that other reusable objects used by speech-language pathologists and audiologists with multiple patients may be contaminated with varying degrees of microbial growth. The relevance of infection control from this perspective cannot be overstated.

IMPLEMENTATION OF INFECTION CONTROL PRINCIPLES

Infection control protocols must be designed to reduce the number of pathogens in the working environment and to eliminate the potential for cross-contamination and cross-infection. To reach this goal, both the WHO and OSHA independently developed specific regulations intended to provide clear direction as to what is expected in terms of infection control. Whereas the WHO represents a branch of the United Nations devoted to health issues that may not have legal jurisdiction in various countries, whereas OSHA's jurisdiction is restricted to the United States. Both organizations adhere to Standard Precautions as a foundational base of infection control. Standard precautions serve as the guideline for how diagnostic and/or rehabilitative procedures and services should be modified to ensure infection control goals are met. The written infection control plan is the document that outlines how a specific clinic will achieve infection control goals. Both are reviewed in more detail below.

Standard Precautions

Generically, standard precautions refer to the premise that every patient is an assumed carrier of and/or susceptible host for an infectious disease. As such, all patients must be treated with the same basic level of established protocol designed to minimize the spread of disease. Specifically, the WHO dictates that the following six standard precautions must be applied to all patients at all times, regardless of diagnosis or infectious status:

■ Hand washing and antisepsis (hand hygiene)
■ Use of personal protective equipment when handling blood, body substances, excretions, and secretions
■ Appropriate handling of patient care equipment and soiled linen
■ Prevention of needle stick/sharp injuries
■ Environmental cleaning and spills management
■ Appropriate handling of waste (WHO, 2004).

In the United States, the CDC issued a number of similar recommendations and guidelines for minimizing cross-infection of blood-borne diseases to health care workers. These pronouncements were officially formalized into the Universal Blood and Blood-Borne Pathogen Precautions (Centers for Disease Control and Prevention [CDC], 1987). The pronouncements originally were intended to protect health care workers from blood and blood-borne pathogens; however, these precautions have since been expanded to include all potentially infectious body substances. The five general pronouncements are as follows:

■ Appropriate personal barriers (gloves, masks, eye protection, and gowns) must be worn when performing procedures that may expose personnel to infectious agents.
■ Hands must be washed before and after every patient contact and after glove removal.
■ Touch and splash surfaces must be precleaned and disinfected.
■ Critical instruments must be sterilized.
■ Infectious waste must be disposed of appropriately (CDC, 1987).

Minor differences exist between the pronouncements outlined by the WHO as compared to the CDC. Although the verbiage differs, conceptually, the standard precautions formalized by the WHO are principally the same as those formalized by the CDC with the exception that the WHO specifically lists the prevention of needle sticks/sharp injuries as a pronouncement whereas the CDC does not. It is important to note that, although the CDC does not list needle sticks/sharp injuries as a standard pronouncement, OSHA, which integrates the CDC's standard precautions within their infection control guidelines, addresses the issue of needle sticks/sharp injuries in a separate section of their guidelines.

The critical issue at this junction is to recognize that the standard precautions represent a critical component of an infection control plan. These pronouncements are relatively straightforward; however, using the CDC's pronouncements as a template, each is reviewed in more detail with specific attention placed on its application to clinical management of patients with communication, hearing, and swallowing disorders.

Appropriate Personal Barriers

Appropriate personal barriers refer to gloves, masks, eye protection, and/or gowns, which must be worn during the provision of services and/or procedures that may expose health care providers working with communication, hearing, and swallowing disorders to potentially infectious agents or substances.

Gloves

Appropriately fitting gloves are indicated during invasive procedures or procedures where open wounds and/or visible blood are present. Wearing gloves is indicated when hands are likely to become contaminated with potentially infective material such as blood, body fluids, secretions, excretions or mucous membranes, as well as in those situations to prevent gross microbial contamination of hands (CDC, 2002; WHO, 2004). Outside of the operating room environment, clean, nonsterile gloves may be used when touching potentially infective material (WHO, 2004); however, certain clinical procedures may require the use of sterilized gloves. For example, sterile gloves should be used when using sterile instruments for purposes of making direct contact with the pharynx or

Table 4–1. Instances for Which Gloves Should Be Worn by Speech-Language Pathologists and Audiologists

- In the presence of an open wounds and/or visible blood

- When handling hearing instruments or ear molds that have not been cleaned and disinfected including but not limited to accepting such instruments from patients, during cleaning and disinfecting procedures, during ear mold or hearing instrument modification procedures

- When inserting or handling removed from the nose, mouth, or ears

- When cleaning instruments contaminated with saliva, cerumen, mucus, or other bodily substances

- When submerging or removing reusable instruments into or from a cold sterilant

- When hands are likely to become contaminated with potentially infectious material including cerumen, saliva, mucous membranes

- In the operating room environment during patient preparation or any other procedures during or after the surgical procedure where hands could potentially come in contact with blood, bodily fluids, or other contaminated materials or contaminated objects

Source: Adapted from Bankaitis et al. (2005) and Bankaitis and Kemp (2005). Reprinted with permission by Auban, Inc.

trachea (Bankaitis et al., 2005). Table 4-1 provides a general guide as to when gloves should be worn by clinicians providing diagnostic or rehabilitative services to individuals with communication, hearing, and swallowing disorders.

The size of the glove is important and should be determined for each clinician separately to ensure an appropriate fit. As shown in Figure 4-1, gloves are considered to fit appropriately when the glove fits the hand tightly, adhering very close to the skin without being too tight. This will allow for effective manipulation of objects, items, or instruments during the provision of services without compromising manual dexterity. Gloves that fit too loosely (Figure 4-2) will hinder the clinician's manual dexterity, creating potential frustration during the execution of procedures and/or increasing the likelihood for an accident to occur that otherwise could be avoided.

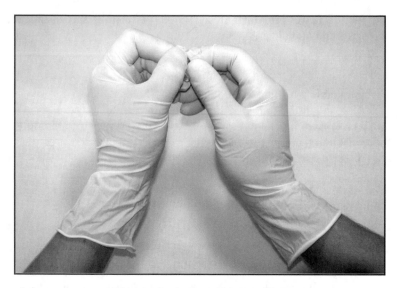

Figure 4–1. *Appropriately sized glove that fits tightly across the fingers, back of hands, palms, and wrists, adhering closely to the skin.*

One-size-fits-all gloves should be avoided as they are not designed to fit most hands appropriately.

Gloves are considered one-time use items and should not be reused. Furthermore, the same pair of gloves should not be used on different patients. After use, gloves should be properly removed and disposed. Unless grossly contaminated with blood or other bodily fluids, gloves may be disposed of in the regular trash or according to the protocol dictated by the hearing care facility. It is highly unlikely for standard clinical procedures related to communication, hearing, and swallowing disorders to result in copious amounts of blood or bodily fluid contamination to require arrangements for hazardous waste removal.

Masks, Eye Protection, and Gowns

Disposable masks, safety glasses, and gowns must be worn when there is a risk of splash or splatter of blood, bodily fluids, secretions, or excretions, or when the clinician may be at risk of airborne contamination. It has been recommended that surgical masks be used in place of cotton masks or masks made of gauze material because

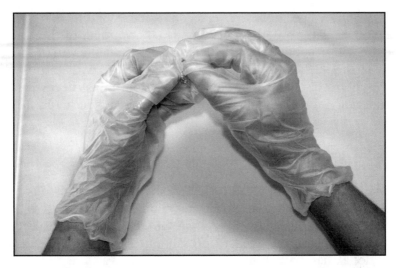

Figure 4–2. *Loosely fitted gloves that reflect an inappropriate fit as the gloves do not adhere tightly to the skin and will result in difficulty handling and/or manipulating objects.*

surgical masks are fluid resistant (WHO, 2004). Eye protection may be available in different forms including safety glasses, goggles, and visors/face shields. Gowns or plastic aprons are intended to protect skin and prevent soiling of clothing during high-risk procedures (WHO, 2004). When managing patients with communication, hearing, and swallowing disorders, clinicians using buffing wheels or drills to modify hearing instruments and/or earmolds minimally should wear masks and safety glasses to avoid breathing in or getting dust and other particles generated by the buffing wheel into the eyes. Similarly, clinicians should wear masks, safety glasses, and/or gowns during activities such as tracheal suctioning to safeguard against exposure to fluid splatter, particularly in the event the patient coughs with the production of copious secretions (Bankaitis et al., 2005). Clinicians providing services to hospital patients with tuberculosis (TB) must wear special TB masks when a diagnosed patient has not been on an antibiotic regimen for 10 days.

As with gloves, disposable masks are not reusable and should be disposed of properly. Eye protection may or may not be reusable as dictated by the specific manufacturer's intended design. Disposable eye protection must be disposed of according to the health care facility's established protocol. Conversely, reusable eye protection should be cleaned and properly decontaminated according to the manufacturers' instructions (WHO, 2004). Finally, contaminated or soiled gowns should be removed as soon as possible with disposable gowns being discarded appropriately; reusable gowns necessitating laundering must be routed to the appropriate laundering facility.

Hand Hygiene

At the time standard precautions were issued in the United States, washing hands with soap and water represented the only recognized hand washing technique; therefore, the current verbiage in the CDC's version of standard precautions specifically references traditional hand washing. Traditional hand washing technique involves the use of hospital-grade, liquid soap. Hospital-grade soap is gentler than household soaps and contains special emollients that moisturize the skin and are effective in reducing or minimizing chapping, chafing, or drying of the skin from excessive hand washing (Bankaitis & Kemp, 2003, 2005).

Recently, the CDC endorsed an alternative method of washing hands with the use of antimicrobial "no-rinse" degermers. These products refer to the alcohol-based hand rubs that do not require the use of or access to running water. The availability and accepted use of alcohol-based, no-rinse hand degermers have led to a substantial increase in hand hygiene compliance among health care workers (WHO, 2005). In the United States, alcohol-based hand rubs have been deemed appropriate to use with the caveat that reasonable access to a sink with running water may not be readily available or convenient (CDC, 2002). In addition, the use of "no-rinse" degermers should be restricted to those situations where the hands are not visibly soiled.

With the recent expansion of hand washing to include the use of hand degermers, the terms hand hygiene is used to refer collectively to these techniques. This is evident in the current WHO guidelines whereby their version of standard precautions makes reference to "hand hygiene." Hand hygiene represents the single most important procedure for effectively limiting the spread of infectious disease (Bankaitis & Kemp, 2003, 2005). It is one of the most critical components of a basic infection control program. The frequency in which hand hygiene is considered ideal is generally unknown due to the lack of well-controlled research in this area. Exhaustively listing every potential circumstance that may require execution of hand hygiene procedures would be a significant and somewhat arbitrary task. The CDC specifies that hand hygiene procedures must occur prior to the initiation of invasive procedures, before providing services to patients, and after glove removal (CDC, 2002). The WHO requires hand hygiene in the same instances and further expands indications for hand hygiene immediately after direct contact with patients, prior to handling an invasive device (regardless of whether or not gloves are used) for patient care, after contact with an inanimate object (including medical equipment) in the immediate vicinity of the patient, and if moving from a contaminated body site to a clean body site during patient care (WHO, 2005). In addition, the CDC outlines that hand hygiene procedures should be followed any time that the professional feels it is warranted (CDC, 2002). For professionals providing clinical services to individuals with communication, hearing, and swallowing disorders, Table 4–2 provides a guideline as to when hand hygiene should be performed.

Table 4–2. Guidelines as to When Hand Hygiene Protocols Must Be Performed by Speech-Language Pathologists and Audiologists

• Prior to initial contact with patient, at the beginning of the patient appointment
• At the end of patient contact
• After glove use, immediately after removing gloves
• Prior to eating, drinking, smoking, applying lotion or makeup
• After eating, drinking, smoking, applying lotion or makeup
• After using bathroom facilities
• Any time it is felt necessary and appropriate

Source: Adapted from Bankaitis et al. (2005) and Bankaitis and Kemp (2005). Reprinted with permission from Auban, Inc.

Hand Hygiene Technique

Given the importance of hand hygiene to an infection control program, executing appropriate hand hygiene techniques is equally if not more critical in ensuring the efficacy of minimizing the spread of disease. Table 4–3 provides necessary components of hand hygiene techniques utilizing traditional and alternative hand hygiene techniques. Specific steps outlined in Table 4–3 are further illustrated in Figures 4–3A through Figure 4–3D.

Table 4–3. Outline of Appropriate Hand Hygiene Techniques Utilizing Soap and Running Water, and No-Rinse Hand Degermers

In cases where there is access to a sink with running water:

- Remove all jewelry including rings, bracelets, and watches
- Start water and place an appropriate amount of hospital-grade, liquid antibacterial soap in the palm of the hand
- Lather the soap, scrubbing the palms, backs of hands, and wrists for a minimum of 10 seconds
- Thoroughly rinse hands with running water
- With the water running, retrieve an accessible clean disposable paper towel and dry hands with the paper towel
- Turn the water off with the used paper towel and without making direct contact with the faucet with clean, bare hands
- Dispose of the paper towel in the appropriate waste container

In cases where there is not access to sink with running water:

- Remove all jewelry
- Squeeze an appropriate amount of "no-rinse" antibacterial hand degermer into the palm of your hand
- Cover both hands with the solution, rubbing palms together
- Rub solution in between fingers on both hands
- Do not dry hands with a towel, as the "no rinse" solution is self-drying

Source: Adapted from Bankaitis et al. (2005) and Bankaitis and Kemp (2005). Reprinted with permission from Auban, Inc.

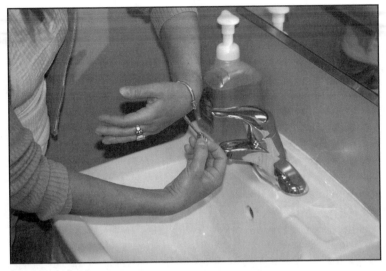

A

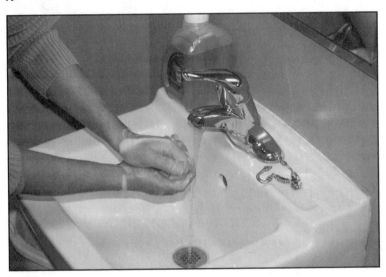

B

Figure 4–3. **A.** *Removal of jewelry prior to initiating hand hygiene procedures.* **B.** *Lathering with hospital-grade liquid soap for a minimum of 10 seconds.* continues

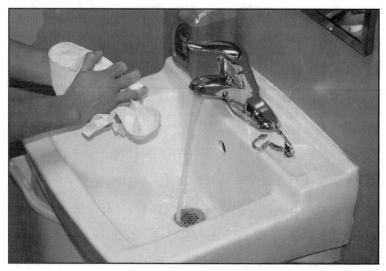

C

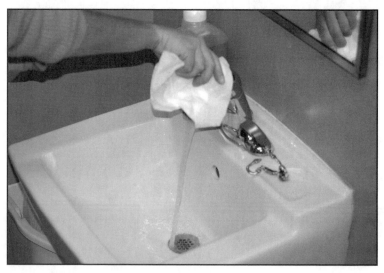

D

Figure 4–3. continued *C.* Wiping hands with readily accessible paper towel. *D.* Using paper towel to turn off water faucet to avoid direct contact of faucet with bare hands.

Cleaning and Disinfecting

Surfaces that come in regular direct or indirect contact with patients and/or clinicians such as countertops, tables, service areas, and the armrest of chairs are referred to as touch surfaces. Splash surfaces essentially are the same thing but involve surfaces that have been contaminated by particles expelled by a patient or clinician, such as when a patient coughs, sneezes, or drools on a surface. Both surfaces must be cleaned and then disinfected between patient appointments.

As outlined in Table 4–4, cleaning refers to procedures in which gross contamination is removed from surfaces or objects without killing germs (Bankaitis & Kemp, 2003, 2005). It does not necessarily involve any degree of germ killing; rather, it serves as an important precursor to disinfecting. Cleaning must occur prior to disinfection; the absence of precleaning a surface will diminish the effectiveness of disinfecting techniques (Kemp & Bankaitis, 2000).

In contrast, disinfection refers to a process in which germs are killed (see Table 4–4). The degree of disinfection that can occur expands across a fairly wide continuum and depends on the specific type and number of microorganisms a product kills. Whereas household disinfectants kill a relatively limited number of microorganisms, hospital-grade disinfectants are much stronger and kill a larger number and variety of germs (Bankaitis & Kemp, 2003). As such, hospital-grade disinfectants should be incorporated in infection control protocols implemented in patient care settings, including clinics, hospitals, or private practice facilities where speech-language pathology, audiological and other related services are provided (Rutala, 1990). As indicated earlier, surfaces must be cleaned first, and then disinfected.

Table 4–4. Differentiation of Common Terms Related to Infection Control Procedures

Cleaning:	removal of gross contamination without necessarily killing germs
Disinfecting:	process in which germs are killed
Sterilizing:	process in which 100% of germs are killed, including associated endospores

Critical Instruments and Sterilization

Critical instruments refer to instruments or objects that meet at least one of the following three criteria: (1) reusable item introduced directly into the bloodstream (e.g., needles), (2) reusable, noninvasive instrument that comes in contact with intact mucous membranes or bodily substances (e.g., blood, saliva, cerumen, mucous discharge, pus), or (3) a reusable, noninvasive instrument that potentially can penetrate the skin from use or misuse (instruments used for cerumen removal, instruments inserted in the nose, mouth, etc.). Within the context of speech-language pathology and audiology, reusable items that make contact with mucous membranes, saliva, or cerumen and are intended to be used with multiple patients should be cleaned first and then sterilized. Although not necessarily an exhaustive list, examples of instruments include laryngeal mirrors, oral tubes, immittance probe tips contaminated with copious amounts of cerumen and/or drainage, hemostats, flexible and rigid endoscopes, and cerumen management instrumentation.

The term sterilization refers to killing 100% of vegetative microorganisms, including associated endospores (see Table 4–4). The term is not synonymous with disinfecting. When microbes are challenged, they revert to the more resistant life form called a spore (Kemp & Bankaitis, 2000). Sterilants, by definition, must neutralize and destroy spores because if the spore is not killed, it may become vegetative again and cause disease. Whereas disinfection involves killing germs, possibly many, sterilization involves killing all germs and associated endospores every time (Bankaitis & Kemp, 2007).

There are several different sterilization techniques including the use of an autoclave and the application of cold sterilization techniques. As the autoclave involves pressurized heat, most speech-language pathologists and audiologists will be limited to utilizing cold sterilization techniques as reusable rubber, silicone, plastic, or acrylic objects will not withstand traditional heat pressurization sterilization techniques. Cold sterilization involves soaking instruments in liquid chemicals approved by the Environmental Protective Agency (EPA) for a specified number of hours. Only two ingredients have been approved by the EPA as sterilants: (1) glutaraldehyde and (2) hydrogen peroxide. Products containing the active ingredient glutaraldehyde in concentrations of 2% or higher or those containing the active ingredient hydrogen peroxide (H_2O_2) in concentrations of 7.5% or higher may be used to sterilize instruments.

Reusable items to be sterilized must be cleaned first because organic material (e.g., blood and proteins) may contain high concentrations of microorganisms with chemical germicide properties that can negatively impact the sterilization process. In addition, it is imperative for cold sterilization procedures to be followed according to instructions provided by the product manufacturer. Soaking times necessary to achieve sterilization will differ from solution to solution. Whereas most glutaraldehyde-based products require 10 hours of soaking time to achieve sterilization, hydrogen peroxide products typically require 6 hours of soaking time. Removing instruments or objects prior to the necessary soaking time will result in high-level disinfection and not sterilization. Reviewing product information for instruction of use is critical.

Disposal of Infectious Waste

There is no epidemiologic evidence to suggest that hospital-grade waste is associated with a greater potential for cross-contamination as compared to residential waste (CDC, 2002). Therefore, identifying wastes for which special precautions are indicated remains a matter of judgment. The most practical approach to infectious waste is to identify the materials for which some special precautions may be sensible (CDC, 2002). Within the context of communication, hearing, and swallowing disorders, disposable items contaminated with saliva, mucus, discharge, cerumen, blood, or blood byproducts may be disposed of in regular waste receptacles; however, in the event the item is contaminated with copious amounts, it should first be placed in a separate, impermeable bag (i.e., biohazard bag) and only then discarded in the regular trash (Bankaitis & Kemp, 2003, 2005). This practice will separate the contaminated waste from the rest of the trash and minimize the chance of maintenance or cleaning personnel coming in casual contact with it. Disposing of sharp objects such as razors or needles requires special consideration and sharps must be disposed of in a puncture-resistant, disposable container (sharps container).

Written Infection Control Plan

Standard precautions serve as the guideline as to how health care workers who see patients with communication, hearing, and swallowing disorders associated with HIV/AIDS must modify diagnostic and/or rehabilitative procedures for purposes of minimizing the spread of disease. Written infection control plan serves as the guiding cornerstone of the specific clinic's global infection control plan, outlining exactly how infection control goals are to be achieved. Practical guidelines for infection control in health care facilities issued by WHO recognize the importance of a hospital-acquired infection prevention manual made available to all employees, which provides instruction for patient care for purposes of minimize the spread of disease, including education and training of health care staff (WHO, 2004). Similarly, OSHA requires each facility in the United States to have a written infection control plan and for that plan to be available to all workers. As listed in Table 4-5, the written plan must include specific requirements mandated by OSHA. The following sections review each required element in further detail.

Employee Exposure Classification

The first requirement of the written infection control plan involves categorizing employees in one of three different categories according to the potential degree to which a specific employee may be exposed to blood and other infectious substances based on primary work responsibilities. The three categories range from Category 1 to Category 3 with the former representing employees associated with the highest probability of exposure, and the later associated with the lowest probability of exposure. Category 1 employees include personnel whose primary job assignment exposes them to potential

Table 4–5. Required Elements of a Written Infection Control Plan as Required by OSHA

• Employee Exposure Classification
• Hepatitis B (HBV) Vaccination Plan and Records of Vaccination
• Plan for Annual Training and Records of Training
• Plan for Accidents and Accidental Exposure Follow-up
• Implementation Protocols
• Postexposure Plans and Records

cross-infection with blood-borne diseases or other potentially infectious microbes. This category typically includes physicians, nurses, paramedics, and dentists. Speech-language pathologists whose primary job responsibilities include evaluating and treating patients with tracheostomy or audiologists primarily involved in intraoperative monitoring procedures may be categorized as Category 1 employees. Category 2 employees include personnel whose secondary job assignment potentially exposes them to cross-infection. The majority of speech-language pathologist and audiologists will fall in this category, including graduate students in training. Finally, employees classified in Category 3 include personnel whose job requirements in the office never expose them to blood or other bodily fluids including administrators and receptionists who do not provide clinical services.

Hepatitis B (HBV) Vaccination Plan and Records of Vaccination

Employers must offer employees in health care settings the opportunity to receive a HBV vaccination. The HBV vaccination must be offered to all Category 1 and Category 2 employees free of charge. The employee is not required to accept the offer of vaccination; in the event the employee refuses vaccination, a waiver must be signed noting the refusal of the offered vaccine and filed in the employee records. OSHA requires that this record be retained for length of employment plus 30 years (Kemp et al., 1996).

Plan for Annual Training and Records of Training

OSHA requires a plan for annual training and maintenance of records documenting that such training occurred. Specifically, OSHA has outlined that infection control training must include explanations of symptoms and modes of transmission of blood-borne diseases, location and handling of personal protective equipment, information on the HBV vaccine, and follow-up procedures to be taken in the event of an exposure incident. Although the standard does not specify length of training, infection control training must be provided to new employees at the time of initial assignment and then minimally every year thereafter. Each facility is to conduct and document completion of annual infection control training for each employee. During the course of the year, if an update or new procedure is to be implemented, appropriate training must be conducted in a timely fashion to ensure that the new or updated procedures are understood and implemented. Established employees changing exposure classification categories must undergo infection control retraining within 90 days of the change in classification category. Records of these training sessions are to be filed with the infection control plan in a designated location.

Plan for Accidents and Accidental Exposure Follow-Up

The fourth requirement of the written infection control plan involves outlining specific steps to be taken in the event an accident occurs within the clinical environment, which can expose individuals to blood-borne pathogens or other potentially infectious agents, and steps to be taken in the event an employee accidentally is exposed to blood-borne pathogens or other potentially infectious agents. For example, in the event a patient falls and suffers a nosebleed, or becomes sick, every staff member should know what steps to take to address the accident. In addition, accidental exposures to blood-borne pathogens require follow-up. Although these encounters may be relatively rare in speech-language pathology and audiology environments, an emergency plan must be created and put in place. The goals in this instance are to confirm that a disease has or has not been transferred and, in the event of a transfer, to treat the disease effectively and efficiently.

Implementation of Protocols

The fifth requirement of the written infection control plan involves outlining specific protocols that will dictate how specific procedures will be executed in the clinical environment for purposes of minimizing exposure to potentially infectious agents. One important element of implementation of protocols involves the development and execution of work practice controls. Work practice controls are written procedures that outline how a health care professional will execute a diagnostic or rehabilitative procedure for purposes of minimizing or eliminating the likelihood of cross-contamination or exposure to a potentially infectious agent. For example, a work practice control can address tracheal suctioning procedures or ear-mold impression procedures, outlining how a clinician will conduct a specific procedure in such a manner to ensure appropriate infection control standards are met. It is important to note that work practice controls are not intended nor should be designed to outline how a clinician is to perform technically a specific procedure; rather, it represents a step-by-step guide as to what infection control procedures will be followed at specific times during the tracheal suctioning procedures or earmold impression procedures to ensure cross-contamination is avoided. As this is such a critical element of implementing an effective infection control plan, work practice controls associated with specific speech-language pathology and audiology procedures are addressed in greater detail.

Postexposure Plans and Records

Finally, the last requirement of an infection control plan as dictated by OSHA involves record keeping of documents related to treatment and subsequent outcomes associated with exposure to potentially infectious pathogens, including HIV.

IMPLEMENTATION OF WORK PRACTICE CONTROLS

As previously mentioned in the section on infection control plan in this chapter, an effective infection control plan includes the development and implementation of work practice controls. Work practice controls are profession-specific, written protocols as to how a health care professional such as a speech-language pathologist or audiologist will execute a specific diagnostic or rehabilitative procedure for purposes of minimizing or eliminating the likelihood of cross-contamination or exposure to a potentially infectious agent. As the extent of services provided by a specific employer will differ from clinic to clinic, the types of work practice controls outlined will differ from clinic to clinic depending on what diagnostic and or rehabilitative services are being provided. For example, a clinic employing speech-language pathologists who provide only feeding and swallowing assessments will maintain different work practice controls in their infection control plan than a public school employing speech-language pathologists who mainly assess and treat articulation disorders.

Furthermore, clinicians with the same knowledge base inherently will execute diagnostic or rehabilitative procedures differently. For example, audiologists may apply different techniques to obtain earmold impressions. Certainly, there are definite right and wrong ways as well as arguably more effective versus less effective ways to executive a clinical technique. Assuming, however, that assessment and therapy procedures are performed in a technically accurate manner, there exists a certain amount of flexibility as to how a diagnostic procedure can be appropriately executed. Similarly, infection control is based on a series of foundational principles and its procedural execution is not necessarily associated with only one correct way of executing a work practice control. With that in mind, the work practice controls addressing specific speech-language pathology or audiology procedures presented in this chapter serve as teaching tools that are designed to further illustrate the concept of a work practice control. The examples are not intended to dictate universal clinical procedure. Considering the different circumstances of each clinician, the work practice control examples provided most likely will need to be modified to meet the unique needs of a specific clinic. Although modifications can be expected, it is critical for the clinician to recognize that modifications must not compromise infection control principles (Bankaitis & Kemp, 2003, 2005; Bankaitis et al., 2005). Modifying a procedure that compromises infection control for the objective of saving money and reducing overhead costs is not appropriate.

Developing Work Practice Controls

The most challenging aspect associated with developing work practice controls involves the process of consciously dissecting a procedure that has otherwise become an unconscious aspect of clinical routine. For example, an experienced speech-language pathologist will not have to stop and think about what step comes next in conducting endoscopy procedures. Similarly, an audiologist will not have to stop and think about masking during the audiologic assessment. In developing work practice controls, it will be necessary for clinicians to stop and think about each step in the clinical process in order to identify whether infection control principles need to be applied.

An effective technique in developing work practice controls is to first outline the general steps associated with executing a diagnostic or rehabilitative procedure. Once the general steps are outlined, each standard precaution should be individually reviewed to determine if that particular pronouncement must be accounted for in the work practice control. For example, speech-language pathologists may be involved in performing oral-facial mechanism or oral motor examinations. This general procedure involves visually inspecting the face and oral cavity, performing general sensory testing, observing various speech and nonspeech movements of the lips, tongue, velum, and jaw and palpation of the oral structures. To visualize the oral cavity, the clinician typically will use a tongue depressor on, or alongside, the tongue. It may be necessary for the clinician to use his or her hands to move the cheek aside for optimal visualization. To assess sensation, the clinician typically will touch the patient's face and neck with the hand, a swab, or cotton ball. To assess resistance, the clinician will need to hold the patient's jaw open or closed. Observation of speech and vegetative oral movements does not require direct contact.

With the general steps in the procedure outlined, the next step involves identifying which of the five pronouncements outlined in the standard precautions must be accounted for and incorporated in a work practice control addressing oral-motor examinations. To illustrate this step, the next section addresses each pronouncement individually in terms of its relevance and application to performing an oral-motor examination.

Appropriate Personal Barriers and Oral-Motor Examinations

During oral motor examinations, the speech-language pathologist generally will insert a tongue depressor into the oral cavity to view the oral mechanism. Because the walls of the oral cavity are mucous membranes, once the tongue depressor is inserted into the mouth its surface will become contaminated with saliva and secretions of the mucous membranes. In addition, the clinician may place his or her fingers into the oral cavity to palpate the structures for submucous clefts or other anomalies (Kummer, 2001). From this perspective, the use of gloves is indicated during the oral-motor examination because contact with saliva and mucous membranes is expected. Specifically, it will be necessary for the speech-language pathologists to wear gloves during portions of the oral-facial examination that involve insertion of the clinician's fingers into the oral cavity and during any procedures assisting the patient in oral care.

The extent to which gloves are to be worn during other portions of the oral-motor examination is less straightforward. As described by Bankaitis et al. (2005), the clinician may choose to wear gloves during procedures that involve insertion of a tongue depressor into the patient's mouth as that action will result in making indirect contact with the oral cavity and handling an instrument that, once removed from the patient's mouth, is contaminated. Alternatively, as only the medial tip of the tongue depressor will be contaminated, the clinician may choose not to wear gloves during this portion of the oral motor examination, justifying that there is sufficient uncontaminated space on the lateral section of the tongue depressor to enable the clinician to simply remove the tongue depressor from the patient's mouth and properly dispose of it. The clinician who chooses to wear gloves throughout the entire oral motor examination has selected the more conservative approach, whereas the clinician who chooses to wear gloves only when it is necessary to insert fingers into the oral cavity has selected a less conservative approach. From an infection control perspective, either approach is considered appropriate. Regardless of which approach is taken, gloves use will be required at some point during the oral-motor examination and must be accounted for in the work practice control.

Hand Hygiene and Oral-Motor Examinations

The CDC clearly states that hand hygiene procedures must occur prior to the initiation of invasive procedures, before providing services to patient, and after glove removal (CDC, 2002). Hand hygiene procedures must occur prior to initiating an oral-motor examination (i.e., before providing services to patient) and then repeated immediately after the clinician removes gloves. In other words, prior to initiating the oral-motor exam, hands must be washed. In addition, during the examination, if the clinician uses gloves halfway through the procedure, as soon as the gloves are removed, the clinician must commence with hand-hygiene procedures even if he or she is not finished with the entire examination. Both of these instances must be accounted for when developing a work practice control for oral-motor examinations.

Cleaning, Disinfecting, and Oral-Motor Examinations

Horizontal surfaces that come into regular direct or indirect contact with patients during the provision of clinical services such as countertops, tables, and other surfaces must be cleaned first and then disinfected. Speech-language pathologists must first clean and then disinfect such surfaces after patient appointments, prior to the next appointment. If a specific clinician conducts an oral-motor examination in a patient-care room with such surfaces, it will be necessary to commence with these procedures; otherwise, this aspect is not necessarily required to be accounted for when developing a work practice control for oral motor examinations. For illustrative purposes, this element will be assumed unnecessary in this particular case.

Critical Instrument Sterilization and Oral-Motor Examinations

Oral-motor examinations involve the use of a disposable tongue depressor. Because this item is a one-time, one-time use only instrument, there is no need to account for sterilization of critical instruments in the oral-motor examination work practice control.

Infectious Waste Disposal and Oral-Motor Examinations

Oral-motor examinations involve the use of items that may become contaminated with saliva and/or mucus. The disposal of gloves and tongue depressor must be addressed in the oral-motor examination work practice control. These items are not anticipated to become contaminated with copious amounts of bodily fluids and may, therefore, be disposed of in the regular waste. Nevertheless, this action must be reflected in the work practice control.

Oral-Motor Examination Work Practice Control Example

Based on the previous section, the following must be accounted for in developing an oral-motor examination work practice control: appropriate personal barriers in the form of gloves, hand hygiene, and infectious waste disposal. Although it was clear that gloves were unequivocally required when inserting fingers into the patient's oral cavity, the extent to which gloves should be used throughout the entire oral-motor examination remained less clear. This situation may be addressed in several ways. First, the clinic can make it policy to approach infection control very conservatively and require the use of gloves throughout the entire examination, even if it involves using several different pairs of gloves with the same patient. In contrast, the clinic may decide to implement a decision-matrix approach whereby the clinician inspects the patient to identify the presence or absence of visible discharge from the eyes, ears, nose, and/or mouth, and/or the presence of open wounds and then uses his or her discretion as to the extent in which gloves will be required. In the presence of visible discharge and/or open wounds, the clinician must proceed with a more stringent work practice control that incorporates the use of gloves throughout the examination. In the absence of such, the clinician may proceed with a modified work practice control. To illustrate these points, Table 4–6 outlines two separate oral-motor examination work practice controls as it relates to the absence versus presence of visible discharge.

Additional work practice controls individually addressing other common speech-language pathology procedures such as feeding/swallowing assessments, examination of resonance and voice disorders, the use of computer-assisted treatment materials with direct contact interfaces, and reusable assessment need to be developed by specific clinics involved in provided such procedures. Specific examples outlining these procedures are beyond the scope of this chapter. For more detailed information on infection control work practice controls and access to infection control templates, other texts can be consulted (e.g., Bankaitis et al., 2005).

Table 4–6. Example of Work-Practice Control for Executing Oral-Motor Examinations with the Integration of Appropriate Infection Control Principles

In the absence of visible discharge from the eyes, ears, nose, and/or mouth, and/or presence of open wounds:
• Visually inspect the face
• Initiate hand hygiene procedures
• Conduct sensory testing
• In preparation for the oral mechanism examination, put on an appropriately sized pair of gloves

Table 4–6. *continued*

- Use a disposable tongue depressor, as needed, to facilitate depression of the tongue, to pull the cheek(s) to the side, and/or to test for the gag reflex
- Dispose of tongue depressor in the regular waste container
- If palpation of oral structures is necessary, conduct procedure with gloved hand*
- At the conclusion of oral palpation, remove gloves and dispose of in regular waste container and immediately initiate hand hygiene procedures

In the presence of visible discharge from the eyes, ears, nose, and/or mouth, and/or presence of open wounds:

- Put on an appropriately sized pair of gloves
- Visually inspect the face
- Conduct sensory testing[+]
- In preparation for the oral mechanism examination, put on a fresh pair of appropriately sized pair of gloves
- Use a disposable tongue depressor, as needed, to facilitate depression of the tongue, to pull the cheek(s) to the side, and/or to test for the gag reflex
- Dispose of tongue depressor in the regular waste container
- If palpation of oral structures is necessary, conduct procedure with gloved hand[++]
- At the conclusion of oral palpation, remove gloves and dispose of in regular waste container and immediately initiate hand hygiene procedures

*Oral mechanical examinations typically are performed with a light source, such as a penlight or flashlight. It is advisable to conduct necessary palpation with the gloved hand that has not been used to handle the light source.

[+]Depending on the extent of drainage, it is possible that gloves may become contaminated with bodily fluids secreted from the eyes, ears, nose, and mouth, and/or open head/neck wounds. Prior to proceeding with oral mechanism examination which will require the insertion of a gloved hand into the oral cavity, it is recommended that the clinician remove the gloves used during sensory testing, proceed with hand-hygiene procedures, and put on a new pair of gloves.

[++]Oral mechanical examinations are typically performed with a light source, such as a pen light or flash light. It is advisable to conduct necessary palpation with the gloved hand that has not been used to handle the light source.

Source: Adapted from and reprinted with permission from Auban, Inc.

Developing audiology work practice controls incorporates the use of the same techniques described in the previous section. First, the general procedural steps associated with the audiology procedure need to be assessed followed by the identification of which pronouncements outlined in the standard precautions must be accounted for that specific work practice control. Additional work practice controls individually addressing other diagnostic and rehabilitative audiological procedures such as cerumen removal, electrophysiological assessments, audiometry, dispensing hearing instruments, earmold impression techniques, and the like must be developed as needed by each clinic based on the scope of services provided in that clinic. The provision of additional work practice controls for these and other audiologic procedures is beyond the scope of this chapter. For more detailed information on infection control work practice controls for audiology and access to infection control templates, other texts can be consulted (e.g., Bankaitis & Kemp 2005).

SUMMARY

HIV/AIDS has had a tremendous impact on infection control, making it a critical component in the delivery of health care services, including diagnostic and rehabilitative procedures conducted by both speech-language pathologist and audiologists. Although the discovery of HIV elevated infection control to the conscious forefront of the medical community, infection control extends far beyond the confines of HIV to any and all potentially infectious microorganisms. Clinicians must adhere to the mindset that every patient, bodily substance, bodily fluid, or agent is potentially infectious.

Health care professionals concerned with communication, hearing, and swallowing disorders conduct a variety of diagnostic and rehabilitative procedures that pose a potential risk of exposure to saliva, mucous membranes, mucosal secretions, bodily fluids, cerumen, blood, and blood by-products. It is important recognize the risks associated with exposure to such substances as well as the consequences of cross-contamination to the potential health of both the clinician and the patient. As reiterated throughout this chapter, these risks can be significantly minimized with the implementation and execution of appropriate infection control protocols.

The goal of an infection control plan is to consciously manage the clinical environment for the specific purposes of eliminating or minimizing the spread of disease. To achieve this goal, standard precautions issued by the CDC must be considered and appropriately applied. Developing and implementing a written infection control plan is critical in this endeavor as it establishes well-defined work practice controls designed to ensure that speech-language pathology and audiology procedures are delivered to patients in a manner consistent with CDC guidelines. The written plan also ensures that other critical aspects of infection control are identified and addressed including the implementation of training, planning for accidents, and coordinating necessary vaccinations of health care workers. These steps are necessary to ensure that infection control goals may be met during the delivery of services to individuals with communication, hearing, and/or swallowing disorders.

REFERENCES

Bankaitis, A. U. (2002). What's growing on your patients' hearing aids? *Hearing Journal, 55*(6), 48–56.

Bankaitis, A. U., & Kemp, R. J. (2002). Hearing aid-related infection control. In M. Valente (Ed.), *Strategies for selecting and verifying hearing aid fittings* (2nd ed., pp. 369–383). New York: Thieme Medical.

Bankaitis, A. U., & Kemp, R. J. (2003). *Infection control in the hearing aid clinic.* St. Louis, MO: Auban.

Bankaitis, A. U., & Kemp, R. J. (2005). *Infection control in the audiology clinic.* St. Louis, MO: Auban.

Bankaitis, A. U., & Kemp, R. J. (2007). Infection control in the audiology clinic. In K. Campbell (Ed.), *Pharmacology and ototoxicity for audiologists* (pp. 124–137). Clifton Park, NY: Thomson Delmar Learning.

Bankaitis, A. U., Kemp, R. J., Krival, K., & Bandaranayake, D. W. (2005). *Infection control for speech-language pathology.* St. Louis, MO: Auban.

Bankaitis, A. E., & Schountz, T. (1998). HIV-related ototoxicity. *Seminars in Hearing, 19*(2), 155–163.

Breathnach, A. S., Jenkins, D. R., & Pedler, S. J. (1992). Stethoscopes as possible vectors of infection by staphylococci. *British Medical Journal, 305*, 1573.

Brooks, I. (1985). Bacterial flora of airline headset devices. *American Journal of Otology, 6,* 111–114.

CDC. (1987). Recommendations for prevention of HIV transmission in health-care settings. *Morbidity and Mortality Weekly Report, 36*(Suppl. 2), 1–18.

CDC. (2002). Guideline for hand hygiene. *Morbidity and Mortality Weekly Report, 51*(RR16), 1–44.

Kemp, R. J., & Bankaitis, A. U. (2000). Infection control. In H. Hosford-Dunn, R. J. Roeser, & M. Valente (Eds.), *Audiology: Practice management* (pp. 257–272). New York: Thieme Medical.

Kemp, R. J., & Roeser, R. J. (1998). Infection control for audiologist. *Seminars in Hearing, 19*(2), 195–204.

Kemp, R. J., Roeser, R. J., Pearson, D. W., & Ballachanda, B. B. (1996). *Infection control for the professions of audiology and speech-language pathology.* Olathe, KS: Iles.

Kummer, A. (2001). *Nasopharyngoscopy.* In A. Kummer (Ed.), *Cleft palate and craniofacial anomalies: The effects on speech and resonance* (pp. 378–398). San Diego, CA: Singular Thomson Learning.

Murray, P. R., Kobayashi, G. S., Pfaller, M. A., & Rosenthal, K. S. (1994). Staphylococcus. In P. R. Murray (Ed.), *Medical Microbiology* (2nd ed., pp. 166–179). St. Louis, MO: Mosby-Year Book.

Rutala, W. A. (1990). APIC guideline for selection and use of disinfectants. *American Journal of Infection Control, 17*(52), 99–117.

Strugulweski, S., Bankaitis, A. U., Klodd, D., & Haberkamp, T. (2006). What's still growing on your patient's hearing aids? *Hearing Journal, 59*(9), 45–48.

World Health Organization. (2002). *Prevention of hospital acquired infections—a practical guide* (2nd ed.) Available at http://whqlibdoc .who.int/hq/2002/WHO_CDS_CSR_EPH_2002.12.pdf

World Health Organization. (2004). *Practical guidelines for infection control in health care facilities.* Available atwww.searo.who.int/Link Files/Publications_PracticalguidelinSEAROpub-41.pdf

World Health Organization. (2005). *WHO guidelines on head hygiene in health care (advanced draft): A summary.* Available at http://www .who.int/patientsafety/information_centre/ghhad_download_link/en/

CHAPTER 5

Psychosocial Impact of HIV/AIDS in Communication Disorders

Irma Eloff

INTRODUCTION

The psychosocial impact of HIV/AIDS in a variety of populations such as orphans and vulnerable children, mothers, migrant workers, and individuals with high-risk behaviors such as drug and alcohol-use is well-documented (Broun, 1999; Bungener, Marchand-Gonod, & Jouvent, 2000; Campbell, 1997; Kadivar, Garvie, Sinnock, Heston, & Flynn, 2006; Liedlie, 2001; Organista & Kubo, 2005; Wingood & DiClemente, 1998). However, the psychosocial impact of HIV/AIDS on vulnerable groups within vulnerable groups, or minorities within minorities, is less well known. A number of studies (Bam, Kritzinger, & Louw, 2003; Bat-Chava, Martin, & Kosciw, 2005; Gaskins, 1999; Groce, Yousafzai, & van der Maas, 2007) have specifically pointed to the need for research and intervention in deaf and hard-of-hearing populations, individuals with communication disorders, as well as broader disability groupings.

This chapter explores the psychosocial impact of HIV/AIDS on individuals with communication and hearing impairments. It starts with a general orientation toward the psychosocial risks and challenges experienced by individuals with communication and hearing impairments and then proceeds to make recommendations for clinical practitioners in terms of psychosocial support and intervention.

PSYCHOSOCIAL RISKS AND CHALLENGES FOR INDIVIDUALS WITH COMMUNICATION AND HEARING DISORDERS

Communication Barriers

Individuals with communication and hearing impairments often are at greater risk for HIV infection due to communication barriers. Normally, the distribution of information about HIV/AIDS is not specifically tailored for deaf and hard-of-hearing communities, thereby increasing their vulnerability. In fact, several authors (Groce, Yousafzai, & van der Maas, 2007; Yousafzai, Edwards, D'Allesandro, & Lindström, 2005) found that significant knowledge gaps exist between individuals with communication and hearing impairments and their nondisabled peers. In a 1992 study, Bares (1992) pointed out an 8-year delay in HIV/AIDS awareness and knowledge of the deaf population in comparison to hearing populations. A study by Bat-Chava, Martin, and Kosciw (2005) even found significant differences between deaf and hard-of-hearing individuals with regard to their knowledge of HIV/AIDS.

Although the immediate implications of communication barriers within these vulnerable groups appear to be obvious, the effect on psychosocial coping may perhaps be less obvious—both for individuals with hearing impairments, as well as those with communication disorders. Limited information and established knowledge disparities are intricately linked to psychological resilience and an individual's ability to respond to psychological challenges. In individuals with HIV/AIDS, these become even more prominent. Knowledge often forms the basis of decision making and the activation of coping mechanisms for dealing with psychological challenges. Within the context of HIV/AIDS, it becomes a life-or-death decision and discrepancies in the transfer of knowledge and information may have dire effects for individuals with communication and hearing impairments. A study by Druck and Ross (2002) confirmed that patients living with HIV/AIDS are increasingly becoming a part of the case loads of speech-language therapists and audiologists in hospital settings—illustrating the intersection between disability support, health care, and HIV/AIDS treatment.

Educational Barriers

Related to communication barriers are the educational barriers experienced by individuals with communication and hearing impairments. Even when communication barriers are overcome (or compensated for), further educational barriers often emerge. In a study conducted in the African countries of Rwanda and Uganda, Yousafzai et al. (2005) illustrated that inappropriate teaching techniques and inaccessible information had hampered adolescents with different disabilities. The study revealed that health care workers were unable to communicate with deaf adolescents through sign language and explained the ways in which educational barriers affected adolescents with different disabilities. The authors indicated strong links between the severity of impairment and the educational barriers that were experienced. They cautioned specifically against the "invisibility" factor in educational programs on HIV/AIDS, for example, when adolescents with disabilities are not acknowledged in the development of HIV awareness programs (Yousafzai et al., 2005). Whereas All and Fried (1994) pointed out that women are the invisible group in the AIDS epidemic, current indications are that such invisibility may have shifted from women to disability groupings (Groce, Yousafzai, & van der Maas, 2007). Complexities within disability groupings further exacerbate educational barriers that contribute to the psychosocial impact of HIV/AIDS. Language disorders, learning disabilities, stuttering, voice disorders, aphasia, dysphagia, articulation and phonological disorders, as well as motor speech disorders (Fogle, 2008), all add unique challenges in terms of the emotional and social effects of the disorders, which, in turn, complicate the educational messages around HIV/AIDS.

The psychological responsibilities of individuals infected and affected by HIV/AIDS can entail several psychological acts, for example, actively seeking quality of life or effectively dealing with assumptions about death and dying. It also may include mediating the effects of diagnosis on immediate friends and families, actively cultivating hope, and also creating functional support for dealing with the future. When educational barriers are not overcome, however, as may be the case with individuals with communication and hearing impairments, all these psychological processes are impeded.

Sociocultural Barriers

Gaskins (1999) elucidates some of the cultural barriers that increase the risk for HIV exposure for deaf and hard-of-hearing individuals. These include dependence on supplemental income, decreased access to care, and parents who find it difficult to accept hearing impairment in their child. Bat-Chava, Martin, and Kosciw (2005) specifically found that participants who live in larger Deaf communities and/or urban areas are exposed to more information about HIV/AIDS than comparable participants in rural communities. They refer to the "Deaf grapevine," which can serve the purpose of communicating information about HIV/AIDS, but caution against the potential detrimental effects of informal sources that may lead to misinformation, gaps in knowledge, and concerns about confidentiality and the maintenance of privacy.

A study by Gore-Felton, Koopman, Turner-Cobb, Duran, Israelski, and Spiegel (2002) strongly recommends that HIV/AIDS prevention programs need to consider the social, psychological, and cultural context in which sexual risk behavior occurs, in order to intervene on this psychosocial level. Within the Deaf and hard-of-hearing community, this would entail acknowledgment of a complex intersection of cultural and psychological factors that relate to HIV/AIDS risk behavior (Bat-Chava et al., 2005; Gaskins, 1999). The sociocultural influences of disability in Deaf and hard-of-hearing populations is evident when it comes to increased risk factors for HIV/AIDS. However, similar but inverted sociocultural risks also are at stake for individuals with other communication disorders. The Global Survey of HIV/AIDS and Disability conducted by Groce (2004) challenges the assumption that individuals with sensory, physical, or intellectual disabilities are not at high risk of HIV/AIDS infection, because it often is believed that they are not sexually active. Furthermore, she points out that disability is often approached as a medical concern, whereas the greatest challenges faced by individuals with disabilities are often social or socioeconomic in nature. Groce (2004) also cautions that the AIDS epidemic (pandemic in some countries) may increase overall disability rates worldwide—yet we know very little about HIV/AIDS within disabled populations.

Self-Esteem

Self-efficacy in relationships, self-esteem, and the ability to negotiate safe lifestyles have been prominent in psychosocial research on HIV/AIDS (Broun, 1999; Cash, Anansuchatkul, & Busayawong, 1999). It also has been explored with specific reference to individuals with communication and hearing impairments. Individuals with communication disorders such as language learning disabilities, stuttering, and traumatic brain injury may have poor self-esteem and are therefore vulnerable within relationships (Fogle, 2008). The study by Yousafzai et al. (2005), for instance, specifically explored the limited power of negotiation that sometimes is afforded individuals with disabilities within a relationship, especially within a disabled/ nondisabled partnership. Their findings indicated strong perceptions that individuals with disabilities cannot be insistent in relationships and that they are vulnerable to the behaviors of their (nondisabled) partners. These findings were confirmed in another study by Groce, Yousafzai, Dlamini, Zalud, and Wirz (2006), which indicated a significant gap in the knowledge of Swazis with hearing impairments, which in turn leads to feelings of inadequacy when they need to negotiate safer lifestyles. In their study on migratory female workers, Cash, Anansuchatkul, and Busayawong (1999) reached a similar conclusion, namely, that the negative social consequences of negotiating safe sex outweighed the negative health consequences.

In addition, the combination of hearing impairment and possible HIV/AIDS infection can have severe isolating consequences for the individual involved, which in turn can contribute to depression, fears about the future, and a lack of psychosocial support. A study by Bogart, Catz, Kelly, Gary-Bernhardt, Hartmann, Otto-Salaj, et al. (2000) points to the optimism that is often experienced by HIV-positive individuals on HAART (highly active antiretroviral treatment), but also shows the negative effects of staying at home. The optimism referred to in the study relates to when participants are responding well to treatment, when perception about quality of life is improving, and when they do not structure their lives around treatments. Feelings of inadequacy related to anticipated rejection in romantic relationships and discrimination by family and friends. As a result, these respondents often felt isolated and depressed.

Within the context of hearing impairment, Gaskins (1999) states that the potential poor self-esteem, learned dependence, isolation, and limited social skills of individuals with hearing impairments often are risk factors for developing social problems. She also mentions that the fairly high incidence of rape/incest, substance abuse, and domestic violence within the Deaf community may put many individuals with communication and hearing impairments at risk for HIV infection. Swartz, Schneider, and Rohleder (2006) share a concern that the challenges posed by HIV/AIDS include all disability groupings, which also may include individuals with a range of communication disorders in the absence of hearing loss.

Depression

The incidence of depression among individuals affected by HIV/AIDS is noted worldwide (Buchanan, Wang, & Huang, 2002; Leserman, 2003). A study by Williams, Narciso, Browne, Roberts, Weir, and Gafni (2005) showed that depression was highly prevalent in people living with HIV/AIDS and that it did not relate to demographic variables. Depression, however, was associated with health-related quality of life, diminished health status, and coping strategies. The study also showed that people living with HIV/AIDS made use of community-based services to a significantly greater extent than did comparative nondepressed participants (Buchanan et al., 2005). Although the study shows the importance of effective treatment for depression in people living with HIV/AIDS—to improve their quality of life and overall coping—it also has indirect implications for individuals with communication and hearing impairments. If the need for accessing community-based services increases for an individual living with HIV/AIDS who has depression, the barriers around education and communication (discussed earlier in this chapter) become compounded for individuals with hearing and communication impairments. Nonmedication treatments for depression often involve verbal therapy, which may be difficult for individuals with hearing and communication impairments to access fully.

The intersection created by depression, positive HIV status, and communication and hearing impairment creates unique challenges for health professionals in terms of providing functional support to individuals who are affected in this triangular way. Studies (e.g., Williams, Narciso, Browne, Roberts, Weir, & Gafni, 2005) have shown that individuals with depression make more use of health care services and have overall poorer health, which means that the barriers to individuals with hearing and communication impairments are even more profound and need to be addressed. Furthermore, chronic depression and stressful life events also have been shown to affect HIV/AIDS disease progression (Leserman, 2003), so the long-term effects of depression in individuals living with HIV/AIDS has a significant impact on their overall health and well-being. Conversely, a study by Moskowitz (2003) found that *positive* affect predicts a significantly lower risk of AIDS mortality. Actively treating depression in individuals with hearing and communication impairments, and vigorously seeking sustainable positive affect, may become a priority for health care professionals.

Resilience

Although the literature is dominated by a preponderance of studies that focus on the "negative" aspects and psychosocial factors associated with HIV/AIDS (O'Dowd, 1995; Strode, 2003), in recent years, a growing number of studies have focused on the "positive" aspects linked to HIV/AIDS, such as resilience, quality of life, asset-based coping, hope, and optimism (Ferreira, 2008; Mohangi, 2008; Phaladze, Human, Dlamini, Hulela, Hadebe, Sukati, et al. 2005).

This trend indicates the need to refrain from the discourse that frames HIV/AIDS only in terms of detrimental factors. On a psychosocial level, it always has been important to strengthen psychosocial coping by focusing on strengths and capacities, while trying to deal with life's challenges. Within disability literature (Kochhar, West, & Taymans, 2000; Smuts, 2004), similar trends are evident when individuals with disabilities are defined in terms of their *abilities* rather than their disabilities. This shift occurred concurrently with the movement to emphasize social inclusion (rather than exclusion) for individuals with disabilities.

Despite the fact that a strong focus on psychosocial strengths can easily be interpreted as a denial of the severity of the psychosocial challenges that are faced, substantial evidence is emerging that indicates that this strength-based focus carries both theoretical and pragmatic value (Ebersöhn, 2008a; Ferreira, 2008). The theoretical value resides in the deepening understanding of the complexities faced by individuals affected by HIV/AIDS. The pragmatic value can be found in the sustainability of interventions that are less dependent on outsider intervention and more responsive to what is needed in a particular context.

Poverty, Stigma, and Discrimination

HIV/AIDS, poverty, stigma, and discrimination often intersect and, in the case of individuals with communication and hearing impairments, another layer of psychosocial complexity is added. Gurung, Taylor, Kemeny, and Meyers (2004) show how social context has become critical in understanding issues of impact, treatment, and a psychosocial nature pertaining to HIV/AIDS. The number of low-income women who are infected with HIV, for instance, is increasing. They face persistent stressors that may contribute to early mortality and subsequently to dismal consequences for their children. Gurung et al. (2004) specifically found that, although increased psychosocial resources are associated with decreased levels of depression, they did not moderate changes in depression over time.

Yousafzai et al. (2005) indicate how HIV/AIDS prevention is often difficult within a context of poverty due to limited financial resources. This is even more so the case for individuals with disabilities. The latter's available resources, which potentially could allow the use of prevention strategies (e.g., condom use, HIV testing), are severely limited and the levels of dependence on others are even higher than in other vulnerable groups such as women, orphans, and vulnerable children. Dos Santos and Pavlicevi (2006) discuss the strains of taking care of orphans and vulnerable children on the kinship system. They state that the greatly increasing numbers of orphans, decreasing numbers of caretakers and increased financial strain on families render it necessary to consider not only the socioeconomic, but also the psychosocial impact of HIV on families. It is safe to say that, in families where there are individuals with disabilities, the available resources are even more thinly spread.

Coping with Loss, Death, and Dying

Some evidence (World Health Organization, 2005) suggests that it is equally detrimental in terms of long-term psychological outcomes for children living with infected parents and for those orphaned by HIV/AIDS. The children are coping with the loss of a healthy parent and the abstract idea of death and dying at a time when their cognitive development does not necessarily allow full understanding of the future implications of death. Often, their basic developmental needs are not being met. The psychological impact of coping with impending death, severe health implications for the parent or caregiver, and limitations on the quality of care to children have been identified (Rochat, Mitchell, & Richter, 2008) as major concerns in this regard. Although some studies (Foster, 2005) emphasize the importance of networks of support, the study by Rochat et al. (2008) shows that most caregivers utilize only two sources of support while coping with the effects of HIV/AIDS, namely, their family and health services. Alarmingly though, the "family" support often consists of a single person, which may increase the caregiver's risk of isolation and subsequent limited psychosocial support. Fragmentation of families due to parents working away from home—often found in developing countries such as South Africa and India—further erodes available support. The implications for health care professionals remain important, however. If health services are one of only two points of access to support for vulnerable and/or HIV-positive individuals, it is crucial that the health services that *are* provided are effective.

Psychosocial Resources

Psychosocial resources such as effective coping strategies, hope, optimism, social support, active problem-solving, and strong relationships can mediate the effects of HIV/AIDS. However, the chronic burden carried by those affected by HIV/AIDS contributes significantly to psychological distress (Gurung et al., 2004) and may increasingly deplete the available psychological resources. The increased burden on individuals with communication disorders and hearing loss, who suffer a silent disability, is not always obvious to those around them. However, it severely restricts their interaction with their community, as well as their access to psychological resources.

For this reason Visser (2005) has broadened the understanding of psychosocial resources to also include resources present within peer groups. In her study, peer support was mobilized to build connections with and among health clinic staff, teachers, and social workers. In this way, high-risk behaviors of adolescents in secondary schools can be addressed.

The mobilization of psychosocial resources to address the challenges around HIV/AIDS is fast becoming the preferred format for successful interventions (Ferreira, 2008). Not only is sustainability increased, but opportunity is provided for unique manifestations of support that is tailor-made for specific needs and challenges. The following two studies are excellent examples of resources being mobilized for the purpose of support: In a study by Viljoen (2004), resources were marshalled from the immediate surroundings in a group of vulnerable children affected by HIV/AIDS. This was done by conducting a process of memory-box making. In a similar fashion, Smuts (2004) used psychosocial resources to redefine the ways in which intervention is planned for a young child with a disability.

RECOMMENDATIONS AND CLINICAL IMPLICATIONS

The preceding discussion highlights the mounting need for health professionals to heed the distinctive challenges presented by individuals with hearing and communication impairments who may be affected by HIV/AIDS. The need for a holistic approach to health care and clinical assistance seems more vital than ever before. A sensitive understanding of health care and support within an ecologic framework seems equally crucial, as health professionals need to be able to work in teams across traditional disciplines to provide optimal care and support to individuals with hearing and communication impairments. Educational, pediatric, and clinical psychologists often focus on psychosocial aspects of patient care. Recent developments in psychology have tended toward strength-based approaches to optimize the efficacy of interventions. However, this generic approach is easily transferable within wider health professions as well. When a psychologist is not available, health professionals can adopt the positive approach with similar effect in patient care. The next section provides guidelines on dealing with the discrete challenges that individuals with hearing and communication impairments cope with within the context of HIV/AIDS.

Acknowledge Psychological Strengths

The psychological challenges faced by individuals with communication and hearing impairments and affected by HIV/AIDS are substantial. However, an emphasis on psychological strengths can serve as a valuable platform from which to address the psychosocial impact of HIV/AIDS. The rationale for this approach is similar to the strength-based movement, which started to include the abilities of individuals with disabilities in order to design interventions for overcoming and compensating for barriers created by such disabilities. The weight that is assigned to psychological strengths can function as a protective factor, while also creating opportunities for positive psychological effect to be created. For instance, people's capacity for compassion, their sense of humor, or their propensity for hope and optimism can have a broadly positive effect on their psychological well-being, which in turn can impact positively on coping with the effects of HIV/AIDS.

Acknowledgment of psychological strengths can be effected through active dialogue and intervention strategies on psychological strengths. This strategy can be used effectively with all age groups —from children to adults. Health professionals can integrate awareness of psychological strengths through interviews, play activities, drawings, feedback sessions, and the planning of interventions. Most importantly, though, the acknowledgment of psychological strengths happens within the mind of the health professional. It is a conscious choice to acknowledge that people are defined by more than their disability, their impairment, their environment, or their health status.

Develop Strength-Based Interventions

The departure point for interventions by health professionals often is the needs of the vulnerable group with which they are engaging. However, to successfully address the psychosocial impact of HIV/AIDS on individuals with communication and hearing impairments, it is crucial to develop interventions that stretch beyond their immediate needs and disabilities. Fully fledged interventions can include a focus on a wide array of psychological strengths, the mobilization of available resources and capacities from the external environment, as well as strong indications of connections being drawn between existing accessible resources and individual capabilities. Strength-based interventions seek out the strengths of individuals, as well as the available capacities in the environment where the intervention is taking place. As an example, Pretorius (2007) connected community resources to develop an 8-month intervention for a group of 28 women in correctional services. She emphasized skills development (much like one finds in HIV interventions), mental health, and collaborative learning. The intervention was found to significantly increase the hope and optimism in the group of participants and to positively impact on the overall psychosocial well-being of these women participants—even though their incarcerated situation often is associated with hopelessness and psychological strain. Although direct parallels cannot necessarily be drawn to interventions for individuals with hearing and communication disorders, some associations can perhaps be made in terms of the potential of mobilizing existing resources to provide support during times of duress.

This approach yielded considerable positive outcomes with South African school children (Ebersöhn, 2008b), even in situations of severe psychological strain. The Ebersöhn study (2008b) was conducted with 2,391 South African children from 78 schools in the Limpopo province. The study shows how a conceptual framework that focuses on strength and resilience broadens and enriches the knowledge that is created. She contends that the strength-based focus of the study also contributed to greater insights into school safety and protective factors in the lives of the children. Protective factors are crucial in understanding the ways in which to support vulnerable children in the context of HIV/AIDS.

A study by Ferreira (2008), in turn, shows how a focus on strengths and capabilities in South African schools can lead to sustainable interventions that provide effective support, regardless of the presence of health professionals. This approach signals an inclusiveness of understanding psychological resilience broadly. It also provides a subliminal message regarding the value of strength within adversity and of the psychological need to look beyond the immediate moment and challenge in order to cope with hardship.

Design Accessible Materials and Strengthen Sensitivity Toward Psychosocial Impact Factors

The need to design tailor-made educational materials for individuals with communication and hearing impairments in raising awareness about HIV/AIDS involves more than the pragmatism of creating materials that are understandable and accessible. Although the pragmatic implications of designing accessible materials for individuals with communication and hearing impairments are evident, the implicit psychosocial effects should also be acknowledged. Individuals with communication and hearing impairments and affected by HIV/AIDS are a vulnerable group within a vulnerable group, where pre-existing psychosocial complexities are already present. Social relationships may be strained, access to resources may be complicated, and self-esteem may be challenging. Depression may be present, but still could be undiagnosed and untreated. Within the context of HIV/AIDS, these complexities are further amplified and yet more levels of psychosocial strain are introduced.

Although all health professionals need to become knowledgeable about different communication needs in vulnerable populations, sensitivity to psychosocial factors is equally important. HIV/AIDS is an emotionally laden concept where high levels of convolution are often present, as it impacts on individuals. Fear and misinformation among the uninformed, as well as stigma and extreme caution, all are aspects that may impede the quality of assistance given to individuals with hearing and communication impairments who are dealing with HIV/AIDS.

Include and Integrate Disability Awareness and HIV/AIDS Awareness in Teacher Training

Worldwide, individuals with disabilities have been included in mainstream schools for more than a decade, and in some instances for even longer. In turn, HIV/AIDS has increasingly been included thematically in teacher training in recent years—also on a global scale, but more so in areas with higher incidence rates, such as Sub-Saharan Africa and other developing countries. Although commendable, the inclusion of HIV/AIDS awareness in teacher training often takes a blanket approach that assumes a high level of homogeneity among recipients of training. Teachers subsequently may have an equal assumption of homogeneity about the children who will be participating in the HIV/AIDS training and awareness that they provide—thereby neglecting the need for differentiation of educational materials.

The concurrent movements of increased inclusion of children with disabilities and increased HIV/AIDS awareness training in teacher training have not necessarily resulted in integrated HIV/AIDS materials that allow accessibility by children with disabilities. It is vital to acknowledge the specific needs of individuals with communication and hearing impairments when it comes to effectively accessing HIV/AIDS materials and information. Incorporating this further layer of awareness in teacher training may have a positive impact on a systemic level. Collaborative teamwork is viewed to be one of the most vital terrains for cooperation between health professionals, as training may be significantly enriched through input from a variety of health professionals. It also may impact positively on prevention strategies, which could help to reduce the spread of the pandemic.

SUMMARY

Individuals with communication and hearing impairments have been shown to have elevated risk levels in terms of HIV/AIDS awareness and subsequent lifestyle choices. This increased vulnerability is compounded by the unique psychological armory of individuals with communication and hearing impairments. It may leave them challenged in terms of social support and social relationships and also prone to fragmented information processing if their particular vulnerabilities remain unacknowledged. The psychosocial impact of HIV/AIDS is considerable—and in combination with the psychological makeup of individuals with communication and hearing impairments, it creates distinctive challenges for health professionals.

REFERENCES

All, A. C., & Fried, J. H. (1994 April/May/June). Psychosocial issues surrounding HIV infection that affect rehabilitation. *Journal of Rehabilitation*, pp. 8-12.

Bam, I., Kritzinger, A., & Louw, B. (2003) Die vroeë kommunikasie-ontwikkeling van 'n groep babas met pediatriese MIV/VIGS in sorgsentrums. *Health SA Gesondheid, 8*, 34-47.

Bares, B. (1992). Facing disease: How prevalent is this deadly disease in the deaf population? *Hearing Health, 8*, 12-16.

Bat-Chava, Y., Martin, D., & Kosciw, J. G. (2005). Barriers to HIV/AIDS knowledge and prevention among deaf and hard of hearing people. *Aids Care, 17*(5), 623-634.

Bogart, L. M., Catz, S. L., Kelly, J. A., Gary-Bernhardt, M. L., Hartmann, B. R., Otto-Salaj, L. L., . . . Bloom, F. R. (2000). Psychosocial issues in the era of new AIDS treatments of persons living with HIV. *Journal of Health Psychology, 5*(4), 500-516.

Broun, S. N. (1999). Psychosocial issues of women with HIV/AIDS. *AIDS Patient Care and STDs, 13*(2), 119-126.

Buchanan, R. J., Wang, S., & Huang, C. (2002). Analyses of nursing home residents with human immunodeficiency virus and depression using the minimum data set. *Aids Patient Care and STDs, 16*(9), 441-455.

Bungener, C., Marchand-Gonod, N., & Jouvent, R. (2000). African and European HIV-positive women: psychological and psychosocial differences. *AIDS Care, 12*(5), 541-548.

Campbell, C. (1997). Migrancy, masculine identity and AIDS: The psychosocial context of HIV transmission on the South African gold mines. *Social Science and Medicine, 45*(2), 273-328.

Cash, K., Anansuchatkul, B., & Busayawong, W. (1999). Understanding the psychosocial aspects of HIV/AIDS prevention for northern Thai single adolescent migratory women workers. *Applied Psychology: An International Review, 48* (2), 125-137.

Dos Santos, A., & Pavlicevic, M. (2006). Music and HIV/AIDS orphans: Narratives from community music therapy. *Muziki, 3*(2), 1-13.

Druck, E., & Ross, E. (2002). Training, current practices and resources of a group of South African hospital-based speech-language therapists and audiologists working with patients living with HIV/AIDS. *Die Suid-Afrikaanse Tydskrif vir Kommunikasie-afwykings, 49*, 3-16.

Ebersöhn, L. (2008a). *From microscope to kaleidoscope*. Rotterdam, The Netherlands: Sense Publishers.

Ebersöhn, L. (2008b). Children's resilience as assets for safe schools. *Journal of Psychology in Africa, 18*(1), 11-17.

Ferreira, R. (2008). Culture at the heart of coping with HIV and AIDS. *Journal of Psychology in Africa, 18*(1), 97-103.

Fogle, P. T. (2008). *Foundations of communication sciences and disorders.* Clifton Park, NY: Thomson Delmar Learning.

Foster, G. (2005). *Bottlenecks and dripfeeds: Channelling resources to communities responding to orphans and vulnerable children in Southern Africa.* London: Save the Children.

Gaskins, S. (1999). Special population: HIV/AIDS among the deaf and hard of hearing. *Journal of the Association of Nurses in Aids Care, 10*(2), 75-78.

Gore-Felton, C., Koopman, C., Turner-Cobb, J. M., Duran, R., Israelski, D. & Spiegel, D. (2002). The influence of social support, coping and mood on sexual risk behavior among HIV-positive men and women. *Journal of Health Psychology, 7*(6), 713-722.

Groce, N. (2004). *HIV/AIDS and disability: Capturing hidden voices.* The World Bank/Yale University Global Survey on HIV/AIDS and Disability.

Groce, N., Yousafzai, A., Dlamini, P., Zalud, S., & Wirz, S. (2006). HIV/AIDS and Disability: a pilot survey of HIV/AIDS knowledge among a deaf population in Swaziland. *International Journal of Rehabilitation Research, 29*(4), 319-324.

Groce, N. E.; Yousafzai, A. K. & van der Maas, F. (2007). HIV/AIDS and disability: Differences in HIV/AIDS knowledge between deaf and hearing people in Nigeria. *Disability and Rehabilitation, 29*(5), 367-371.

Gurung, R. A. R., Taylor, S. E., Kemeny, M., & Meyers, H. (2004). "HIV is not my biggest problem": The impact of HIV and chronic burden on depression in women at risk for AIDS. *Journal of Social and Clinical Psychology, 34*(4), 490-511.

Kadivar, H., Garvie, P. A., Sinnock, C., Heston, J. D. & Flynn, P. M. (2006). Psychosocial profile of HIV-infected adolescents in a Southern U.S. urban cohort. *AIDS Care, 18*(6), 544-549.

Kochhar, C. A., West, L. L., & Taymans, J. M. (2000). *Successful inclusion: Practical strategies for a shared responsibility.* Columbus, OH: Merrill.

Leserman, J. (2003). HIV & AIDS disease progression: Depression, stress, and possible mechanisms. *Society of Biological Psychiatry, 54*, 295-306.

Liedlie, S. W. (2001). Commentary: The psychosocial issues of children with perinatally acquired HIV disease becoming adolescents: A growing challenge for providers. *AIDS Patient Care and STDs, 15*(5), 231-236.

Mohangi, K. (2008). *Finding roses amongst thorns: How children negotiate pathways to well-being while affected by HIV and AIDS.* Unpublished Ph.D. thesis, University of Pretoria, South Africa.

Moskowitz, J. T. (2003). Positive affect predicts lower risk of AIDS mortality. *Psychosomatic Medicine, 65*, 620-626.

O'Dowd, M. A. (1995). Psychopathology and psychotherapy in the dying AIDS patient. *Psychiatry and Clinical Neurosciences, 49*(Suppl.), 117-121.

Organista, K. C., & Kubo, A. (2005). Pilot survey of HIV risk and contextual problems and issues in Mexican/Latino migrant day laborers. *Journal of Immigrant Health, 7*(4), 269–281.

Phaladze, N. A., Human, S., Dlamini, S. B., Hulela, E. B., Hadebe, I. M., Sukati, N. A., . . . Helzmer, W. L. (2005). Quality of life and the concept of "living well" with HIV/AIDS in sub-Saharan Africa. *Journal of Nursing Scholarship, 37*(2), 120–126.

Pretorius, T. (2007). *Internship in partnership with community resources as peer support for women in correctional services.* Unpublished M.Ed. dissertation, University of Pretoria, South Africa.

Rotchat, T., Mitchell, C., & Richter, L. (2008). *The psychological, social and development needs of babies and young children and their caregivers living with HIV and AIDS.* Human Sciences Research Council, UNICEF, Department of Health; South Africa.

Smuts, E. (2004). *'n Narratiewe lewensgeskiedenis oor die manifestasie van bates by 'n kleuter met spina bifida miëlomeningoseel.* Unpublished M.Ed. dissertation, University of Pretoria, South Africa.

Strode, A. (2003). *The nature and extent of problems facing child-headed households within the Thandanani Programme.* Pietermaritzburg, South Africa: Thandanani Children's Foundation.

Swartz, L., Schneider, M., & Rohleder, P. (2006). *HIV/AIDS and disability: New challenges.* Pretoria, South Africa: HSRC Press.

Viljoen, J. (2004). *Identifying assets in the memory-box making process with vulnerable children.* Unpublished M.Ed. dissertation, University of Pretoria, South Africa.

Visser, M. (2005). Implementing peer support in secondary schools: Facing the challenges. *South African Journal of Education, 25*(3), 148–155.

Williams, P., Narciso, L., Browne, G., Roberts, J., Weir, R., & Gafni, A. (2005). The prevalence, correlates, and costs of depression in people living with HIV/AIDS in Ontario: Implications for service directions. *AIDS Education and Prevention, 17*(2), 119–130.

Wingood, G. M., & DiClemente, R. J. (1998). The influence of psychosocial factors, alcohol, drug use on African-American women's high-risk sexual behavior. *American Journal of Preventive Medicine, 15*(1), 54–59.

World Health Organization. (2005). *What is the impact of HIV on families?* Copenhagen, Denmark: Health Evidence Network.

Yousafzai, A.; Edwards, K.; D'Allesandro, C.; Lindström, L. 2005. HIV/AIDS information and services: The situation experienced by adolescents with disabilities in Rwanda and Uganda, *Disability and Rehabilitation, 27*(22), 1357–1363.

CHAPTER 6

Ethical Challenges in HIV Research and Clinical Care

Ann Bartley Williams

INTRODUCTION

All health disciplines profess a code of ethical conduct whose goal is to provide guidance to members of the profession in challenging situations, where the "right" course of action is unclear. In addition to the values outlined in their professional codes, individual health care workers also bring personal beliefs and values to their work.

The HIV/AIDS epidemic, by virtue of the common routes of HIV transmission, the natural history of infection, the clinical manifestations, and the populations most often affected, historically has triggered difficult ethical dilemmas for health care workers. These include dilemmas related to the duty to care versus fears of personal risk, dilemmas related to the duty to protect patients and to warn others, as well as dilemmas related to HIV testing and participation in research. Patients' rights regarding autonomy and confidentiality are of particular concern in the context of HIV testing and disclosure of test results.

Established ethical concepts primarily address health care dilemmas that arise in relationships between individuals, such as patients and individual clinical care providers (Gruskin & Dickens, 2006; Mann, 1997). These ethical concepts have proved less useful in the context of the HIV/AIDS epidemic. The reason is that in every part of the globe the HIV/AIDS epidemic inevitably is concentrated among the most socially and economically vulnerable members of society (Mann, 1996). Codes for ethical conduct that are limited to individual patient-provider relationships fail to adequately address the glaring disparities in health status and vulnerability that have been laid bare by the HIV/AIDS epidemic (Alcabes & Williams, 2002). One response to this omission has been a call to integrate human rights concepts into the ethical framework for HIV/AIDS research and clinical care (Alcabes & Williams, 2002; Loue & Pike, 2007; Mann, 1997). Relevant human rights concepts include the right to a standard of living adequate to health and well-being (United Nations General Assembly, 1948), the right of women to be free from discrimination based on gender (United Nations General Assembly, 1981), and the right of every child to the highest attainable standard of health (United Nations General Assembly, 1989). A framework comprising ethical and human rights concepts acknowledges the dynamic relationship between health and human rights and provides a common language with which to describe the impact of human rights abuses on the ability of individual health care professionals to practice ethically.

> *Human rights abuses—including lack of resources—obstruct professional practice in that they compromise these [patient-provider] relationships through limiting the ability to provide care. The difference between care that is unaffordable or inaccessible, and care that is inadequate or intermittent, is no real difference at all. Health professionals who care for those on both sides of the divide—the impoverished and the privileged—are thus held hostage by such abuses.* (Alcabes & Williams, 2002, pp. 232–233)

Integrating human rights concepts into a framework for ethical HIV/AIDS research and care requires attention to both the individual and societal level complexities of preserving the human right of each individual to receive care. Adopting such a framework means that health care workers, including researchers, are responsible not only for the care they deliver to individuals, but also for the actions they do or do not take to dispel disparity.

BASIC HEALTH CONCEPTS AND APPLICATION IN PRACTICE

Currently established standards for the ethical conduct of clinical care and research derive from Western philosophical thought. Three basic principles—respect for persons, beneficence, and justice—are discussed at length in an influential document from the United States, known as the Belmont Report (National Commission for the Protection of Human Subjects of Biomedical and Behavioral Research, 1979). The HIV/AIDS epidemic, which calls attention to socially and politically sensitive issues including death, suffering, sex, power, and poverty, has engendered extensive controversy and debate regarding the application of ethical concepts to clinical and research practice. The basic concepts reviewed generally are not controversial. However, application of these concepts is often complex; and highly ethical individuals can disagree about practical implications for a health care setting.

Respect for Persons

Maintaining respect for persons requires attention to two dimensions of the patient-provider relationship. First, health care professionals have an obligation to respect the patient's right to make decisions about his or her own body. Therefore, the practice of obtaining informed consent derives from the principle of respect for persons. The requirement for informed consent applies to treatment decisions as well as to decisions regarding participation in research.

Second, we are obliged to protect those who are vulnerable and not able to exercise their autonomy (National Commission for the Protection of Human Subjects of Biomedical and Behavioral Research, 1979). How best to protect the vulnerable is the dilemma at the root of many ethical clinical challenges. Poverty, illiteracy, gender discrimination, social discrimination, concomitant illness, and the clinical manifestations of HIV/AIDS itself ensure that the vast majority of the world's population of HIV-infected people faces significant obstacles to exercising the right to autonomy.

Consent

Respect for persons includes the obligation to respect the autonomy of individuals. This principle underlies the assertion that one must obtain consent from a patient before providing clinical interventions or involving the patient in research. The patient or potential subject must understand the elements of the procedure or research study, the risks of participating in the procedure or study, and the benefits of participation. This principle applies to the side effects of treatments as well. For example, some antiretroviral agents may be ototoxic (Bankaitis & Schountz, 1998). The audiologist is most likely to be aware of this risk, particularly if the patient's hearing is already compromised, and should alert both the patient and the prescribing clinician, so that an informed decision can be made.

For consent to be "informed," the patient must be competent. That is, the patient must be able to understand the information presented, to evaluate the risks and benefits, and to communicate a choice. If the patient does not understand the essential elements of the decision and its consequences, the health care professional is obliged to take the steps necessary to help the patient develop an adequate understanding. Obtaining informed consent is, in effect, a dynamic process of communication across significant physical, social, and cultural divides. Obstacles to effective communication include language and class differences, hearing disorders, speech and language disorders, and cognitive dysfunction resulting from HIV/AIDS.

In spite of the most sensitive and valiant efforts of health professionals, some individuals will not be competent to give informed consent. Possibly incompetent individuals include young children and those with cognitive impairments. Children are assumed incapable of understanding what is being asked and of protecting their own best interests. Further, children do not have legal capacity to consent to treatments or research participation (Levine, 1988). As a result, parental or proxy-decision makers are required. Unfortunately, in a community hit hard by the AIDS/AIDS epidemic, many HIV-infected children will have lost both parents, raising the question of who is the appropriate proxy.

Neurologic manifestations of advanced HIV/AIDS include cognitive slowing, AIDS dementia, central nervous system infections, and neoplasm. All of these conditions potentially render the patient incapable of providing informed consent. Not all patients with a psychiatric diagnosis are incompetent, but those who are demented or severely psychotic are vulnerable. If the mental illness compromises the patient's ability to understand and communicate, the consent is likely not to meet the standard for informed consent.

Obtaining truly informed and competent consent is highly dependent on adequate communication between the patient, the family, the clinician, and the researcher. Informed consent requires that the patient or his surrogate receive the necessary information and possess the ability to ask questions and communicate his or her choice. Establishing clear communication across linguistic, cultural, and class lines is a significant challenge in many parts of the world (Louw & Delport, 2006). In most societies, health care professionals are members of the educated and socially advantaged class, while the majority of people living with HIV/AIDS are less well educated, have limited social power, often speak a different language, and are relatively unfamiliar with medical and scientific concepts.

The audiologist and speech-language pathologist/therapist need to assess whether patients' hearing, speech, or language dysfunction limits their ability to receive information and to communicate preferences clearly. In many instances, recognition of the nature of the obstacle suggests the remedy. For example, treatment of medical causes of auditory system impairment, such as otitis media, can improve hearing in some instances and improve the patient's ability to communicate. When this is not possible, linguistically and culturally competent translators provide essential services to improve communication between professionals, patients, and families.

It is generally accepted that consent must be voluntary (CIOMS, 2002; National Commission for the Protection of Human Subjects of Biomedical and Behavioral Research, 1979; World Medical Association, 2000). Coercion or unjustified pressure compromises the voluntary nature of consent. This can occur when there is a power disparity between the patient and the professional, when the patient or family fears retaliation for withholding consent (such as less attentive care in the future), and when the inducements to agree are disproportionate in the situation. For example, for impoverished individuals, a small monetary reward may lead the patient to agree to a procedure or participate in a study that he or she otherwise would decline. Another source of undue influence on patient consent is present in circumstances where clinical resources are limited and the patient perceives that agreeing to a procedure or study will ensure access to otherwise unavailable care (de Zulueta, 2001).

Ethically, health care professionals are required to ensure that patients fully understand the implications of participating in research. Before participating in a research protocol or referring patients to a study, one should be confident that the study will be conducted ethically, that it does not pose an unreasonable risk of harm to the patient, and that there will be no undue coercion involved in recruiting of patients into the study.

Researchers from outside the institution or clinic are likely to have a more impersonal attitude toward the patient population than the health care workers who are providing ongoing care. The researchers' goal is to further medical knowledge, not to alleviate individual suffering. This is a difficult concept and most people, even highly educated individuals, require help from a trusted professional to grasp the options on offer. The health care worker who is on the front line, who is familiar with the patients and with the social and cultural context, is well placed to serve as a patient and community advocate.

Confidentiality

Respecting patients as persons requires that the privacy of patient information is maintained. The consequences of failing to maintain the confidentiality of HIV/AIDS-related patient information can be quite severe, due to the social stigma that continues to be associated worldwide with the disease. In most countries, there are legal regulations related to disclosure of HIV/AIDS status and many hospitals and health care institutions have established procedures to implement these regulations. However, official regulations and procedures are not always followed in practice; therefore, health care professionals should take responsibility for learning and being guided by the requirements, regardless of the behavior of others.

Maintaining confidentiality means that patients should not be identified as HIV-infected through any type of external indicator, such as special signs on patient rooms or beds or noticeable labels on the outside of medical records. HIV/AIDS-dedicated clinics, hospital wards, and home visiting programs present an obvious threat to confidentiality, leading some patients to avoid these services. The dilemma is that by concentrating skilled clinicians and resources in one location, these facilities improve the quality of care for patients and provide coordinated access to a range of services. They offer an efficient structure within which to deliver comprehensive and multidisciplinary care. On the other hand, in most instances, the community quickly learns that the facility is dedicated to HIV/AIDS and individuals seen entering or leaving are vulnerable to discrimination. Patients who find this risk unacceptable must seek care from more generalized health care facilities, which often cannot offer the same quality of care. Institutions for the care of children with HIV/AIDS or for children orphaned by the HIV/AIDS epidemic present a special challenge. In most instances, the children have no choice about whether or not they reside in such a center and options for survival level care, such as food and shelter, often are limited.

Discussions about patient status should be restricted to those who need to know and should be held in private clinical areas. Curious health care colleagues as well as the patient's family members and friends are not entitled to information about the patient's diagnosis, treatment, or prognosis. Maintaining confidentiality is quite difficult and even uncomfortable when the patient is unable to communicate his or her preferences in the matter, when the clinical condition is advanced and the prognosis is poor, or when the patient is a child whose parent denies or wishes to conceal the results of an HIV test.

Disclosure of an individual's personal medical information to another person who is not engaged in providing clinical care to the individual is rarely justified, but may be acceptable in circumstances where the risk to an identifiable individual is clear. When a patient with documented HIV infection is placing another person at risk through his or her behavior, the health care worker should encourage the patient to inform the partner directly. If this fails, and if local laws and institutional policies permit, the health care worker may seek another method to inform the person at risk of the risk. In many instances, the local health department will take responsibility for notification and will attempt to do so in a manner as to protect the identity of the HIV-infected person.

Right to Autonomy: HIV Testing

Knowledge of HIV status offers patients the opportunity for a longer life and a better quality of life as a result of the remarkable strides that have been made in clinical science over the past 2 decades. Although antiretroviral medications are not available yet for everyone who needs them in all parts of the world, basic clinical monitoring and prevention of opportunistic infections are more widely available and can improve outcomes. Individuals should be encouraged to accept HIV testing and testing should be considered a routine part of clinical care in the 21st century.

Nevertheless, the persistence of stigma and discrimination associated with HIV-infection means that an HIV test carries significant psychological meaning. When even seeking testing can lead to negative social consequences, respect for persons requires that patient consent be obtained before an HIV test is ordered. Patients have the right to decline to be tested.

When the patient is unable to grant consent as a result of physical incapacity, and if the results of the HIV test are central to the provision of adequate clinical care, it is ethically permissible to proceed with testing, although legal regulations may vary and may require the consent of a proxy. Most institutions also permit HIV testing without the patient's consent when a health care worker suffers an occupational exposure to potentially infected patient blood or tissue.

The results of HIV tests should be presented to patients privately, with attention to the patient's need for emotional support. Patients have a right to the information necessary to understand the results of the HIV test and to make informed decisions about treatment. It is unethical to give a patient a positive test result without accompanying support and information.

Accurate communication of test results and the provision of supportive services are essential, but present an extremely complicated challenge in most societies. Cultural, linguistic, and educational barriers mean that what is said is often not what is heard by either clinicians or patients. Health care workers need training in strategies to convey the diagnosis effectively and to evaluate patient understanding of the situation and treatment options (Druck & Ross, 2002). Patients with hearing and communication disorders are clearly at a disadvantage and clinicians who specialize in working with these groups have an obligation to ensure that their patients fully comprehend their situation and that they have the information necessary to make informed decisions.

Beneficence and Nonmalfeasance

The Hippocratic oath requires physicians to strive to benefit their patients and to do no harm. All direct service health professions accept this essential ethical obligation. Health care professionals have an obligation to use their skills and expertise to promote the well-being of each patient. Conversely, health care professionals have an obligation not to harm a patient.

Duty to Care

The principle of beneficence comprises both the obligation to maximize benefit and a proscription against doing harm (National Commission for the Protection of Human Subjects of Biomedical and Behavioral Research, 1979). It is clearly and universally unacceptable for health care workers to refuse to care for patients based on presumed HIV status. When choosing a health care profession as a career, some risk is adopted. In reality, there is less risk associated with caring for a patient with HIV infection than with other infectious diseases, such as hepatitis or tuberculosis. However, in the initial years of the HIV/AIDS epidemic, health care workers in the developed world who were not infectious disease specialists had limited recent experience with the psychological consequences of professional risk from infectious agents. In addition, fear of the unknown combined with the social stigma of presumed sexual promiscuity or drug abuse provoked some health care workers to shun patients believed to harbor HIV infection (Meisenhelder & LaCharite, 1989). Fear of acquiring HIV continues to haunt health care workers and is most effectively addressed with comprehensive education regarding transmission of infectious agents such as HIV, hepatitis viruses, and tuberculosis.

The duty to care includes the duty to provide the best possible care. This means that all indicated procedures should be performed, including invasive diagnostics, therapeutic procedures, and hands-on care. Treatment plans should be determined by the clinical needs of the patient. However, in situations where clinical resources are limited, it may be necessary to ration services, based on clinical assessment of the likelihood of benefit. Prioritizing patients to receive care is extremely challenging, resting as it does on assumptions about prognosis. It also is emotionally stressful, requiring health care workers to select some patients before others. At its core, this is not an ethical dilemma, but an injustice done to patient and provider alike by gross disparities in wealth and health care resources.

Although health care workers have a duty to respond to those in need of clinical care, they are not required to place themselves at unreasonable risk of harm. Transmission of HIV and other blood-borne pathogens can be reduced significantly with the use of appropriate barriers and with the application of the principles of universal precautions in the clinical setting. Health care workers have the right to access to the supplies they need to protect themselves and their patients and to implementation of institutional policies and procedures that mandate universal precautions.

Caring for patients with HIV disease is demanding both intellectually and emotionally. Caring for the caregiver, including family caregivers and health care workers, is essential. Family members and health care workers need a safe venue in which to express feelings of frustration, grief, and loss. Unfortunately, in a context of limited resources and inadequate staffing, opportunities for debriefing, mentoring, and mutual support are rare. Health care workers can form informal support networks with colleagues. When support is available, the duty to care may be perceived less as an individual burden and more as a mutual challenge. There is a social and ethical responsibility for all health care professionals to participate in responding to the HIV/AIDS epidemic. This responsibility includes providing support to colleagues who are on the front lines of HIV prevention and care.

Duty to Protect: Universal Precautions

Health care workers caring for people with HIV infection have a duty to protect patients from nosocomial transmission of infectious agents, including HIV. Implementation of appropriate precautions, such as the use of gloves when examining the oral cavity, with all patients addresses the risk posed by the patient who is unaware of his or her HIV infection and who is assumed by health care workers to be uninfected by virtue of age, gender, or social class.

Health care workers also have a duty to protect patients from discrimination and stigma related to HIV infection. By implementing precautions with all patients, those with known or presumptive

HIV infection are not singled out for the special attention that could lead to negative treatment.

Duty to Protect: HIV-Infected Health Care Workers

Health care workers who are themselves HIV-infected must consider carefully whether the nature of their contact with patients presents a risk for HIV transmission to patients. In the great majority of cases, there is no risk because the patient is not exposed to the blood or bodily secretions of the health care worker in the course of delivering care. Health care workers whose work requires manipulation of sharp instruments during invasive procedures may feel ethically bound to change specialties. A few instances of HIV transmission from a health care worker to patients have occurred, most likely as a result of inadequate infection control procedures.

Health care workers should know their HIV status, although requirements for HIV testing of health care workers vary across countries, institutions, and professions. There is no ethical duty for health care workers to reveal their HIV status to patients or colleagues, although individual professional organizations and institutions may have policies requiring disclosure to supervisors or professional committees.

Justice

The ethical principle of justice requires that risks and benefits, burdens, and advantages be shared equally among individuals and groups. This principle raises the question of "fairness" and equality (National Commission for the Protection of Human Subjects of Biomedical and Behavioral Research, 1979). We live in an unfair world, a world in which equals are not treated equally and benefits are not distributed fairly. Many dilemmas in HIV/AIDS clinical practice reflect this essential injustice. When health care professionals are forced to select who is offered access to antiretroviral medications, who is admitted to the hospital, who receives expensive intravenous treatment, and who is sent home based on the availability of resources rather than clinical need, ethical professional practice is being held hostage by an unjust world.

Access to Care

Inequities in the world's health care systems mean that many people with HIV/AIDS have limited access to care, particularly to state-of-the-art advances in HIV/AIDS care. Research projects often are better funded and offer access to supportive services that are not available in the local public health system. Many clinical trials include supportive counseling and adjunctive health services to entice and retain subjects. Furthermore, in some instances, new therapies are available only through research protocols. Justice requires equal access to care, including the opportunity to participate in research.

The quality of care provided to research subjects is a thorny ethical dilemma for researchers and clinicians alike. The Declaration of Helsinki (Medical Association, 2000) suggests that additional standards apply when research is combined with clinical care. Researchers must be attentive to the quality of care provided to their subjects. However, if research subjects receive access to care that is not available to members of the same community who are not part of the study, then an undue inducement to participate is present. In resource-limited settings, well-funded research projects may represent the only source of high quality care for people with HIV/AIDS. This situation both reflects and furthers injustice.

Justice also requires that research subjects receive fair benefit from their study participation. The Declaration of Helsinki explicitly requires that every patient participating in a study receive access to the "best proven" methods identified by the study at its conclusion (World Medical Association, 2000). The statement on *International Ethical Guidelines for Biomedical Research Involving Human Subjects* (CIOMS, 2002) moderated that position, suggesting "reasonable availability" of the products of research to the local population. However, determination of exactly what constitutes "best proven," "reasonably available," and "local" remains challenging and controversial, particularly in the international research arena.

Purely descriptive research, such as that often conducted in audiology and speech-language pathology, aims to identify symptoms and group characteristics in order to understand the natural history of disease and with the long-term objective of improving care. The principle of fair benefit dictates that there must be a reasonable assurance that any improvements in patient care developed as a result of the information collected in the descriptive study will be available to the original study participants. Clearly, this standard is difficult to meet but, equally clearly, it is unacceptable to collect data from vulnerable, impoverished subjects only to improve the care of wealthier and less vulnerable populations. For example, the Tuskegee Syphilis Study, a descriptive study that observed poor, African-American men with syphilis for decades in order to describe the natural history of the disease, is widely acknowledged to have become unethical when the researchers failed to offer treatment after penicillin became available (Reverby, 2000).

PUBLISHED GUIDELINES

Many of the world's wealthiest countries have invested substantial resources into HIV/AIDS research conducted in less fortunate regions. Although these endeavors bring substantial value, they are sometimes associated with questions regarding best practices in clinical research. For example, a study conducted in the United States and France demonstrated that zidovudine, administered for 6 months during pregnancy, intrapartum, and to the newborn, significantly reduced the probability of transmission of HIV from mother to infant (Connor et al., 1994). The regimen, which was quite expensive, quickly became standard of care in the developed world, but was considered unaffordable for the developing countries. To address the problem, shorter, less expensive interventions were studied in Asia and Africa, using placebo controls. U.S. investigators and institutions in collaboration with foreign investigators sponsored most studies of the shorter, simpler regimens.

In a widespread and vehement controversy, objections were raised to the use of placebos in view of the fact that an effective therapy had been demonstrated. There was no doubt that the second wave of studies would not have been approved for conduct in the United States or Europe, but collaborators in the host countries argued that, in view of the realities in the developing world, the potential for the studies to generate important information that could lead to practical, affordable interventions justified the use of placebo.

Researchers are required to adhere to ethical standards established in their home country, which may not be consistent with the culture and values of the host country. For example, the principle that individuals should be treated as autonomous agents conflicts with cultures that emphasize a person's membership in a group over individual decision-making (Louw & Delport, 2006). Western researchers may be required to obtain individual consent from village women before enrolling them in a study, whereas the local practice may dictate that consent must be obtained from a local elder. In this situation, the local health care professionals, who are familiar with local culture and customs, have a key role to play by ensuring that not only international ethical standards, but also local standards are acknowledged and respected.

Behavior that would be considered highly ethical in one country or culture may be unacceptable in another. It is useful for the clinician and researcher involved with individuals with HIV/AIDS to be aware that this range exists when negotiating or participating in an international collaboration. The challenge in these circumstances is to fashion an approach that meets the ethical standards of both sides. A number of documents adopted by national and international bodies are intended to guide ethical behavior of clinicians and researchers in health care settings.

Nuremberg Code

Chief among the international guidelines is the Nuremberg Code, created as part of the Nuremberg doctors' trial that followed the Second World War (Nuremberg Code, 1946). The Nuremberg Code speaks directly to the ethical requirements for the conduct of research with human subjects and establishes the need for voluntary consent, the responsibility of the researcher to ensure the quality of the consent and the quality of the research design, as well as the need to avoid suffering and injury. The tenets of the Nuremberg Code underlie most of the subsequent consensus statements on ethics in clinical research.

Declaration of Helsinki

In 1964, the World Medical Association adopted the Declaration of Helsinki (World Medical Association, 2000). Revised five times, most recently in 2000, the Declaration of Helsinki addresses issues on which the Nuremberg Code was silent, such as the acceptability of surrogates in the consent process, the need for independent ethical reviews of proposed research, the use of placebos, the need for additional protections when research is combined with clinical care, and the obligation to provide access to the "best proven" methods identified by a study to all subjects at the conclusion of the study. The Declaration of Helsinki is of particular value to clinicians struggling to reconcile the ethical responsibilities of care with the obligations of rigorous research.

CIOMS and WHO Guidelines

Given that the greatest burden of the global HIV/AIDS epidemic is borne by the developing world, the statement on ethical guidelines developed by the Council for International Organizations of Medical Sciences (CIOMS) is of increasing relevance (CIOMS, 2002). The CIOMS guidelines were developed in collaboration with the World Health Organization (WHO) in response to the challenges raised especially by research activities in the less developed countries where populations under study often are economically and politically disadvantaged. The CIOMS guidelines speak to many of the issues raised in the Helsinki Declaration, but with substantially more commentary on each guideline. This very useful document resulted from extensive international collaboration and review and is well worth consulting when a clinician or researcher is uncertain about the ethical acceptability of a research project.

ETHICAL DECISION-MAKING

There are no easy answers to the myriad of ethical dilemmas facing clinicians and clinical researchers. The HIV/AIDS epidemic has not introduced new questions, but it has infused the old questions with new urgency. Professionals who care for individuals with hearing, communication, and swallowing disorders must bring their all their knowledge, experience, and sensitivity to bear when faced with the inevitable ethical quandaries raised by this epidemic.

There is substantial variation in what resources are available to the frontline clinician who is faced with an ethical problem. Professional and institutional guidelines identify important principles. Local laws and regulations describe what is required and what is proscribed. But application of principles and regulations in practice often is not straightforward.

The first step in making an ethical decision is to describe the problem as concretely as possible, including identification of the individuals and institutions that have a stake in the outcome. For example, a child has been sent for evaluation of delayed speech and the speech-language pathologist/therapist suspects HIV/AIDS, but the mother refuses to give permission for HIV testing. The child's care may be altered based on the results of the test, so the child is a stakeholder. In fact, if the child is found to be HIV infected, she or he may qualify for life-saving antiretroviral therapy. But, the mother fears that if the child is known to be HIV positive, both of them will be rejected by the family. So, the mother is also a stakeholder. And the speech-language pathologist/therapist, who is interested in providing the best quality care, is also a stakeholder.

The second step is to identify the range of available options and the consequences of each. What will happen if the child is not tested? If the child is tested with the mother's permission? If the child is tested without the mother's permission? Can the consequences be ameliorated? Can the clinician proceed without this information?

The third step is to consult local professional resources, such as colleagues, professional mentors, and institutional review committees when they exist. Without violating patient confidentiality, discussing the situation allows the clinician to confirm his or her assessment of the situation and brings an additional perspective to the table. When there is an ethical review committee, sharing the burden of decision-making reduces emotional and psychological stress for the clinician.

The fourth step is to select an option, taking into account one's best clinical judgment, the ethical requirements of the profession, the advice of experienced colleagues, and institutional and legal requirements. In this instance, the speech-language pathologist/therapist may decide that the mother's wish to decline HIV testing for her child takes precedence over the professional's recommendation that the child be tested. A consequence of that decision could be that the child's health suffers. To ameliorate this consequence, the speech-language pathologist/therapist may monitor this child closely and provide additional education to the mother about the benefits of HIV treatment, in the hope of persuading her to accept testing in the future. This example demonstrates that there are not easy answers and that the "solution" to an ethical dilemma often leaves no one completely satisfied.

SUMMARY

Professional codes of ethical practice and international guidelines for the ethical conduct of research are grounded in three basic principles derived from Western philosophical thought—respect for persons, beneficence, and justice. However, application of these principles is far from straightforward in the context of the HIV/AIDS epidemic. Well-intentioned professionals can come to quite different conclusions given similar circumstances.

Health care providers who care for individuals with hearing, communication, and swallowing disorders must bring all their knowledge, experience, and sensitivity to bear when faced with the inevitable ethical quandaries raised by the HIV/AIDS epidemic. If the health care provider addresses each unique situation thoughtfully and in an organized, step-by-step fashion, making use of the principles and guidelines available, consulting with respected colleagues, and evaluating the consequences of the eventual course of action, then he or she can feel confidence in the integrity of the process.

However, poverty, illiteracy, gender discrimination, social discrimination, gross disparities in wealth, and uneven availability of health care resources often are at the root of ethical challenges in HIV research and clinical care. In a world in which equals are not treated equally and benefits are not distributed fairly, health care workers, including researchers, are responsible not only for the care they deliver to individuals, but also for the actions they do or do not take to dispel disparity and injustice.

REFERENCES

Alcabes, P., & Williams, A. (2002). Human rights and the ethic of care: A framework for health research and practice. *Yale Journal of Health Policy, Law, and Ethics, 11*(41), 229–254.

Bankaitis, A. E., & Schountz, T. (1998). HIV-related ototoxicity. *Seminars in Hearing, 19*(2), 155–163.

Connor, E. M., Sperling, R. S., Gelber, R., Kiselev, P., Scott, G., O'Sullivan, M. J., . . . Jacobson R. L. (1994). Reduction of maternal-infant transmission of human immunodeficiency virus type 1 with zidovudine treatment. *New England Journal of Medicine, 331*, 1173–1180.

Council of Organizations for Medical Sciences. (2002). *International ethical guidelines for the conduct of biomedical research involving human beings.* Geneva, Switzerland: CIOMS.

de Zulueta, P. (2001). Randomized placebo-controlled trials in HIV-infected pregnant women in developing countries: Ethical imperialism or unethical exploitation? *Bioethics, 15*(4), 289–311.

Druck, E., & Ross, E. (2002).Training, current practices and resources of a group of South African hospital-based speech-language therapists and audiologists working with patients living with AIDS. *South African Journal of Communication Disorders, 49*, 3–16.

Gruskin, S., & Dickens, B. (2006). Human rights and ethics in public health. *American Journal of Public Health, 96*(11), 1903–1905.

Levine, R. E. (1988). *Ethics and regulation of clinical research* (2nd ed.) New Haven, CT: Yale University Press.

Loue, S., & Pike, E. C. (2007). HIV/AIDS and human rights. In S. Loue & E. C. Pike (Eds.), *Case studies in ethics and HIV research* (pp. 1–14). New York: Springer.

Louw, B., & Delport, R. (2006). Contextual challenges in South Africa: The role of a research ethics committee. *Journal of Academic Ethics, 4*, 39–60.

Mann, J. (1996). Human rights and AIDS: The future of the pandemic. *John Marshall Law Review, 30*, 195–206.

Mann, J. (1997, May/June). Medicine and public health, Ethics and human rights. *Hastings Center Report*, pp. 6–13.

Meisenhelder, J. B., & LaCharite, C. L. (1989). *Comfort in caring: The client with AIDS.* Boston: Little & Brown.

National Commission for the Protection of Human Subjects of Biomedical and Behavioral Research. (1979). *The Belmont Report: Ethical principles and guidelines for the protection of human subjects of research.* Washington, DC: United States Department of Health, Education, and Welfare [DHEW Pub.No. OS 78-0012].

Nuremberg Code. (1946). Ethical and regulatory guidance for research. In E. J. Emanuel, R. A. Crouch, J. D. Arras, J. D. Moreno, & C. Grady (Eds.), *Ethical and regulatory aspects of clinical research* (p. 29). Baltimore and London: Johns Hopkins University Press.

Reverby, S. M. (Ed.). (2000). *Tuskegee's truths*. Chapel Hill: University of North Carolina Press.

United Nationals General Assembly. (1948). *Universal declaration of human rights*, Resolution 217 A (III), article 25. Available at http://www.un.org/Overview/rights.html

United Nations General Assembly. (1981). *Convention on the elimination of all forms of discrimination against women*. Available at http://www.unhchr.ch/html/menu3/b/e1cedaw.htm

United Nations General Assembly. (1989). *Convention on the rights of the child*. Available at http://www.unhchr.ch/html/menu3/b/k2crc.htm

World Medical Association. (2000). *Declaration of Helsinki*. 52nd World Medical Association General Assembly, Edinburgh, Scotland: Author.

CHAPTER 7

Communication Disorders in Children with HIV/AIDS

Thomas L. Layton
Jianping (Grace) Hao

INTRODUCTION

The purpose of this chapter is to describe various cognitive, behavior, and communicative manifestations in young children with HIV/AIDS. We begin with the prevalence of the disease, then a description of its transmission, and finally a discussion of the potential and serious manifestations of the disease as well as its effects on communication.

OVERVIEW

Pediatric acquired immunodeficiency syndrome (AIDS) initially was reported in 1982, or approximately 1 year after the first adult cases were reported (Rogers, 1988, p. 324). Globally, the number of children living with HIV/AIDS has increased from 1.5 million, in 2001, to 2.5 million in 2007 (UNAIDS, 2007). HIV remains a global problem.

Table 7–1 presents a breakdown in the number of children with HIV/AIDS across different regions of the world for the year 2005. As can be seen in the table, the Sub-Saharan Africa region contains most of the children living with HIV/AIDS (2 million), followed by Asia and the Pacific region with some 170,000 children. North America and Europe combined have reported only 15,000 children under age 13 years who are living with HIV/AIDS. Thus, nearly 88% of the world's children with HIV/AIDS are located in the Sub-Saharan Africa region.

Reported data also indicate that mother-to-child transmission rates within the Sub-Saharan region is 25 to 35 % (WHO, 2005), whereas only 2% transmission exists in developed countries like North America (WHO, 2006). Ninety-five percent of the affected children have acquired HIV from their mothers in utero, during delivery, or from breast feeding; whereas only a small number are infected from unsafe injections, transfusions, or sexual abuse (WHO, 2006). These findings suggest that, although pediatric HIV/AIDS is a global problem, economic, and social conditions within specific regions play an important role in the acquisition of the disease (Popich et al., 2007).

Table 7–1. Number of Children Living with HIV/AIDS Reported Globally in 2005

Area	Number of Children	Percent of Cases
Sub-Saharan Africa	2, 000,000	87.8%
Latin America	32,000	1.4%
Caribbean	22,000	0.9%
North America and Europe	15,000	0.7%
North Africa and Middle East	31,000	1.4%
Eastern Europe and Central Asia	6,900	0.3%
Asia and Pacific	170,000	7.5%
Total	2,276,900	

Source: WHO (2006).

Within the confines of specific regions, the disease also can vary. For instance, in the United States, different regions of the country vary in prevalence of the disease. The prevalence does not seem to be related strictly to population alone. This is represented in Table 7–2 for the United States. This table presents the most recent data, reported at the end of 2005. Due to confidentiality, many of the states do not report children living with HIV infection. For clarity, rather than viewing overall population of a state, it is more important to consider the rate of HIV/AIDS in children per 100,000 population (i.e., the last column in Table 7–2). Such a rate yields a more accurate estimate of the prevalence of the disease. It appears that using rates per 100,000 population yields data that are

Table 7–2. Number of Children Under Age 13 Years Living with HIV/AIDS Reported in the Top 10 States and District of Columbia at the End of 2005

State	Number of HIV Infection[a]	Number of AIDS Cases[b]	Rate of AIDS to Child 100,000 Population[c]
District of Columbia	—	246	206.4:100,000
New York	920	220	4.8:100,000
California	—	118	1.2:100,000
Pennsylvania	—	88	4.2:100,000
New Jersey	247	74	3.4:100,000
Texas	282	66	1.0:100,000
Illinois	—	56	1.7:100,000
Florida	—	54	1.3:100,000
Maryland	—	52	3.7:100,000
Delaware	—	38	19.0:100,000

[a]Some states have laws or regulations requiring confidential name-based HIV infection reporting since at least 2001.

[b]From HIV/AIDS Surveillance Report (CDC, 2007).

[c]Based on estimated child population data reported by U.S. Census Bureau 2005 (U.S. Census, 2008).

Source: CDC revised (June 2007).

different from using overall populations. We contend, as do Popich et al. (2007), that this variance is related to social, economic, and racial conditions rather than overall population per se. To our knowledge, these criteria of social, economic, and racial conditions have not been documented in relation to the prevalence of the disease in children per 100,000 population.

What percentage of these children eventually will convert to full AIDS is unclear. Current investigations indicate that proper treatment and early management have slowed the progression of HIV/AIDS (Howland et al., 2000). Unfortunately, in Sub-Saharan Africa, as well as other underdeveloped countries, fewer than 13% of the children who need antiretroviral therapy are receiving it (WHO, 2006). According to the WHO (2006) several factors may explain why this occurs. Many developing countries are struggling with human resource constraints and weak health systems; limited screening programs in these countries exist for HIV/AIDS in children; diagnosing HIV/AIDS in infants is unaffordable or absent; misconceptions exist regarding the effectiveness of antiretroviral therapy for children; limited experience exists with simplified, standardized treatment guidelines; and finally practical pediatric antiretroviral treatment (ART) is limited or unaffordable.

Any effort to provide proper treatment in all parts of the globe obviously would make a significant difference in the number of children living with HIV/AIDS. The positive results in developed countries have altered the prevalence and progress of the disease. Such efforts are needed in developing countries.

Interestingly, new annual infections of pediatric HIV/AIDS have declined globally from 460,000 in 2001 to 420,000 in 2007 (UNAIDS, 2007). Table 7–3 shows the decline in the United States for the number of new HIV/AIDS cases and cumulative cases between the

Table 7–3. Number of Cases of HIV/AIDS in the United States from 2001 Through 2005

	2001	*2002*	*2003*	*2004*	*2005*
New	368	294	212	179	168
Cumulative[a]	4834	4605	4199	3744	3336

[a]Cumulative totals since the beginning of the epidemic.
Source: CDC (revised June 2007).

years 2001 and 2005. As can be seen from Table 7–3, there has been more than a 50% decrease in new cases from 2001 to 2005, with a 20% decrease from 2001 to 2002, a 28% decrease from 2002 to 2003, and a 15.6% decrease from 2003 to 2004. Between the years 2004 to 2005, the decrease was merely 6%. Still, the overall decrease across these 5 years clearly demonstrates that the current prevention approaches are working.

Some developing countries also had a decrease in new cases between the years 2001 and 2007 (UNAIDS, 2007). In Sub-Saharan Africa, newly infected cases of adults and children have decreased from 2.2 million in 2001 to 1.7 million in 2007. In the Middle East and North Africa, new cases decreased from 41,000 in 2001 to 35,000 in 2007; whereas in Asia and Southeast Asia, the decrease went from 450,000 in 2001 to 340,000 in 2007. These decreased findings in developing countries, may be the result of improved population-based surveys (UNAIDS, 2007); that is, results from population-based surveys generally indicate lower national HIV/AIDS prevalence than do extrapolations from sentinel site surveillances, as used in 2001. Furthermore, changes in HIV/AIDS prevalence could be due to an expansion of surveillance systems that typically yield more representative data. Also, additional adjustments to antenatal clinic data from urban areas have resulted in a lowering of estimates of national prevalence, like in Angola, Congo, the Gambia, Guinea-Bissau, Mozambique, Namibia, Nigeria, Somalia, and Sudan (UNAIDS, 2007).

Thus, whether there has been an actual decrease in new cases or merely an adjustment due to improved population-based surveys is inconclusive. Regardless, in the United States, it has been well documented that early prevention works. Such steps are still needed in all regions of the globe (UNAIDS, 2007).

VIRUS TRANSMISSION

Children acquire HIV/AIDS in four ways namely parenterally by shared contaminated needles or sharp objects, accidental blood exposure, blood transfusion, and tissue or organ transplantation; sexually by infected semen, genital secretion, or blood; perinatally, through exposure to the infected mother via maternal fetal or maternal-infant transmission; and through breast feeding (Ammann, 1994).

Perinatal transmission accounts for nearly 80% of all pediatric HIV/AIDS cases (Oxtoby, 1991; Scott & Layton, 2000). All children born of mothers infected with HIV are also HIV-positive at birth, but the majority (60–75 %) will lose their maternally acquired antibodies and serovert or change their HIV antibody status from positive to negative within in a year (Lepage et al., 1992).

Children who are perinatally infected with HIV/AIDS are now surviving much longer, often into adulthood, with improved quality of life due to ART (Howland et al., 2000). Transmission rates have been found to drop from 25 to 40% to approximately 2 to 8% if the mother receives antiretroviral therapy like zidovudine during pregnancy (azidothymidine [AZT]) (Connor et al., 1994; WHO, 2006).

Children who are immunocompromised are reported to experience a variety of medical conditions (Layton & Davis-McFarland, 2000; Layton & Scott, 2000). The most common nonspecific symptoms include failure to thrive, recurrent fever, anorexia or decrease in appetite, and generalized lymphadenopathy (disease of lymph node); organ system-related diseases such as progressive encephalopathy (i.e., atrophy of the brain), peripheral neuropathy, and lymphocytic interstitial pneumonia; infection complications such as tuberculosis (usually in the lungs), *Candida* esophagitis (yeastlike fungus), and cytomegalovirus (group of herpes viruses); and malignancies such as non-Hodgkin's lymphomas (Hoyt & Oleske, 1992).

As can be seen in Table 7–4, children and adults show different patterns of opportunistic infections. For example, lymphoid interstitial pneumonitis (LIP) occurs quite frequently in children (i.e., 21%), but is rare among adults. It can cause oxygen deprivation and permanent lung damage. In contrast, Kaposi's sarcoma, which has been reported to occur in 12.5 % of adult males, is found less often in adult females, but rarely occurs in children (see Table 7–4). It may be necessary for children with LIP to be treated with antibiotics to prevent pneumonia, and they may need to be placed on oxygen or use inhalers to open their bronchial tubes.

The most common associated disease in children is *Pneumocystis carinii* pneumonia (PCP), which occurs in approximately 32% of the cases (CDC, January 1993). PCP is a lung infection that can cause fever, dry cough, and difficulty breathing. Potentially, all children with HIV/AIDS are at high risk for PCP and should receive prophylactic medications during the first year of life.

Being exposed to HIV-infection appears to have a detrimental effect on the child. It is important for the professional to understand the various manifestations that are associated with the disease in order to treat and establish appropriate management strategies.

Table 7–4. Frequency of CDC-Defined AIDS Related Opportunistic Infections in Children* and Adult+ Men and Women

Disease	Children (Frequency %)	Adult Men (Frequency %)	Adult Women (Frequency %)
Pneumocstis carinii pneumonia (PCP)	32	35.7	33.7
Lymphoid interstitial pneumonitis (LIP)	21	rare	rare
Recurrent bacterial infections	15	2.3	7.1
HIV encephalopathy	15	4.2	3.2
HIV wasting syndrome	14	7.8	9.0
Candida esophagitis	14	11.9	19.9
Kaposi's sarcoma	rare	12.5	1.1
Mycobacterium avium-intracellulare complex	rare	6.4	6.8
Pulmonary tuberculosis	rare	4.8	6.6
Cytomegalovirus retinitis	rare	3.8	3.4
Cytomegalovirus disease	rare	3.4	2.1
Chronic herpes simplex	rare	2.0	4.1

*Child data adapted from CDC (January 1993). +Adult data adapted from *MMWR Weekly Report* (1999). Adapted from Layton and Davis-McFarland, (2000).

RELATED MANIFESTATIONS

HIV/AIDS-associated diseases differ between adults and children and, therefore, should be addressed by different intervention strategies. HIV/AIDS is a multisystemic disease in children. The most frequent findings are neurodevelopmental abnormalities (Diamond & Cohen, 1992; Krikorian & Wrobel, 1991; Rubinstein, 1989), where the disease can invade the brain directly, producing HIV/AIDS encephalopathy (any type of brain disorder), or it can affect the development of the maturing nervous system, resulting in microencephaly (small brain) and possible atrophy. HIV/AIDS infection can lead to cryptococcus (yeastlike fungus) and cytomegalovirus (group of herpes viruses), opportunistic infections of the central nervous system. These opportunistic infections are secondary to the compromised immune system.

HIV/AIDS-related neuropathologies often produce cognitive, behavior, and motor deficits (Nozyce et al., 1994). These deficits may translate into possible feeding problems or dysphagia, articulation disorders, dysarthria (a disturbance of speech due to paralysis, incoordination, or spasticity of oral musculature secondary to progressive encephalopathy), and inadequate respiratory support for speech (Davis-McFarland, 2000; Pressman, 1992). In addition, various otopathologies may exist, such as recurrent otitis media, which may occur in 45% of the pediatric group (Falloon et al., 1989). Finally, subsequent candidiasis (yeast infection) may cause hoarseness in the voice or odynophagia (painful swallowing), as well as an oral language dysfunction. The remainder of the chapter details these communicative deficits in young children with HIV/AIDS.

Oral Manifestations

The most common oral manifestation in HIV/AIDS infected children is candidiasis. Candidiasis is a yeastlike infection of the mouth and esophagus with white plaquelike lesions, reddened mucous membranes resulting in hoarseness and discomfort in chewing and swallowing (Peiperl, 1993; Tami & Lee, 1994; Thomas, 1993). Candidiasis affects up to 12% of HIV-infected children (CDC, 1992, 1993).

Another common oral manifestation is salivary gland disease. This includes xerostomia (a dryness of the mouth), diffuse glandular swelling, or benign lymphoepithelial cysts (Tami & Lee, 1994). Parotid enlargement due to lymphocytic infiltration occurs in about 30% of infected children (Williams, 1987). Pressman (1992) has reported both herpes gingivostomatitis (inflammation of the gingival and oral mucous membranes) and cytomegalovirus esophagitis (herpes virus) in children.

Impairment in oral manifestation can have detrimental effects on speech, language, and swallowing (Davis-McFarland, 2000). Children may choose not to speak due to the discomfort or pain in the oral cavity or a discoordination of the oral mechanism. Oral discomfort needs to be addressed medically.

Otologic Manifestations

Singh et al. (2003) reported ear, nose, and throat (ENT) illnesses in 50% of the 107 confirmed HIV/AIDS-infected children in the United Kingdom. The most common ENT manifestations were cervical lymphadenopathy, otitis media, oral candidiasis, adenotonsillar disease, salivary gland hypertrophy, and rhinosinusitis. Singh et al. (2003) found that only 50% of their patients presented with ENT illnesses. They contributed this to early identification and improved antiretroviral therapy. Their findings support the work of Chem et al. (1996) in Texas and Chaloyoo et al. (1998) in Thailand, suggesting a global concern, but with an understanding that early intervention has excellent benefits.

Singh et al. (2003) reported that otitis media is a common otologic manifestation among children with HIV/AIDS; namely, in their study of 107 children, 46% presented with otitis media. This ratio has been documented in many previous investigations (Barnett, Klein, Pelton, & Luginbuhl, 1992; Falloon et al., 1989; Kohan, Rothstein & Cohen, 1988; Principi et al., 1991; Smith & Canalis, 1989). Otitis media presents itself in children with HIV/AIDS infection similar to most children of the same age, due to eustachian tube dysfunction and/or depressed cell-mediated immunity (Kohan, Rothstein, & Cohen, 1988). Otitis media responds well to oral antimicrobial therapy such as amoxicillin (Gold & Tami, 1998). However, failure of response may require tympanocentesis and a fluid culture; similar to most children presenting with recurrent otitis media (Poole, Postma, & Cohen, 1984).

Hearing loss of any kind can have a serious consequence in the pediatric HIV population (Scott & Layton, 2000). A hearing loss, along with other developmental delays, can interfere with speech and language development (Williams, 1987) and have a long-term effect on academic learning. Gold and Tami (1998) recommended routine audiologic examinations including an auditory brainstem response test for all children with HIV/AIDS.

Developmental Manifestations

Delays in cognitive and motor skills are common among children with HIV/AIDS infection (Calvelli & Rubinstein, 1990; Diamond &

Cohen, 1992; Indacochea & Scott, 1992; Levinson et al., 1992). Cohen and Diamond (1992) reported that mental retardation, cerebral palsy, and attention-deficit hyperactivity disorder (ADHD) are part of the manifestations that characterize HIV/AIDS infection. Gay et al. (1995) reported that mental and motor deficits developed as early as 3 months of age. In essence, developmental delays are common among children with HIV/AIDS infection.

Children with progressive encephalopathy appear more likely to have developmental abnormalities (Ultmann et al., 1985), including pseudobulbar palsy, truncal hypertonia, spastic diplegia or quadriplegia, hyperreflexia, and focal or more generalized seizures (Armstrong et al., 1993).

Levinson et al. (1992) found that HIV-infected and seroverted children demonstrated no differences on the motor scale of the McCarthy Scales of Children's Abilities (McCarthy, 1972). In other words, having been exposed to the HIV infection at birth affected the motor performance of children with HIV/AIDS similar to perinatally exposed seroverted children. Being exposed to the virus can have a serious effect regardless of whether the individual develops the disease or remains free of the antibodies.

Swallowing and Feeding

Dysphagia is a common oral manifestation in HIV/AIDS-infected children. In a study of 150 children, Pressman (1992) reported 20.8% of HIV/AIDS children experienced feeding difficulties that were demonstrated in coughing on solid-foods or liquids, slow feeding, failure to thrive, and gagging on solids or chewable foods. According to Pressman (1992), all phases of swallow can be affected, including oral, pharyngeal, and esophageal phases. Etiologies consisted of encephalopathy, neuromuscular discoordination, and odynophagia related to candida esophagitis, herpes gingivostomatitis, and CMV esophagitis.

Gazzard (1988, 2008) reported that gastrointestinal (GI) and hepatabiliary symptoms are common in patients with HIV/AIDS. It is estimated that up to 93% of patients will have significant GI symptoms at some point during their HIV/AIDS illness.

Bentler and Stanish (1987) reported HIV-positive children frequently had other GI symptoms such as diarrhea, malabsorption, constipation, and nutrient loss. Davis-McFarland (2000) suggests that adequate oral-motor and swallowing is important because many of these children need to take medicines orally. If impaired oral-motor and swallowing skills affect medical care and nutritional intake, enteral feedings may need to be done (Bentler & Stanish, 1987). Treatment of dysphagia should be aimed at addressing the various etiologies.

Language Functions

Only a limited number of studies have been reported on the language functions in pediatric children with HIV/AIDS (Table 7-5). There are no consistent protocols for measuring the cognitive and language functions across studies, whereas age differences across the studies also have varied from 1 year to 10 years. This makes contrasts of receptive and expressive language skills somewhat difficult to interpret within and across investigations.

Condini et al. (1991) found HIV-infection had an effect on language skills. In their study, Condini et al. compared the language functions in a group of 36 children, of which 18 were HIV-positive and 18 were seroverters. They found that the HIV-positive children were more delayed in language production than were the seroreverters. The mean length of utterance (MLU) was also significantly lower for the HIV-positive group than for the uninfected children. The researchers concluded that being infected by the HIV virus had a detrimental effect on language functions, especially on expressive language.

In a second longitudinal study, Copland et al. (1998) administered the Early Language Milestone Scale-Second Edition (ELMS-2) (Copland, 1993) and the Bayley Scales of Infant Development (Bayley, 1993) every 3 months to a group of 9 HIV-positive, 69 seroverters, and 26 infants younger than 6 months of age who had indeterminate infection status. Coplan et al. (1998) found that the ELMS-2 global score was significantly lower for the HIV-infected children than for the seroreverters or the indeterminate group. They also found that 7 of 9 of the HIV-positive children demonstrated deterioration in skills over time. They concluded that language deterioration may precede deterioration in global cognitive ability (Coplan et al., 1998).

Table 7–5. Studies Reporting Language Dysfunction in Children with HIV

Source	Population	Age/Grouping	Cognitive Function
Condini et al. (1991)	36 18 HIV+ 18 seroverters	18–30 months	3/15 HIV+ Showed cognitive deficits
Copland et al., (1998)	9 HIV+ 69 seroverters 6 unknown	1.5–45 months longitudinal	Bayley
Davis-McFarland & Cowan (1998)	54 11 HIV+ 43 seroverters	6–25 months longitudinal	
Havens et al. (1993)	60 26 HIV+ 14 seroverters 20 controls	5–12 years	Stanford-Binet
Hodson, Mok, & Dean (2001)	40	36 months– 10 years	Reynell Develop; TROGG
McCardle et al. (1991)	27 8 HIV+ blood 19 perinatal (7 infected 12 seroverters)	Not given	Not specified

Language Tests	Receptive Language	Expressive Language	Conclusions
Brunet-Lezine Scale 20-min language sample			HIV+ had more delayed language production HIV+ lower MLU
ELMS-2 3-month intervals			ELMS score lower for HIV+ 7/9 showed decline in language skills
ELMS-2	HIV+ 6–9 mo, 114 10–15 mo, 93 16–25 mo, 80	HIV+ 6–9 mo, 102 10–15 mo, 92 16–25 mo, 77	HIV+ more delayed in expressive and receptive language milestones
	Seroreverters 6–9 mo, 118 10–15 mo, 97 16–25 mo, 87	Seroreverters 6–9 mo, 105 10–15 mo, 97 16–25 mo, 83	
Gardner One-Word Picture Test Reception and Expression			All groups low average language scores
			Motor control less over time Child B: regression and died 11 months later Child C: not affected motor; grammar improved Child D: not affected motor; grammar improved
	5/7 perinatal had language deficits 6/7 had expressive deficit		No definite pattern of language deficit Expressive language more affected 25% seroverters showed language deficits

continues

Table 7–5. *continued*

Source	Population	Age/Grouping	Cognitive Function
McNeilly (1998)	30 HIV+ moderate HIV+ mild seroreverters	15–30 months	
Pressman (1992)	96	4 months to 17 years	ELAP HELP
Scott (1995)	3 seroverters	3;8 years 5;2 years 7;8 years	
Wachtel et al. (1994)	HIV+ seroverters controls	6, 12, and 18 months	Bayley
Wolters (1992) Dissertation Wolters et al. (1995)	36 20 uninfected siblings	1–10 years	

In a similar study, Davis-McFarland and Cowan (1998) used the Early Language Milestone Scale-Second Edition (ELMS-2) (Copland, 1993) to measure a group of 54 children: 11 who were HIV-positive and 43 seroverters. The infected children were seen longitudinally every month from 6 weeks to 36 months of age. The seroverters were evaluated every 3 months. They found no difference in language

Language Tests	Receptive Language	Expressive Language	Conclusions
PLS-3			Mild exposed less infected Moderate exposed had lowest scores Expressive language affected more than receptive
Birth to 3 PLS PPVT Expressive One-Word			69% had receptive/expressive language deficits
PVT EOWPVT Reynell			Receptive vocabulary deficit Expressive deficit One child overall language deficit
CAT/CLAMS			No difference 6m Differences at 12 mo Correlation between Bayley and CAT/CLAMS
Reynell Developmental Language Scale CELF			HIV+ lower expressive than receptive language Children with encephalitis performed lowest

function between the groups at 6 to 9 months, nor at 10 to 13 months, but several differences occurred at the 22- to 25-month age level (Davis-McFarland & Cowan, 1998). At the 22- to 23-month age level, the HIV-positive children performed less well than the seroverters on the expressive, receptive, and global scores. Furthermore, for both groups, performances deteriorated across the three age levels, with the mean scores being consistently and significantly lower as the children aged. Davis-McFarland and Cowan (1998) concluded that, at early ages, HIV-positive and seroreverters perform similarly, but at around age 22 to 25 months, the performance of the HIV-positive group worsened.

Another investigation, by Havens et al. (1993), provided information on the Receptive One-Word Picture Vocabulary Test (Gardner, 1985) and the Expressive One-Word Picture Vocabulary Test (Gardner, 1990). A group of HIV-positive children were compared with a group of children with no history of HIV/AIDS. The investigators found no difference between the two groups of children. Havens et al. (1993) concluded that other factors, such as genetics and background, were more important to language functions than was exposure to the HIV infection.

Hodson et al. (2001) administered the Reynell Developmental Scales (Reynell & Huntley, 1987) and the Test for Reception of Grammar (Bishop, 1983) to a group of four HIV-positive children at different ages. Each child was tested several times, and each child varied in age from the others. For instance, child A was first seen at age 3 years and was tested again at ages 4;0 years, 4;11 years, and 5;0 years. Child A's speech motor control became worse over time, but his expressive language demonstrated continued growth. Child B was assessed at age 5 years but died within one of the initial studies. Before his death, he demonstrated deterioration of both expressive and receptive language functions. Child C was first seen at 7;10 years, and then again at 8;00 years, 8;11 years, and 9;00 years. Her receptive language scores were low but fairly consistent (low 80s standard score) across the measures. Her expressive language function also appeared to remain consistent. The fourth child, child D, was seen twice at age 9 years and twice at age 10 years. Her receptive scores improved and remained stable across the four testing condition, as well as her expressive language functions. Hodson et al. (1987) concluded that thorough and regular assessments are needed to ensure accurate speech and language management strategies.

McNeilly (1998) assessed the receptive and expressive language functions of 30 children, ages 15 to 36 months, exposed perinatally to the HIV infection. The children were divided into three groups: HIV-positive and moderately symptomatic (group 1), HIV-positive and mildly symptomatic (group 2), and seroverters (group 3). McNeilly (1998) administered the Preschool Language Scale-3 (PLS-3) (Zimmerman et al., 1979) and found, as expected, that the HIV-positive, moderate symptom (group 1) performed less well than the HIV-positive, mild symptom (group 2) on the PLS-3. Furthermore, both of the HIV-positive groups (1 and 2) did less well than the seroverters (group 3) on the PLS-3. Expressive language functions were affected more than receptive language functions.

Pressman (1992) administered several language and developmental tests to a group of 96 children living with HIV/AIDS. She found that 69% of the children demonstrated moderate to profound deficits in both receptive and expressive language functions. However, Pressman (1992) did not provide the details of her test results. She concluded that factors such as prenatal development, medical history, environment, and psychological factors appeared to have important influences on the children's language functions (Pressman, 1992).

Scott (1995) measured the receptive and expressive vocabulary and language functions of three children who were all seroverters. One of the children was age 3 years 8 months, the second was age 5 years 2 months, and the third was 7 years 2 months. Scott (1995) found that receptive vocabulary was impaired in all three children; two of the children demonstrated problems in expressive vocabulary; and one of the children (i.e., the 5-year-old) demonstrated problems on the Reynell Developmental Language Scales-Revised (Reynell & Gruber, 1990). Scott (1995) concluded that children who had been exposed, but were HIV-negative, can present with receptive and expressive language impairments.

In a longitudinal investigation, Wachtel et al. (1994) administered the Clinical Adaptive Test/Clinical Linguistic and Auditory Milestone Scale (CAT/CLAMS) (Capute et al., 1983) and the Bayley Scales of Infant Development (Bayley, 1993) to three groups, namely, a group of HIV-positive, seroverters, and a healthy control group between the ages of 6 and 18 months. They found no differences between the three groups at 6 months of age. In contrast, there were significant differences between the groups of children at 12 and 18 months of age (Wachtel et al., 1994). Unfortunately, the investigators did not provide details regarding the language functions that were responsible for the significant differences.

Wolters (1992) and Wolters et al. (1995) provided a good deal of information regarding testing protocol for a group of 36 HIV-positive and 20 seroverted children, ages 1 to 12 years. Wolters et al. (1992, 1995) found that HIV-positive children presented with lower expressive language scores than receptive language scores. In addition, they found that children with encephalopathy performed less well than children without encephalopathy. Wolters (1992) concluded that HIV-infection clearly affects the expressive language skills in children. Furthermore, advanced stages of the disease yielded significantly more impairments in both receptive and expressive language functions.

Summary of Language Functions

Taken together, the above studies reveal some interesting findings. First, several of the studies reported on children from a longitudinal paradigm (Copland et al., 1998; Davis-McFarland & Cowan, 1998; Wachtel et al., 1994), or across different ages (Hodson et al., 2001). The findings were that early exposure to the HIV-infection had little effect on language function, but as the child grew, or lived with the infection longer, the HIV-infection tended to have more of an effect, with language function skills deteriorating. These deteriorating skills tended to occur more often in expressive language than receptive language, with vocabulary being less involved than global language functions. This suggests that children exposed to the HIV-infection need to be tested early and followed carefully over several years to document any changes in language functions. Furthermore, HIV-positive children with more serious symptoms (McNeilly, 1998; Wolters, 1992; Wolters et al., 1995) tend to have more serious cognitive and language impairments than do HIV-positive children with milder symptoms. This suggests that control of the infection, through medical treatment, is important in reducing or preventing a deterioration of the child's speech and language functions. Finally, several of the studies (Condini et al., 1991; Davis-McFarland & Cowan, 1998; Havens et al., 1993; McNeilly, 1998; Scott, 1995; Wachetel et al., 1994) found that children who had been exposed but not infected by the disease (i.e., seroreverters) also had impairments in language functions, but not as severe as the children who were HIV-positive. This suggests that even children who are just exposed to the disease are at risk for language impairments. Why this occurs is uncertain. It can be contributed to either the long-term effects of the disease itself or the environment in which the child is being raised. For one thing, most children living with HIV/AIDS have only a single parent in the home, a parent who also has HIV/AIDS, or are placed in a foster care environment (Popich et al., 2007). Regardless of the reason, it is important that all children exposed to HIV/AIDS be assessed for cognitive and language function and followed up routinely to make sure that proper treatment services are provided.

ASSESSMENT

The nature and progression of the disease clearly indicate that a multidisciplinary team approach is recommended (Davis-McFarland, 2000; Layton & Scott, 2000, Scott & Layton, 2000). General medical management is necessary to determine the status of the mother's health and/or infection during pregnancy, the amount of prenatal care, and monitor the development of the infant's HIV antibody status. In addition, pediatric medical assessment is needed to measure baselines and follow up regarding nutrition, weight gain, growth history, and recurrent illnesses. Immunologists and infectious disease specialists are needed to diagnose and treat the opportunistic infections. Other specialists are needed as consultants to treat pulmonary diseases and otolaryngologic issues. The child living with HIV/AIDS also may experience failure to thrive and feeding difficulties due to dysphagia. A swallowing assessment is needed to determine the child's diet, feeding techniques, and feeding schedule (Cohen & Diamond, 1992).

A neurodevelopmental assessment is needed to identify possible developmental delays and potential neuropathologies. Psychological testing is recommended to determine the level of cognitive function and should be routinely completed to show progression or regression of cognitive function as the disease progresses. Motor impairment may influence cognitive assessment results. For example, motor impairments such as visual-motor coordination, drawing, or block design also can affect performances on cognitive assessment.

Social services, by a social worker, as part of the assessment team are important as living with HIV/AIDS means living with stress that is associated with the disease. The child may experience painful medical treatments, occasional hospitalizations, and various side effects from the antiretroviral therapy or medications. In addition, the child may demonstrate various psychiatric symptoms and dementia that require special services. Parents of the child also may be chronically ill, making them less available to provide appropriate and necessary child care.

Educational assessment will determine preliteracy, academic skills, and special education interventions that may be necessary (Cohen & Diamond, 1992). Because of developmental delays and disorders, the child may require special education and/or early intervention services (Scott & Layton, 2000).

Physical and occupational therapy are also recommended to assess the motor difficulties, especially the oral-motor complications. Occupational therapy also can assist in the fine motor skills that are related to daily living activities, dysphagia, and feeding difficulties. Physical therapy can help in the development of large muscle coordination and fine motor activities.

Speech-language pathologists/speech-language therapists (SLPs/ SLTs) and audiologists are important team members. Speech, language, and hearing evaluations are needed. Because of various otopathologies, like otitis media, an audiologic evaluation is recommended (Layton & Scott, 2000; Scott & Layton, 2000.) A full assessment battery of speech, language, and pragmatic skills is recommended (Davis-McFarland, 2000; Layton & Scott, 2000).

According to Layton and Scott (2000), the initial step is to examine the child's oral mechanism to identify the gross cranial nerve dysfunction. The Robbins and Klee (1987) oral-motor skills protocol can be used to assess the oral mechanism. This protocol assesses oral-motor functions as rapid coordination movements (i.e., diadochokinetic tasks), blowing, lip closure, and tongue mobility with and without speech function.

Pitch and vocal qualities can be measured through acoustic analysis including baseline measurements of fundamental frequency, pitch perturbation (jitter), and an s/z ratio. Subjective measures are needed for ratings of voice quality including hoarseness, nasality, and breathiness.

Davis-McFarland (2000) recommends screening for speech and language development on a regular basis to determine changes in performances from visit to visit. She recommends two language screening measures for infants and toddlers. The Early Language Milestone Scale (ELMS-2) (Copland, 1998) can be administered on a pass/fail basis for language. Both typical developing children and HIV-positive children were included in the ELMS-2 standardized population. The other is the Clinical Adaptive Test/Clinical Linguistic and Auditory Milestone Scale (CAT/CLAMS) (Capute et al., 1983). This screening tool is used to determine neurologic and language development that most likely can be compromised in children living with HIV/AIDS.

Both standardized and nonstandardized diagnostic measures for speech and language should be considered. Several standardized tests have been used in the literature, but the most frequently reported instruments were the Reynell Developmental Language Scales-Revised (RDLS-R) (Reynell & Huntley, 1985) and the Clinical Evaluation of Language Fundamentals-4 (CELF-4) (Semel et al., 2003). In addition, the Peabody Picture Vocabulary Test (PPVT-4) (Dunn & Dunn, 2007) and the Expressive One Word Picture Vocabulary Test (EOWPVT) (Brownell, 2000) may be used to assess receptive and expressive vocabulary. The Goldman-Fristoe Test of Articulation (GFTA-2) (Goldman & Fristoe, 2000) and the Khan-Lewis Phonological Analysis (KLPA-2) (Khan & Lewis, 2002) are recommended to assess the child's sound system and phonological processes.

Nonstandardized approaches include obtaining a spontaneous language sample (Lund & Duchan, 1988) with a scoring system like the Systematic Analysis of Language Transcripts (SALT) (Miller & Chapman, 2008). From the SALT, mean length of utterance, a general index of grammatical development, Type Token ratio, a general semantic measure, and number of mazes (i.e., false starts, reformulated utterances, etc.) can be determined. A behavior observational scale is also recommended, like the CELF-4 Observational Rating Scale (Semel et al., 2003) that requires parents or teachers to rate the child's listening, speaking, reading, and writing behaviors.

Often, it is difficult to select appropriate diagnostic tests in other countries and cultures because cultural, linguistic, and test-standardization issues may interfere in test results. Cultural differences occur when the child is not prepared to take tests as followed in the protocol. For instance, children may be reluctant to answer a question that is directly addressed to them because in certain cultures they are told not to talk to adults. Similarly, children of one race may be reluctant to talk to individuals from another race. These issues directly affect test results (Kohnert, 2008). Linguistic differences are a problem when selected vocabulary items may not be part of the child's cultural experience (Brice, 2002). For instance, the word "cowboy" is a North American term for someone who "roamed the west during the late 1800s." Children from Africa may not know the term because it is not part of their history. Another example is the word "pineapple," a fruit that is common among warm weather climates but less common among cold climate environments. Syntactic differences also can affect test results; for instance, the pronouns "he" and "she" are not differentiated in oral language in Mandarin and this often causes confusion in spoken language. Test-standardization issues are a problem in that a reliable and valid test needs to be standardized on the population for which it was designed. To adjust for cultural, linguistic, and standardization issues, Damico (1991) has presented guidelines for adaptation of tests.

First, Damico (1991) suggests there be a content modification of existing English tests. This is done by altering the content to remove biased items or change items in conflict by omitting or redoing them. This is done by changing the stimuli items so that culturally sensitive items are included. It also means that performance criteria need to be changed such as allowing more time, more repeats, and potential code switching. Second, Damico (1991) recommends that the modifications to exiting tests be made by changing the scoring criteria such as not penalizing a Mandarin speaker who does not use a proper subjective pronoun. Third, Damico (1991) recommends modifying existing norms. This can be accomplished by including group stratification in the normative data, establishing new local norms, or developing a new set of norms for the population under study. These guidelines, as well as those suggested by others (Battle, 2002; Franklin, 1992; Hanson, 1992), help to guide unbiased and more accurate assessments in culturally and linguistically diverse children.

ASHA (2004) also recommends appropriate use of alternative approaches for assessment besides standardized testing. One preferred approach is termed "dynamic assessment." Dynamic assessment (DA) has evolved from Vygotsky's (1986) "zone of proximal development" (ZPD). ZPD suggests that initially a child needs maximal assistance for learning but later becomes more independent. ZPD lies between where the child needs assistance and where the child can work independently. DA follows this model and is an alternative to traditional standardized testing with children. DA methods include testing the limits, graduated prompting, and test-teach-retest. In testing the limits, traditional test procedures are modified with elaborated feedback. Elaborated feedback is providing elaboration on the correctness of the answer, a reason why the answer was correct or not, and an explanation of the principles applied. Graduated prompting is providing the child with a hierarchy of predetermined prompts. Prompts vary in the contextual support that is needed. Thus, a child's response to the test is used to predict how well the child will respond to intervention. Test-teach-retest consists of first testing the child to determine deficient skills. Then the examiner provides an intervention to modify the child's level of functioning. The retest serves as determinant of the child's behavior following training. Lidz and Peña (1996) used the test-teach-retest on a standardized assessment of vocabulary among a group of bilingual preschoolers. They found that the preschoolers performed better in the test-teach-retest paradigm than under the standard approach (Lidz and Peña, 1996). In a related study, Gutiérrez-Clellen and Peña (2001) used the test-teach-retest model and found it useful in differentiating the language skills of two bilingual children, one child was found to have a true language impairment while the other had only a language difference.

TREATMENT

Davis-McFarland (2002) and McNeilly (2000) have helped to explain the issues and strategies necessary for intervention with children with HIV/AIDS. Both suggest that intervention strategies do not differ from the approaches that are used with other speech and language impaired children, except that many other complications are associated with the disease. A team effort is necessary. The team needs to take into account the stage of the illness as well as the concerns presented by the parents or caregiver. Family resources and dynamics need to be considered when developing realistic treatment programs (McNeilly, 2000). As indicated in the assessment section, a similar team of specialists is needed for treating the oral motor disorders (McNeilly, 2000), dysphagia (Pressman, 1995), and hearing impairment (Layton & Scott, 2000).

Most common speech disorders among children living with HIV/AIDS are in articulation and language (Davis-McFarland, 2002; Layton & Scott, 2000; McNeilly, 2000). Unfortunately, little efficacy data is available on the clinical interventions with communication disorders among children with HIV/AIDS. Clearly, there is a need for good research that documents efficacy treatment service delivery models. Davis-McFarland (2002) suggests that clinicians need to approach the child based on the severity of the disorder and type of impairment. The goal, according to Davis-McFarland's (2002), is to provide for communication first and then intelligibility and/or speech and language skills second. McNeilly (2000) similarly recommends using proven treatment approaches that have been effective with non-HIV-infected children presenting similar impairments. For instance, McNeilly (2000) used the Hodson and Paden (1983) approach for phonological impairments, and a traditional approach for children with articulation errors. She also suggests that speech intelligibility can be improved in children with HIV/AIDS by slowing the speech rate, using a syllable-by-syllable attack, and exaggeration of consonants (Darley et al., 1975).

Voice and phonation problems are also a concern (McNeilly, 2000). It is important to help improve the child's loudness level and voice quality (Darley et al., 1975). These children often display a weak, breathy voice and lack of pitch variation. Using a loudness level meter or a tape recorder is useful biofeedback for increasing loudness (McNeilly, 2000). The current authors have used the computer software program PRAAT (Boersma & Weenik, 2007) and IBM SpeechViewer II (1995) to visually help the child practice pitch changes, intensity, and duration.

Language Intervention

As with speech intervention strategies, language intervention for children living with HIV/AIDS is similar to approaches used for children with specific language impairments. The concern is to determine whether receptive and/or expressive language skills should be targeted; whether vocabulary, morphology, syntax, or pragmatics needs to be targeted; or whether to work on oral speech or alternative and augmentative communication skills. These concerns are made by a "decision tree" to assist the clinician, parent, or teacher in making appropriate choices. We have adopted a flow chart (Figure 7–1) from Lahey (1988), which we use to determine the needs for specific interventions for children with HIV/AIDS.

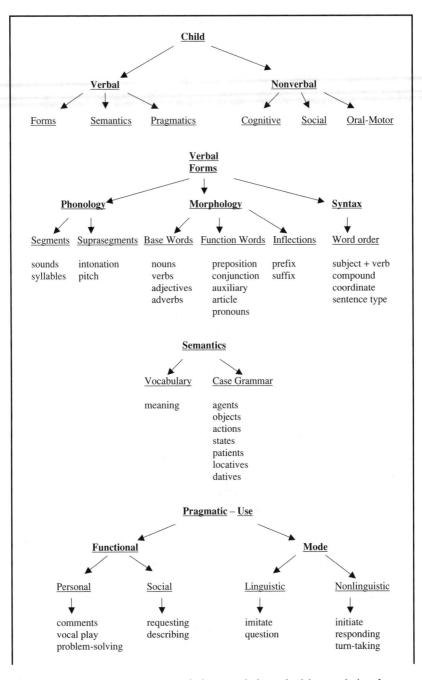

Figure 7–1. Language content and elements (adapted with permission from Lahey, 1988. Copyright 1988 Macmillan).
continues

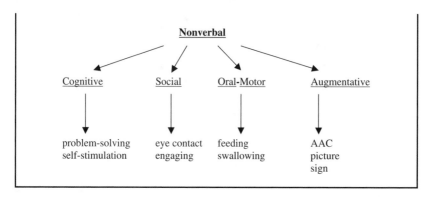

Figure 7–1. continued

Figure 7-1 generally speaks to the various language elements acquired by most children. As can be seen from Figure 7-1, the first level is divided between verbal and nonverbal elements of language. Thus, when deciding on appropriate language approaches for a child with HIV, we would consider the verbal ability of the child as well as the nonverbal ability. In the verbal area, Lahey (1988) suggests that language should be subdivided into phonology, morphology, and syntactic elements. Thus, articulation treatment would be recommended, as indicated in the previous section, if the child has problems with his or her sounds. If the problem lies in the suprasegmental features of the child's speech, such as intonation, pitch, and stress, the intervention would be to work directly on these areas. These areas, as previously suggested, may well be related to the child's oral-motor deficiencies, such as candidiasis. If so, then medical treatment is needed. However, if a functional problem is observed in volume output, monotone speech, or an abnormal pitch occurs, then direct speech therapy addressing these concerns is recommended.

Morphology is the second section of Lahey's (1988) verbal forms of language. Sometimes morphology is tied to syntax, as in such situations as third person agreement or plural subjects which requires no addition to the verb form. If a child with HIV/AIDS has a problem in any of these areas, a direct language intervention approach can be useful.

One of the original direct language approaches reported by Lee et al. (1975) is the "interactive language development teaching" approach. In this approach, receptive and expressive language teaching is emphasized in a natural environment, but in a highly structured setting. The approach begins with the clinician selecting the morphology feature that needs to be improved. The child's production is never imitated, but is incorporated in a meaningful context. The clinician gradually incorporates new structures into a narrative/story routine. The story routine typically contains a theme. The story or theme is read with normal prosody and the clinician asks probing questions throughout. The topic or theme of the story is always appropriate for the child and contains the morphologic elements under consideration. The clinician-child interchanges elicit creative thinking and appropriate responses. The interchanges fall into six techniques (1) Completion: Child: "They hot." Clinician: "They are hot."; (2) Reduction: Child: "They hot." Clinician: "were . . . "; (3) Expansion: Clinician: "Tell me more"; (4) Repetition Request: Child: "Him goed to town." Clinician: "What did you say? Tell me again."; (5) Repetition of Error: Child: "He goed to town." Clinician: "Goed?"; and (6) Self-Correction Request: Clinician: "Is that answer right?"

Owens (2004) expanded these procedures and outlined several similar techniques. The first of his techniques he calls "modeling": a procedure "where the clinician produces a rule-governed utterance at appropriate junctures in conversation or activities but does not ask the child to imitate" (Owens, 2004, p. 266). This approach is similar to the Lee et al. (1975) approach in that question-answers are frequent and require responses from the child. Owens (2004) recommends that the linguistic target be modeled to the child before eliciting the target. This he calls focused stimulation. The clinician produces several of the targets in a meaningful context that requires the child to respond; for instance, the pronoun "she" could be the target. The child might say, "Mommy made a salad." Clinician would then state, "*She* must be a good cook. What else did *she* make?" Through this modeling and focused stimulation, the child with HIV/AIDS learns proper forms of the preposition or other morphological features.

Another technique is "direct linguistic cues," which is sometimes referred to as the mand model (Hart, 1985). Here the clinician directs the child's attention to an attractive toy or object. When the child approaches the object, the clinician states or demands, "Tell me what this is." or "Tell me what you want." If the child does not respond, the clinician provides a direct-model for the child to imitate. The clinician may also prompt within this step by elaborating the mand, for example, "Give me a whole sentence" and then the clinician provides a model, for example, "I want more juice."

Often, a clinician will move from one of these approaches to another in order to elicit and stabilize the targeted morpheme being taught to the child with HIV/AIDS. All of these approaches have one thing in common. They are all considered clinician-directed approaches, in which where the clinician is controlling or directing the treatment session. It has an advantage in that targeted morphemes are being practiced. The disadvantage is that children do not necessarily learn language from a direct teaching model. Children, especially younger children, learn language skills typically from incidental adult-child interchanges (Owens, 2004).

Incidental teaching, also called milieu treatment (Hart & Risley, 1978), is a child-initiated approach to language intervention. Here the learning occurs by following the child's lead or interest. This is a good approach for developing base vocabulary words. Any child production is explicitly prompted. Consequences for the child's productions include association with specific linguistic forms and being natural to the context in which the learning occurs. The approach is as follows: materials are displayed for the child; child begins to interact with the materials; when the child initiates, the clinician focuses full attention on the child, creating a joint attention; clinician requests elaboration; if no elaboration occurs, clinician models; and finally, clinician confirms the correctness of the child's language.

Approaches similar to incidental teaching have been developed for children with special needs. It is useful and appropriate for young children living with HIV/AIDS at early stages of language development. For instance, the program DIR/FloorTime (Greenspan, 2008; Greenspan & Wieder, 1998) is a functional developmental approach. The purpose of Greenspan's program is to identify whether or not the child integrates all of his or her abilities (e.g., emotional, language, sensory modulation, spatial, and motor skills) to the social and cognitive world in a purposeful, emotional, and meaningful manner. Relevant areas of functional communication include shared attention, engagement, purposeful and effective communication, social problem-solving interactions, creative and meaningful use of ideas, and building logical connections between ideas and symbols (Greenspan, 1992). The clinician is expected to follow the child's lead of his or her emotional and cognitive interests to engage the child at his or her functional development. Other areas of verbal elements (see Figure 7–1) are semantics and pragmatics. Semantics are meaning of words, but are also related to case grammar (Bloom et al., 1975). An example of a case grammar form would be agent + action: here the noun form is referred to as an agent, or doer, and the verb form is referred to as the action completed by the doer. The auxiliary is meaningless for semantic-syntactic relations, but is necessary for complete adult syntax.

Pragmatics is the social use of language (Arwood, 1983; Gallagher & Prutting, 1983). In essence, pragmatics is how understanding is accomplished. According to Prutting and Kirchner (1983), this understanding is accomplished by the act of speaking, the propositional act of speaking, the illocutionary act, and the perlocutionary act.

One social-pragmatic intervention program that is recommended for use with children with HIV/AIDS is Gutstein and Sheely's (2003) Relationship Development Intervention (RDI). RDI is for younger developing language learners (preschool early elementary) as well as older language learners (preteens and teens). RDI is based on social-pragmatic skills that are to be taught within the context of meaning, interventions that are experience based, and interventions with a social learning context. RDI is a systematic intervention program that divides the early learners into three categories: Novice, Apprentice, and Challenger. The Novice curriculum covers the prerequisites for learning about relationships and feelings. The child learns to make adults the center of the attention-social referencing. The Apprentice curriculum helps the child acquire the necessary skills for shared regulations and communication repairs. The Challenger curriculum introduces improvization and cocreation. Challengers practice relationships in small groups. The more advanced levels of older learners target perceptions and subjective experiences; inner ideas, interests, beliefs, and emotional reactions; and assist in lifelong relationships (Gutstein & Sheely, 2003).

Returning to Figure 7–1, it can be seen that the other broad area of language falls under the category of nonverbal skills. Nonverbal skills are subdivided into cognitive (i.e., problem-solving, self-stimulation, etc.), social physical skills (i.e., eye contact, engagement, closeness, etc.), oral-motor (i.e., feeding skills, swallowing, tongue-lip-teeth mobility, etc.), and augmentative skills (i.e., augmentative/

alternative communication [AAC], picture exchange, sign language, etc). The first three areas, namely, cognitive, social, and oral-motor, have been discussed extensively throughout the chapter. The latter area, augmentative skills is further described here.

The point is that, regardless of the progression of the HIV-infection, it remains important that the child is able to communicate. The use of AAC devices provides this opportunity. It is important for the child to be independent and to be able to control the situation. AAC devices can assist the child in accomplishing this.

On occasion, a child with HIV/AIDS will become so severely impaired due to the complications of the disease that verbal/oral communication essentially is not possible (McNeilly, 2000; Scott & Layton, 1997). When this occurs, it is important to introduce some form of AAC. The purpose of AAC devices is to assist the child in communicating with family members at home and across other environments, such as hospital personnel, teachers, clinicians, and friends. ACC devices can be used short-term while a child is recovering from a medical treatment and his or her vocal skills are recovering, or they may be required when the child's communication abilities are deteriorating. This was the need for the case study, "Lydia," reported by Scott and Layton (2000). Scott and Layton (2000) reported that as Lydia grew older her disease progressed. Several AAC devices were tried with some failure and success. Initially, a digital voice output device was used, but Lydia showed little interest. Then an electrolarynx was tried, but Lydia was too weak to push the tone generator button. Subsequently, a Passy-Muir device was tried and Lydia was somewhat successful. Still, Lydia relied on gestures and head nods to communicate along with the Passy-Muir. Scott and Layton (2000) did not attempt to use AAC devices like pictures, signs, or an electronic device because Lydia soon died.

McNeilly (2000) suggests that the handbook of Glennen and DeCoste (1997) is a useful resource for assessing and selecting AAC systems. Such devices can be programmed to produce letters for spelling, sounds for words, as well as words combined into sentences. It is important for the clinician to know which devices are easy for the child to use, which are appropriate for the child's communicative setting, and which ones the child is willing to use. This gives the child the opportunity to control his or her environment. Many children become successful communicators with their AAC devices and enjoy interacting with their family, friends, and caregivers.

SUMMARY

The above review indicated that young children exposed to HIV-infection have cognitive and language dysfunctions. The chapter addressed how hearing, oral-motor, swallowing, cognition, and language functions are related to the disease and how they are involved in children who were exposed to the HIV-virus. When considering the influences of the disease on children, a variety of related factors should be considered, such as, age, socioeconomic status, medical history, and culture. These too have an important role in language development and, therefore, need to be taken into account when making treatment decisions. The one thing that prevails, throughout the review, is that early identification and intervention are important for language acquisition in all children exposed to the HIV. It is just as important to follow these children in order to plot progress or loss of cognitive and language functions. The SLP/SLT plays an important role in the assessment and treatment of children exposed to HIV/AIDS. They can document progressive improvement in communication skills, help to determine related services for the child, or demonstrate decreases in speech, language, and/or social communication. The SLP/SLT has a critical role in the treatment for speech, language, cognitive, literacy, and social interaction.

REFERENCES

Ammann, A. J. (1994). Overview of pediatric HIV disease. In P. T. Cohen, M. A. Sande, & P. A. Volberding (Eds.), *The AIDS knowledge base: A textbook on HIV disease from the University of California, San Francisco, and the San Francisco General Hospital* (pp. 1–7). Boston: Little Brown.

Armstong, F. D., Sejdel, J. F., & Swales, T. P. (1993). Pediatric HIV infection: A neuropsychological and educational challenge. *Journal of Learning Disabilities, 26*(2), 92–103.

Arwood, E. (1983). *Pragmaticim: Theory and application.* Rockville, MD: Aspen Publication.

ASHA. (2004). *Knowledge and skills needed by speech-language pathologists and audiologists to provide culturally and linguistically appropriate services.* Available at http://www.asha.org/policy

Bangs, T. E. (1979). *Birth to Three Developmental Scale.* Allen, TX: DLM Teaching Resources.

Barnett, E. D., Klein, J. O. Pelton, S. I., & Luginbuhl, L. M. (1992). Otitis media in children born to human immunodeficiency virus-infected mothers. *Pediatric Infectious Diseases Journal, 11*(5), 360-364.

Battle, D. (2002). Language development and disorders in culturally and linguistically diverse children. In D. Bernstein & E. Tiegerman-Farber (Eds.), *Language and communication disorders in children* (pp. 354-386). Boston: Allyn & Bacon.

Bayley, N. (1993). *Bayley Scales of Infant Development* (2nd ed.). San Antonio, TX: Psychological Corporation.

Bentler, M., & Stanish, M. (1987). Nutrition support for the pediatric patient with AIDS. *Journal of the American Dietetic Association, 87*, 488-491.

Bishop, D. (1983). *Test for Reception of Grammar.* Published by the author and available from Age and Cognitive Performance Research Center, University of Manchester, M13 9PL.

Bloom, L., Lightbown, P., & Hood, L. (1975). Structure and variation in child language. *Monographs of the Society for Research in Child Development, 40*(2), 1-97.

Brice, A. (2002). *The Hispanic child.* Boston: Allyn & Bacon.

Boersma, P., & Weenik, D. (2007). *PRAAT 5.0.* University of Amsterdam, The Netherlands. Available at http://www.fon.hum.uva.nl/praat/

Brownell, R. (2000). *Expressive One-Word Picture Vocabulary Test.* Novato, CA: Academic Therapy Publications.

Brunet, O., & Lezine, I. (1967). *Scala di sviluppo psicomtorio della prima infanzia.* Florence, Italy: OS.

Calvelli, T. A., & Rubinstein, A. (1990). Pediatric HIV infection: A review. *Immunodeficiency Review, 2*, 82-127.

Capute, A., Palmer, F., Shaprio, B., Wachtel, R., & Gunther, A.. (1983). *Clinical Adaptive Test/Clinical Linguistic and Auditory Milestone Scale.* San Antonio, TX: Psychological Corp.

CDC. (1992, January). *HIV/AIDS Surveillance Report, 4*, 1-22.

CDC. (1993, January). *HIV/AIDS Surveillance Report, 5*(3), 1-22.

CDC. (2007, June). *HIV/AIDS Surveillance Report, 17*, 10-13.

Chaloyoo, S., Chotpitayasunondh, T., & Na Chengmaik, P. (1998). AIDS in ENT in children. *International Journal of Paediatric Otolaryngology, 44*, 103-107.

Chem, A., Ohlms, L., Stewart, M., Kline, M. W. (1996). Otolaryngologic disease progression in children with human immunodeficiency virus infection. *Archives of Otolaryngology-Head and Neck Surgery, 122*, 1360-1363.

Cohen, H. J., & Diamond, G. W. (1992). Developmental assessment of children with HIV infection. In A. C. Crocker, H. J. Cohen, & T. A. Kastner

(Eds.), *HIV infection and developmental disabilities: A resource for service providers* (pp. 53–62). Baltimore: Paul H. Brookes.

Condini, A., Axia, G., Cattelan, C., D'Urso, M. R., Laverda, A. M., Viero, F., & Zacchello, F. (1991). Development of language in 18 to 30-month old HIV-1-infected but not ill children. *AIDS, 5*, 735–739.

Connor, E. M., Sperling, R. S., & Gelber, R. (1994). Reduction of maternal-infant transmission of human immunodeficiency virus type 1 with zidovudine treatment. *New England Journal of Medicine, 33*, 1173–1180.

Copland, J. (1993). *Early Language Milestone Scale* (2nd ed.). Austin, TX: Pro-Ed.

Copland, J., Contello, K, Cunningham, C., Weiner, L., Dye, T. D., Roberge, L., et al. (1998). Early language development in children exposed to or infected with HIV. *Pediatrics, 102*, 161–182.

Damico, J. (1991). Descriptive assessment of communicative ability in limited English proficient students. In E. Hamayan & J. Damico (Eds.), *Limiting bias in the assessment of bilingual students* (pp. 157–218). Austin, TX: Pro-Ed.

Darley, F., Aronson, A., & Brown, J. (1975). *Motor speech disorders*. Philadelphia: W. B. Saunders.

Davis-McFarland, E. (2000). Language and oral-motor development and disorders in infants and young toddlers with human immunodeficiency virus. *Seminars in Speech and Language, 21*, 19–36.

Davis-McFarland, E. (March 5, 2002). Pediatric HIV/AIDS-Issues and strategies for intervention. *ASHA Leader*, pp. 10–21.

Davis-McFarland, E., & Cowan, L (1998). Unpublished manuscript. Adapted from L. Cowan, M.Ed. thesis, *Speech and language acquisition in HIV-positive and HIV-seroreverted children, age 6 to 25 months*. North Carolina Central University, Durham, NC. Also cited in Davis-McFarland, E. (2000). Language and oral-motor development and disorders in infants and young toddlers with human immunodeficiency virus. *Seminars in Speech and Language, 21*, 19–35.

Diamond, G., & Cohen, H. (1992). Developmental disabilities in children with HIV infection. In A. C. Crocker, H. J. Cohen, & T. A. Kastner (Eds.), *HIV infection and developmental disabilities: A resource for service providers* (pp. 33–43). Baltimore: Brookes.

Dunn, L. M., & Dunn, L. M. (1981). *Peabody Picture Vocabulary Test-Revised*. Circle Pines, MN: American Guidance Service.

Dunn, L. M, & Dunn, D. (2007). *Peabody Picture Vocabulary Test-Fourth Edition*. Bloomington, MN: Pearson Assessment.

Falloon, J., Eddy, J., Wiener, L., & Pizzo, P. (1989). Human immunodeficiency virus infection in children. *Journal of Pediatrics, 114*(1), 1–30.

Franklin, M. (1992). Culturally sensitive instructional practices for African American learners with disabilities. *Exceptional Children, 59*, 115–122.

Gallagher, T., & Prutting, C. (1983). *Pragmatic assessment and intervention issues in language*. San Diego, CA: College-Hill Press.

Gardner, M. (1985). *Receptive One-Word Picture Vocabulary Test-Revised*. Novato, CA: Academic Therapy Publications.

Gardner, M. (1990). *Expressive One-Word Picture Vocabulary Test-Revised*. Novato, CA: Academic Therapy Publications.

Gay, C. L., Armstrong, D., Cohen, D., Lai, S., Hardy, M. D., Swales, T. P., et al. (1995). The effects of HIV on cognitive and motor development in children born to HIV-seropositive women with no reported drug use: Birth to 24 months. *Pediatrics, 96*, 1078–1082

Gazzard, B. (1988). Disease and the gastroenterologist. *Gut, 29*, 1497–1505.

Gazzard, B. (2008). British HIV Association guidelines for the treatment of HIV-1-infected adults with antiretroviral therapy. *HIV Medicine, 9*, 563–608.

Glennen, S., & DeCoste, D. (1997). *Handbook of augmentative and alternative communication*. San Diego, CA: Singular Publishing.

Glover, M. E., Preminger, J. L, & Sanford, A. R. (1978). *Early Learning Accomplishment Profile (ELAP)*. Winston-Salem, NC: Kaplan.

Gold, S., & Tami, T. (1998). Otolaryngological manifestations of HIV/AIDS. *Seminars in Hearing, 19*, 165–175.

Goldman, R., & Fristoe, M. (2000). *Goldman-Fristoe Test of Articulation-2*. Circle Pines, MN: American Guidance Service

Greenspan, S. (1992). *Infancy and early childhood: The practice of clinical assessment and intervention with emotional and developmental challenges*. Madison, CT: International Universities Press.

Greenspan, S. (2008). *DIR/Floortime Model. Clinical practice guidelines*. Bethesda, MD: Interdisciplinary Council on Developmental and Learning Disorders.

Greenspan, S., & Wieder, S. (1998). *The child with special needs: Intellectual and emotional growth*. Reading, MA: Addison-Wesley Longman.

Gutiérrez-Clellen, V., & Peña, E. (2001). Dynamic assessment of diverse children: A tutorial. *Language, Speech, and Hearing Services in Schools, 32*, 212–224.

Gutstein, S., & Sheely, R. (2002). *Relationship development intervention with young children: Social and emotional development activities for Asperger's syndrome, autism, PDD and NLD*. London: Kingsley, Jessica Publishers.

Hanson, M. (1992). Ethnic, cultural, and language diversity in intervention settings. In E. Lynch & M. Hanson (Eds.), *Developing cross-cultural competence: A guide for working with young children and their families* (pp. 1–18). Baltimore: Brookes.

Hart, B. (1985). Naturalistic language training techniques. In S. Warren & A. Rogers-Warren (Eds.), *Teaching functional language* (pp. 63–88). Baltimore: University Park Press.

Hart, B., & Risley, T. (1975). Incidental teaching of language in the pre-school. *Journal of Applied Behavior Analysis, 8,* 411–420.

Havens, J., Whitaker, A., Feldman, J., Alvardo, L., & Erhardt, A. (1993). A controlled study of cognitive and language function in school-aged HIV-infected children. *Annals of the New York Academy of Sciences, 693,* 249–251.

Hodson, A., Mok, J., & Dean, E. (2001). Speech and language functioning in pediatric HIV disease. *International Journal of Language and Communication Disorders, 36,* 173–178.

Hodson, B., & Paden, E. (1983). *Targeting unintelligible speech: A phonological approach to remediation.* San Diego, CA: College-Hill Press.

Howland, L., Gortmaker, S., Mofenson, L., Spino, C., Gardner, J., Gorski, H., et al. (2000). Effects of negative life events on immune suppression in children and youth infected with human immunodeficiency virus type 1. *Pediatrics, 106,* 540–546.

Hoyt, L. G., & Oleske, J. M. (1992). The clinical spectrum of HIV infection in infants and children: An overview. In R. Yogev, & E. Connor (Eds.), *Management of HIV infection in infants and children* (pp. 227–245). St Louis, MO: Mosby Year Book.

Indacochea, F., & Scott, G. (1992). HIV infection and the acquired immunodeficiency syndrome in children. *Current Problems in Pediatrics, 22,* 166–204.

Khan, L., & Lewis, N. (2002). *Khan-Lewis Phonological Analysis-2.* Bloomington, MN: Pearson Assessment.

Kohan, D., Rothstein, S. G., & Cohen, N. I. (1988). Otologic disease in patients with acquired immunodeficiency syndrome. *Annals of Otology Rhinology and Laryngology, 97,* 636–640.

Kohnert, K. (2008). *Language disorders in bilingual children and adults.* San Diego, CA: Plural Publishing.

Krikorian, R., & Wrobel, A. J. (1991). Cognitive impairment in HIV infection. *AIDS, 5*(12), 1501–1507.

Lahey, M. (1988). *Language disorders and language development.* New York: MacMillan.

Layton, T., & Davis-McFarland, E. (2000). Pediatric human immunodeficiency virus and acquired immunodeficiency syndrome: An overview. *Seminars in Speech and Language, 21,* 7–18.

Layton, T., & Scott, G. (2000). Language development and assessment in children with human immunodeficiency virus: 3 to 6 years. *Seminars in Speech and Language, 21,* 37–48.

Lee, L., Koenigsknecht, R., & Mulhern, S. (1975*). Interactive language development teaching: The clinical presentation of grammatical structure.* Evanston, IL: Northwestern University Press.

Lepage, P., Van de Perre, P., Simonon, A., Msellati, P., Hitimana, D. G., & Dabis, F. (1992). Transient seroreversion in children born to human immunodeficiency virus 1-infected mothers. *Pediatric Infectious Disease Journal, 11*(10), 892–894.

Levinson, R., Mellins, C. A., Zawadzki, R., Zawadzki, R., Kairam, R., & Stein, Z. (1992). Cognitive assessment of human immunodeficiency virus-exposed children. *American Journal of Diseases in Children, 146,* 1479–1483.

Lidz, C., & Peña, E. (1996). Dynamic assessment: The model, its relevance as a nonbiased approach and its application to Latino American preschool children. *Language, Speech, and Hearing Services in Schools, 27,* 367–384.

Lund, N., & Duchan, J. (1988). *Assessing children's language in naturalistic contexts.* Englewood Cliffs, NJ: Prentice-Hall.

McCardle, P., Nannis, E., Smith, R., & Fischer, G. (June 16–21, 1991). Patterns of perinatal HIV-related language deficit. *International Conference of AIDS, 7,* Abstract No. W.B. 2021,

McCarthy, D. (1972). *McCarthy Scales of Children's Abilities.* New York: Psychological Corporation.

McNeilly, L. (1998). *A descriptive analysis of the receptive and expressive language skills of young children born to mothers with human immunodeficiency virus infection.* Doctoral dissertation, Howard University, Washington, DC.

McNeilly, L. (2000). Communication intervention and therapeutic issues in pediatric human immunodeficiency. *Seminars in Speech and Language, 21,* 63–77.

Miller J., & Chapman, R. (2008). *Systematic analysis of language transcriptions.* Muscoda, WI: SALT Software, LLC.

Nozyce, M., Hittelman, J., Muenz, L., Durako, S., Fischer, M., & Willoughby, A. (1994). Effect of perinatally acquired human immunodeficiency virus infection on neurodevelopment in children during the first two years of life. *Pediatrics, 94,* 883–891.

Oxtoby, M. J. (1991). Perinatally acquired HIV infection. In P. A. Pizzo & C. M. Wilfert (Eds.), *Pediatric AIDS: The challenge of HIV infection in infants, children and adolescents* (pp. 3–21). Baltimore: Williams & Wilkins.

Owens, R. (2004). *Language disorders: A functional approach to assessment and intervention.* Boston: Pearson.

Periperl, L. (1993). *Manual of HIV/AIDS therapy.* Fountain Valley, CA: Current Clinical Strategies Publishing International.

Poole, M. D., Postma, D., & Cohen, M. S. (1984). Pyogenic otorhinologic infections in acquired immune deficiency syndrome. *Archives of Otolaryngology, 110,* 130–131.

Popich, E., Louw, B., & Eloff, I. (2007). Caregiver education as a prevention strategy for communication disorders in South Africa. *Infants and Young Children, 20,* 64–81.

Pressman, H. (1992). Communication disorders and dysphagia in pediatric AIDS. *Asha, 34*, 45-47.

Pressman, H. (1995). Dysphagia in children with AIDS. In S. Rosenthal, J. Sheppard, & M. Lotze (Eds.), *Dysphagia and the child with developmental disabilities: Medical, clinical, and family interventions.* San Diego, CA: Singular Publishing.

Principi, N., Marchisio, P., Tornaghi, R., Onoratio, J., Massirioni, E., & Picco, P. (1991). Acute otitis media in human immunodeficiency virus-infected children. *Pediatrics, 88*, 566-671.

Prutting, C., & Kirchner, D, (1983). Applied pragmatics. In T. Gallagher & C. Prutting (Eds.), *Pragmatic assessment and intervention issues in language* (pp. 29-54). San Diego, CA: College-Hill Press.

Reynell, J., & Huntley, M. (1987). *Reynell Developmental Language Scales* (2nd ed.). Windsor, UK: NFER-Nelson.

Reynell, J., & Gruber, C. (1990). *Reynell Developmental language Scales-Revised.* Greenville, SC: Super Duper Publications.

Robbins, J., & Klee, T. (1987). Clinical assessment of oropharyngeal motor development in young children. *Journal of Speech and Hearing Disorders, 52*, 271-277.

Rogers, M. G. (1988). Pediatric HIV infection: Epidemiology, etiopathogenesis and transmission. *Pediatric Annals, 17*(5), 325-331.

Rubinstein, A. (1989). Background, epidemiology, and impact of HIV infection in children. *Mental Retardation, 27*(4), 209-211.

Scott, G. (1995). *Communication skills in three siblings perinatally exposed to HIV or HIV at-risk behaviors.* Master thesis, University of North Carolina-Chapel Hill.

Scott, G., & Layton, T. (1997). Epidemiologic principles in studies of infectious disease outcomes: Pediatric HIV as a model. *Journal of Communication Disorders, 30*, 303-324.

Scott, G., & Layton, T. (2000). Human immunodeficiency virus (HIV) infection in children. In T. Layton, E. Crais, & L. Watson (Eds.), *Handbook of early language impairments in children: Nature* (pp. 317-353). Albany, NY: Delmar Publishers.

Semel, E., Wiig, E., & Secord, W. (1987). *Clinical Evaluation of Language Fundamentals-Revised.* San Antonio, TX: Psychological Corporation.

Semel, E., Wiig, E., & Secord, W. (2003). *Clinical Evaluation of Language Fundamentals-Fourth Edition.* San Antonio, TX: Psychological Corporation, Pearson Assessment.

Singh, A., Georgalas, C., Patel, N., & Papesch, M. (2003). ENT presentations in children with HIV infection. *Clinical Otolaryngology, 28*, 240-243.

Smith, M. E., & Canalis, R. F. (1989). Otologic manifestations of AIDS: The otosyphilis connection. *Laryngoscope, 99*, 365-372.

Speech Viewer II. (1995). IBM Lotus software product.

Tami, T. A., & Lee, K. C. (1994). Otolaryngologic manifestations of HIV disease. In P. T. Cohen, M. A. Sande, U. P. A. Volberding (Eds.), *The AIDS knowledge base: A textbook on HIV disease from the University of California, San Francisco, and the San Francisco General Hospital* (pp. 1–25). Boston: Little & Brown.

Thomas, C. L. (1993). *Taber's cyclopedic medical dictionary* (17th ed.). Philadelphia: Davis.

Ultmann, M. H., Belman, A. L., Ruff, H. A., Novick, B. E., Cone-Wesson, B., Cohen, J., & Rubinstein, A. (1985). Developmental abnormalities in infants and children with acquired immunodeficiency syndrome (AIDS) and AIDS-related complex. *Developmental Medicine and Child Neurology, 27,* 563–571.

UNAIDS. (2007). *AIDS epidemic update.* World Health Organization. Available from http://www.unaids.org

Vygotsky, L. S. (1986). *Thought and language.* Cambridge, MA: MIT Press.

Wachtel, R. C., Tepper, V. J., Houck, D., McGrath, C., & Thompson, C. (1994). Neurodevelopment in pediatric HIV infection. *Clinical Pediatrics, 33*(7), 416–420.

WHO. (2005). *HIV/AIDS epidemiological surveillance report for the WHO African Region: 2005 update.* Harare, Zimbabwe: Asiimwe-Okiror, G., Ntabangana, S., Asamoah-Odei, E., & Garcia Calleja, J.M.

WHO. (2006). *Taking stock: HIV in children.* Reference: WHO/HIV/2006.04.

Williams, M. A. (1987). Head and neck findings in pediatric acquired immune deficiency syndrome. *Laryngoscope, 99,* 365–372.

Wolters, P. (1992). *The receptive and expressive language functioning of children with acquired immune deficiency syndrome.* Unpublished doctoral dissertation, University of North Carolina-Chapel Hill.

Wolters, P., Brouwers, P., Moss, H., & Pizzo, P. (1995). Differential receptive and expressive language functioning of children with symptomatic HIV disease and relation to CT scan brain abnormalities. *Pediatrics, 95,* 112–119.

Zimmerman, I., Steiner, V., & Pond, R. (1979). *Preschool Language Scale.* Columbus, OH: Charles E. Merrill.

CHAPTER 8

Communication Disorders in Adults with HIV/AIDS

Lemmietta McNeilly

INTRODUCTION

Adults living with human immunodeficiency virus/acquired immune deficiency syndrome (HIV/AIDS) can experience an array of communication disorders. HIV/AIDS has important implications for speech-language pathologists/speech language therapists (SLPs/SLTs) (ASHA, 1989). Among the communication problems observed in those infected with HIV/AIDS are speech, language, cognition, and swallowing (Mathew & Bhat, 2008). SLPs/SLTs are essential members of the team of professionals who assess and treat the communication needs of these adult patients. SLPs/SLTs possess knowledge and skills required to effectively address the needs of patients and their families by utilizing culturally appropriate strategies. The progress in medical management of HIV/AIDS, especially the advent of highly active antiretroviral therapy (HAART), is leading to longer and healthier lives for individuals with HIV/AIDS. As a result, the importance of quality of life is becoming more prominent and effective functional communication and feeding skills are central to achieving quality of life. SLPs/SLTs play an important role in medical teams that treat persons living with HIV/AIDS.

SPECIFIC COMMUNICATION DISORDERS EXHIBITED BY ADULTS LIVING WITH AIDS

As early as 1998 representatives of the American Speech-Language Association (ASHA) met jointly with the International Association of Physicians in AIDS Care (IAPAC) to discuss hearing loss and communication disorders in individuals with HIV/AIDS. The best approach to increasing awareness among community physicians and HIV/AIDS specialists regarding the special challenges to HIV/AIDS patients with communication disorders was addressed in that meeting (Zuniga, 1999). The National Institutes of Health estimates that as many as 75% of adults with HIV/AIDS experience some kind of auditory dysfunction as a result of opportunistic infections or treatments with combination therapies that are ototoxic. The National Institute of Neurological Disorders and Stroke (NINDS) fact sheets on neurologic complications of HIV/AIDS also reviews a variety of topics, including the types and causes of hearing loss, pediatric HIV/AIDS, and communication disorders, and the differences between adults and children living with HIV/AIDS. Additionally, central nervous system lymphomas result in speech disturbances. There appears to be little awareness among health care workers of the effects of hearing loss and related language disorders that impact the quality of care among this group of patients. The nature and types of communication disorders seen in children versus adults varies with respect to time of onset, type, and severity.

Communication disorders include areas of speech, language, and dysphagia. The speech disorders include difficulties with sound production, fluency, and vocal quality. The language disorders include problems with organization of ideas to express themselves clearly to others, difficulty understanding utterances spoken by others, as well as pragmatic disorders or problems in the functional usage of language. Feeding and swallowing problems are commonly seen in this population and painful swallowing (odynophagia) and difficulty with food transitions are frequently reported in individuals living with HIV/AIDS. Some antiretroviral (ARV) treatments result in reduced appetites, modification in the way foods taste, nausea, and oral lesions resulting in odynophagia. Assessments should include evaluating each of these areas to rule out or identify problems that warrant intervention or follow-up.

In 1987, Flower, a SLP/SLT and Sooy, a physician, published the first data that addressed communication disorders in adults with HIV/AIDS. Their work was based on 399 cases seen at the University of California-San Francisco. They noted that Kaposi's sarcomas often occur in the mouth, pharynx, and larynx. They found that one in eight patients with AIDS showed such lesions. The communication disorders they identified were attributable to the neurologic components associated with HIV/AIDS and included language disorders and motor speech disorders. They also suggested that functional communication systems are important to individuals and family, friends and caregivers during the late stages of the disease when patients may be intubated or on respirators (Flower & Sooy, 1998).

Individuals living with HIV/AIDS may exhibit communication disorders that are unrelated to their HIV status. Therefore, it is important to perform comprehensive speech, language, and swallowing assessments in these adults. Some individuals may have disorders that were not managed prior to becoming infected with HIV. Additionally, they may, for instance, acquire a communication disorder caused by injuries sustained in a motor vehicle accident that resulted in a traumatic brain injury. Individuals who are HIV positive may present with any of the communication disorders that HIV-negative individuals exhibit, as well as communication and feeding problems that are caused by the disease.

Speech Disorders

HIV/AIDS typically does not lead to articulation or fluency problems. Some adults may have motor speech disorders caused by CNS involvement that can impact articulatory movements resulting in decreased fluid movement of the articulators. Dysarthria or apraxia of speech may be exhibited by slurred and imprecise speech. Vocal quality may be impacted in the late stages of HIV/AIDS for patients with comprised respiratory functioning. Low loudness level and weak, strained vocal quality may be exhibited by individuals with HIV/AIDS in the later stages of the disease. Some may have oral manifestations of the disease but no notable speech problems as a result of presenting symptomatology.

Language Disorders

Central nervous system problems can lead to problems in comprehension of language and the ability to formulate and express clear messages. Memory and executive functioning can also be impacted as a result of damage to the central nervous system.

Although HAART has resulted in improved outcomes for individuals with HIV/AIDS, HIV-related cognitive disorders continue in patients who are treated (Scaravilli, Bazille, & Gray, 2007). HAART has successfully prevented many of the end-stage complications formerly seen in HIV/AIDS. However, the prevalence of minor HIV/AIDS-associated cognitive impairment seems to be on the rise in adults treated over time, thus impacting older individuals (Bell, 2004). The role of the SLP/SLT is to assess and treat any language problems exhibited by the adult that warrant intervention. The SLP/SLT needs to consider the individual's cognitive abilities and stage of the disease to determine if direct intervention for the HIV/AIDS dementia complex is warranted or if augmentative communication strategies are indicated for the patient.

Cognitive Impairments

In young adults, a major neurologic complication of HIV infection is cognitive impairment. Young adults may experience encephalopathy resulting in motor speech impairments and diminished cognitive functioning. Epidemiologic findings suggest that increasing age is a significant risk factor for HIV-1-associated dementia as the AIDS-defining illness. Mixed results have been reported from the few studies that have directly measured cognition in younger and older HIV-infected individuals. Due to small sample sizes and other methodological differences between studies it is challenging to generalize findings (Symes et al., 2003).

Wilkie et al. (1999) presented preliminary findings on cognitive functioning in symptomatic HIV-infected younger (ages 20–39 years) and older (ages 50 years or older) adults. Independent of age, HIV infection was accompanied by learning and memory retrieval deficits, which were significantly associated with high plasma viral loads in the young adults. Relative to the younger and older HIV-1-negative (HIV-1−) groups, only the younger HIV-1-positive (HIV-1+) group had significantly longer reaction times (RTs). Within the older HIV-1+ group, however, longer simple and choice RTs were significantly correlated with higher viral loads and lower CD4 cell counts. Although HIV-1 infection affects cognition independent of age, longitudinal studies involving large numbers of older individuals are needed to determine whether there are age differences in the prevalence, nature, and severity of HIV-associated cognitive dysfunction (Wilkie et al., 1999). SLPs/SLTs working with adults who are infected with HIV should assess both their cognition and communication functioning.

Oral Manifestations

Oral manifestations of HIV/AIDS are exhibited in a number of individuals. The symptoms noted include oral lesions of the tongue and oral cavity, white spots, or candidiasis. Non-Hodgkin's lymphoma, atypical ulcers, necrotizing periodontitis, and hairy leukoplakia are symptoms that may be present in a small number of individuals, but are a major public health problem requiring education about oral hygiene and appropriate management. Oral lesions, candidiasis, and advanced periodontal disease are among the problems adults living with HIV/AIDS may experience. Additionally, some medications may result in oral lesions in patients.

The prevalence of oral manifestations described in clients at The AIDS Support Organization (TASO) of Uganda and their influence on oral functions was studied in 514 subjects ages 18 to 58 from five TASO clinics in Uganda (Tirwomwe et al., 2007). The subjects were clinically examined for oral lesions under field conditions by four trained dentists based on World Health Organization (WHO) criteria. Oral manifestations were recorded in 72% of the subjects, of which 70% had candidiasis of pseudomembranous erythematous, and angular cheilitis variants. Of those identified with oral lesions ($n = 370$), the majority (68.4%) expressed some form of discomfort in the mouth. Tooth brushing, chewing, and swallowing were described as being uncomfortable. Reported forms of discomfort included dry mouth, increased salivation, and burning sensation especially when salty and spicy foods or acidic drinks were ingested.

Only 8.5% (*n* = 44) of the subjects were taking medications specifically for oral lesions, which included antifungal, antiviral, and antibacterial agents. None of the subjects received antiretroviral therapy (Tirwomwe et al., 2007). Thus, oral manifestations can negatively impact feeding and swallowing in adults with HIV/AIDS. SLPs/SLTs need to note these symptoms when performing oral mechanism examinations and conducting clinical swallowing examinations as they provide valuable clinical information.

Feeding/Swallowing Difficulties

Individuals with HIV/AIDS may experience difficulty swallowing a variety of textures safely and painlessly. They may experience odynophagia when placing acidic foods in the mouth. Difficulty transferring foods and liquids to swallow safely and pain free may be observed clinically in adult patients. Individuals may exhibit difficulty clearing boluses that require multiple swallows. They also may exhibit slow transit of the bolus from the oral cavity to trigger a swallow. Individuals may fatigue quickly and not be able to intake adequate amounts of food to sustain them. Additionally, they may experience difficulty with spicy foods or hot foods causing pain or discomfort. Chlebowski et al. (1989) noted that 21% of the adult males with HIV/AIDS studied, exhibited dysphagia. These problems can lead to feeding and swallowing difficulties and are important to consider in the assessment and treatment of dysphagia in this population.

ROLE OF THE SLP/SLT IN ASSESSING COMMUNICATION PROBLEMS IN ADULTS LIVING WITH HIV/AIDS

The role of SLPs/SLTs with this population spans the entire scope of practice for the speech-language pathology profession. Individuals diagnosed with HIV/AIDS may present with a multitude of the diverse array of communication disorders ranging from feeding and speech disorders to language disorders. The differences encountered within this population relate to the complexity of psychosocial and health issues that the adult deals with while receiving treatment for the communication disorder. The incidence and prevalence of HIV/AIDS in adults is increasing globally, especially in Sub-Saharan countries. Individuals are identified with HIV/AIDS across the globe, including rural and urban communities, and all age groups including young adults and the elderly. Thus SLPs/SLTs working in all settings, including health care, community-based clinics, private practices, or primary health care clinics in remote or rural areas, may encounter individuals with HIV/AIDS that exhibit communication disorders.

As individuals with HIV/AIDS continue to live longer lives, they experience challenges associated with the disease as well as side effects of pharmacological intervention. Health care professionals from various disciplines deliver services to individuals living with HIV/AIDS including SLPs/SLTs, occupational and physical therapists to improve their quality of life. As HIV crosses the blood-brain barrier and impacts all aspects of an infected person's life, speech-language and hearing professionals need to be members of the interdisciplinary teams that evaluate and manage patients living with HIV/AIDS (McNeilly, 2005). SLPs/SLTs can specifically enhance the quality of life for patients that experience feeding and swallowing problems and communication disorders. A small number of SLPs/SLTs have expertise in working with large numbers of HIV-positive individuals. However, this is not the case in many parts of the developing world where large numbers of patients with HIV/AIDS are serviced including urban health centers and public health HIV/AIDS centers. Many SLPs/SLTs will see only a few individuals with HIV/AIDS in their practices but they need to be knowledgeable about the course of the disease and how it impacts communication and swallowing. SLPs/SLTs also need to communicate with the other professionals involved in the care of individuals living with HIV/AIDS, including their internists, nurse case managers, and others to convey both the importance of communication and strategies to enhance communication. Family members need support and education regarding the benefits of intervention, the importance of appropriate referrals, and information on the impact of HIV/AIDS on the individual's communication functions.

What are the red flags that indicate that a referral to an SLP/SLT is warranted? Many years ago SLPs/SLTs only received referrals for adults in the final stages of HIV/AIDS. With the success of early diagnosis and pharmacologic intervention, individuals are now being referred to SLPs/SLTs when communication disorders are first recognized by health care practitioners. However, it is important to note that, due to limited numbers of SLPs/SLTs in rural communities and developing countries, referrals may not occur routinely. The treatment of communication disorders can enhance the quality of life for individuals living with HIV/AIDS. People with HIV/AIDS who are receiving HAART are living longer. Unfortunately, this is not necessarily true in developing countries where ARV treatments are not yet available to the majority of people who need it. In adults living with HIV/AIDS, damage to the central nervous system can result in changes in cognition, feeding and swallowing, speech, and language functioning. Additionally, some pharmacologic interventions have side effects that also can impact feeding, swallowing, speech, and hearing.

Assessment of Communication Disorders

Adults living with HIV/AIDS may exhibit communication disorders both associated with the disease and not associated with the progression of HIV/AIDS. Thus, the SLP/SLT should conduct a comprehensive speech, language and feeding assessment to adequately determine the adult's communication functioning. The assessment should include the areas of feeding and swallowing, speech, and language. Hearing also should be screened by the SLP/SLT and referrals made to an audiologist or otorhinolaryngologist if indicated by the screening results. The patient's HIV/AIDS status and ARV treatment need to be factored into the assessment to determine the most appropriate course of intervention.

Speech Assessment

The speech assessment should evaluate the oral mechanism, the fluency of speech, the voice quality, and the articulation of sounds in conversational speech. The oral mechanism is the first component of the assessment for speech. The articulators' structure, functioning, and mobility should be assessed. The individual's ability to produce phonemes that exist in his or her primary language should be assessed and fluency in conversation and reading should be evaluated. Vocal quality while speaking should be assessed for pitch, loudness, and vocal quality. If problems are noted in any of these areas of speech, the SLP/SLT should also check the medications that the individual is taking and possible side effects that may contribute to the symptoms observed during the evaluation.

Language Assessment

The assessment should include language comprehension and language expression by the adult with HIV/AIDS. The SLP/SLT should review the individual's chart for diagnosis of any central nervous system damage and medications taken that may impact communication. The evaluation should be conducted in the primary language spoken by the adult. If there is a question about what that language is, the family should be consulted for verification and, if necessary, the services of an interpreter need to be employed. The adult's ability to organize ideas and thoughts and express them clearly should be assessed. Naming of objects and people, morphology, and pragmatic skills should be evaluated by the SLP/SLT. Comprehension of objects and people's names as well as following directions, answering simple questions, and awareness of surroundings should be included in the assessment. The adult's current level of performance should be compared with previous functioning and discussed with family members for validation. If the individual has experienced a stroke or cerebral vascular accident, or is diagnosed with dementia, these diagnoses should be factored into the assessment process and plans for intervention in speech-language treatment.

Dysphagia Assessment

Clinical assessment is different from an instrumental assessment. The clinical assessment should be done first. An examination of the oral mechanism should be conducted to determine if there are any oral lesions and to observe the structures and functioning of the oral musculature. The individual's feeding history needs to be obtained and his or her ability to propel the bolus and swallow liquids (thin/thick), eat foods including soft foods and foods requiring chewing/mastication should be assessed. Initially, this is done through observation of feeding during the clinical assessment followed by an instrumental assessment to view the structures internally. The SLP/SLT should note coughing that occurs during eating and swallowing as well as a wet gurgling sounding voice, spillage of liquids or food, and slow transit of bolus as indications of dysphagia. The SLP/SLT should obtain the individual's medical history and review the medications that the patient is taking and possible side effects that may contribute to the symptoms observed during the evaluation. Instrumental assessment tools are a component of an overall assessment. Based on the results of the clinical assessment, if pharyngeal swallowing problems are suspected then a modified barium swallow study (MBS) or videofluoroscopic study (VFS) should be conducted to further assess the pharyngeal phase of swallowing. The MBS or VFS should include different textures and different maneuvers to facilitate safe swallows with the individual positioned to facilitate safe swallows. The results of the assessment should provide the SLP/SLT with adequate information to recommend dietary changes or strategies to facilitate safe swallowing practices.

Treatment Considerations

Adults living with HIV/AIDS require intervention and treatment from a number of team specialists. Physicians monitor the individual's response to pharmacologic intervention. Case managers help to coordinate services from other health care professionals including SLPs/SLTs, respiratory therapists, social workers, audiologists, and physical therapists. In other instances, no one person serves as a cohesive point of coordination and individual practitioners assess and deliver services without full knowledge of all other services being rendered to the individual. This fragmented service delivery may result in duplication of efforts or strategies attempted without knowledge of other strategies or medications that may prevent the individual from achieving the goals. SLPs/SLTs are active members of the service delivery team and it is a part of their responsibilities to be aware of the roles of each team member and to communicate effectively with the team to enhance the efficient delivery of appropriate services for the adult living with HIV/AIDS. The SLP/SLT's primary role on the team is to contribute expertise regarding feeding, swallowing, speech, and language functioning for the patient. The progression of the disease in individuals will determine how they respond to intervention and what modifications are necessary to the intervention plans made by the SLP/SLT.

Universal precautions should be practiced by all health care professionals working with other persons. As SLPs/SLTs may not know the HIV status of an individual, it is important to use gloves when conducting oral mechanism examinations and placing hands inside another person's oral cavity. Bodily fluids should not be touched by hands or skin. The HIV-positive status of a person should not be disclosed to another person without consent. If the SLP/SLT has a need to know information located in an individual's medical record, then authorization to review that information should be sought. If a SLP/SLT has an active infection, viral or bacterial, treatment should not be provided to the patient without wearing a mask or covering the area of infection. Postponing treatment until the SLP/SLT is no longer contagious should be considered. This cuts down on spreading germs to others regardless of health status.

Pharmacologic Intervention

Highly active antiretroviral therapy (HAART) is the standard of care for providing pharmacological treatment to HIV symptomatic and asymptomatic individuals. This involves using three or more drugs to suppress the virus. HAART is significantly decreasing the mortality and morbidity rates in individuals infected with HIV. Clinical research has yielded enhanced understanding of the virologic and immunologic markers in the progression of the disease as well as viral resistance to antiretroviral medications (Panos et al, 2008). Many governmental and nonprofit organizations are working to increase individual's access to antiretroviral medications across the globe including developing countries where many individuals do not have resources to access health care facilities or to afford the medications. Asymptomatic HIV-positive individuals with CD 4 counts below 350 per µl and all symptomatic individuals should be managed pharmacologically. The specific medications that are efficacious for a specific patient will be determined by the treating physicians.

Guidelines for antiretroviral (ARV) treatment are available based on expert panels and scientific evidence. "A Guide to Primary Care for People with HIV/AIDS including Antiretroviral Therapy" is available from the Centers for Disease Control (http://www.hab .hrsa.gov/tools/primarycareguide/PCGchap5.htm). The advances with ARV treatment result in individuals living longer without the disease manifesting into AIDS. Many individuals are living with HIV/AIDS with fewer complications that may result in poor health status and symptoms in the area of feeding, swallowing, speech, and language disorders. Adults living in developing countries may have limited access to ARV treatment and as a result they have different profiles of complications and disease manifestation.

Pharmacologic Interactions

The number of medications that adults living with HIV/AIDS may need to take for the complications associated with the disease can be quite high. Several of the medications may produce side effects that impact communication disorders. It is important for SLPs/SLTs to be knowledgeable of the side effects of medications that impact oral cavities, cognitive functioning, stamina, and gastrointestinal functioning. Additionally, the combination of medications may cause side effects, for example, dry mouth, oral lesions, or reflux that need to be monitored and communicated to the physician. In developing contexts or impoverished environments where access to medications is limited, some individuals may not take their medications consistently or as prescribed, thus causing additional side effects that may impact feeding, swallowing, or communication. Counseling of adults and their family members is a role that the SLP/SLT needs to perform in these contexts. SLPs/SLTs require appropriate education and need to develop skills and competencies prior to engaging in these types of tasks.

A study by Hinkin et al. (2002) applied a two-way analysis of variance, which revealed that neurocognitive compromise as well as complex medication regimens were associated with significantly lower adherence rates. Cognitively compromised participants on more complex regimens had the greatest difficulty with adherence. Deficits in executive function, memory, and attention were associated with poor adherence. Logistic regression analysis demonstrated that neuropsychological compromise was associated with a 2.3 times greater risk of adherence failure. Higher age (>50 years) was also found to be associated with significantly better adherence.

HIV-infected adults with significant neurocognitive compromise are at risk for poor medication adherence, particularly if they have been prescribed a complex dosing regimen. As such, simpler dosing schedules for more cognitively impaired individuals might improve adherence (Hinkin et al., 2002).

Insel et al. (2006) studied older adults living in communities to investigate the association between cognitive processes and medication adherence in this group. Ninety-five participants ($M = 78$ years) completed a battery of cognitive assessments including measures of executive function, working memory, cued recall, and recognition memory. Medication adherence was examined over 8 weeks for one prescribed medicine by use of an electronic medication-monitoring cap. In a simultaneous regression, the composite of executive function and working memory tasks was the only significant predictor ($\beta = .44$, $p < .01$). The results indicated that assessments of executive function and working memory can be used to identify older adults living in the community who may be at risk for failure to take medicines as prescribed (Insel et al., 2006). SLPs/SLTs need to take the cognitive abilities of the patient into account in designing appropriate speech-language therapy goals.

Treatment of Communication Disorders

Most of the treatment approaches for communication disorders are appropriate options to consider when treating an adult with HIV/AIDS who exhibits a communication disorder. Health status and stamina are primary considerations for treatment. Gathering information on the medications that the individual is, or is not, taking and the possible side effects thereof are important to determine if there are any implications for the person with respect to the condition that is being treated. It is also important for the SLP/SLT to make appropriate recommendations for adults who are not on ARV treatment and to monitor the progression of the disease as it impacts their communication functioning.

Speech and Language Intervention

There are no additional considerations for speech and language treatment approaches when treating adults living with HIV/AIDS in comparison to those without HIV/AIDS. Treatment decisions should consider the type of problem being treated in conjunction with the targeted outcomes. Health status should be monitored and duration of sessions should consider the individual's stamina. Adults' level of motivation and interest in participating in a speech-language treatment program also must be taken into account by the SLP/SLT. The individual's mental status factors into the intervention planning as well. If adults are not on ARV treatment and their condition is in the final stages of the disease progression, then the SLP/SLT needs to consider this in making recommendations for intervention or palliative care.

Functional Communication Intervention

It is important to set goals that facilitate the individual's functional communication. During the late stages of the HIV/AIDS disease, SLPs/SLTs may need to devise augmentative methods of communication due to the individual's weakness, reduced cognitive functioning, limited speech skills, and compromised respiration. Many adults living with HIV/AIDS become demented and lose abilities to handle food, use speech, comprehend language, or express their ideas and thoughts to others. The course of the disease in adults, whether treated or untreated, is one that requires monitoring and periodic reassessment by the SLP/SLT. Individuals who fatigue easily or have muscle weakness and or limited cognitive functioning will develop different communication disorders as the disease progresses. It is important for SLPs/SLTs to explain the changes in communication functioning to family members so that the individual living with HIV/AIDS and family and friends have a communication system that works well for them at home and in the hospital or other health care settings. The role of the SLP/SLT may involve training of the caregivers about the individual's communication needs. Adults with HIV/AIDS that may have suffered strokes or central nervous system damage will experience changes in their communication function. It is important to explain these changes to the individual and his or her family.

Feeding and Swallowing Intervention

The oral cavity should be checked for oral lesions prior to each feeding session to determine if treatment modifications are indicated. Gloves should be worn when putting fingers inside the oral cavity, which holds for all individuals, regardless of their HIV/AIDS status. Moisture options that have a low acidic quality need to be considered. Individuals need to be consulted regarding their level of discomfort with oral stimulation and any medications that may result in oral lesions need to be noted. For adults who exhibit active oral lesions cold liquids or pureed foods may be indicated to reduce their pain and discomfort. Monitoring of the individual's stamina and level of fatigue is indicated so that the consultation with dieticians to increase caloric density is warranted as well. The introduction of swallowing techniques such as multiple swallows and increased time to clear the bolus are other strategies for feeding adults with dysphagia and should be investigated on a trial basis, as needed. For those who are not able to safely engage in oral feeding, nonoral feeding options should be explored with the physician. The amount of time that the individual will not be able to eat safely orally, his or her medical status, and availability of feeding tubes, particularly in developing countries, are considerations in taking the decision of nonoral feeding. Oral hygiene and oral stimulation during the time that food is not being swallowed are important elements that the SLP/SLT needs to include in the intervention plan.

Collaboration with Other Professionals

The complexity of HIV/AIDS causes problems or changes in many areas of functioning, thus requiring assessment and intervention from a team of professionals representing different disciplines. SLPs/SLTs collaborate with members from a variety of health professions as they deliver services to individuals with HIV/AIDS. Communication is important in all activities for adults. It is important for SLPs/SLTs to collaborate with all of the service providers and be aware of the services that are being provided to facilitate functional communication for adults living with HIV/AIDS.

Physicians often are the team leaders. They diagnose the disease, monitor the progression of the disease, and discuss and prescribe ARV treatment options. It is important for physicians to be made aware of the information that SLPs/SLTs identify with their assessments that may connect to the extent of central nervous system involvement of the disease. SLPs/SLTs also can share information regarding the impact of oral manifestations of the disease that may compromise the individual's eating. Changes in memory and cognitive functioning are also important elements for the physician to be aware of from communication intervention outcomes.

Nurses often serve as case managers for adults living with HIV/AIDS and they coordinate or are aware of services that are rendered in health care settings. As SLPs/SLTs deliver services in a variety of settings, including health care settings and community-based clinics as well as private practices, physicians and nurses may not always be aware that an individual is receiving speech-language therapy. They also may not be aware of the communication or swallowing problems that the individual is exhibiting or of the changes in communication function that results from the therapeutic intervention. A SLP/SLT can provide in-service training to physicians, participate in ward rounds, share printed information with other members of the medical team and family members, as well as share and explain the strategies to enhance effective communication skills.

Social workers are germane to assisting adults living with HIV/AIDS and their families with accessing services in the community and providing them with financial and housing assistance as needed. SLP/SLT are knowledgeable about communication skills with families within culturally appropriate contexts and may offer information to social workers that will assist families an accessing services that meet their needs.

Dieticians address caloric intake and the SLP/SLT needs to consult with them with respect to information regarding feeding and swallowing disorders that may limit the amount of food or liquids that are taken safely as well as types of foods that may cause them oral discomfort.

Physical therapists and occupational therapists intervene with expertise in fine and gross motor skills and ambulation and transferring and mobility of adults with HIV/AIDS. They are also helpful with rib cage movement and elongation necessary to facilitate respiration that is needed for adequate breath supply for speech production.

Family members often serve as caregivers to the individual living with HIV/AIDS and they are essential members of the team. They are knowledgeable about the adult's pre-HIV status, daily changes, and progression of the disease. They are critically important to the successful execution of intervention plans, not only in communication and feeding, but in all aspects of the individual's functioning.

Communication with Patients and Family Members

SLPs/SLTs know that it is important to share the purpose, goals and targeted outcomes of speech-language therapy with individuals with communication disorders and their family members. This is also important and can be challenging for adults and families affected by HIV/AIDS because SLPs/SLTs typically are not the only professionals delivering services. Families can feel overwhelmed by the amount of information they need to understand, monitor, and follow-up weekly. It is important for the SLP/SLT to consider the culture of the family and provide information that is culturally appropriate. In developing contexts, the role of the SLP/SLT is not always clearly understood and this is an opportunity to educate other professionals and the public about the competence they have in this area.

Cultural Values, Beliefs, and Practices

Cultural values, beliefs, and practices impact how individuals deal with illnesses and access services from health care professionals. It is not possible for one SLP/SLT to be knowledgeable about all cultural groups. It also is dangerous for health care professionals to assume that they know the values, beliefs, and practices that individuals follow. It is important for SLPs/SLTs to be aware that these are topics to discuss with the team members and the patients/families to ensure the ease of service delivery. It is also important for the individual living with HIV/AIDS and his or her family to feel that their needs are being addressed with sensitivity to their cultural beliefs. It is necessary for the SLP/SLT to ask the individual or family members to validate that their needs are being addressed in ways that are consistent with their cultural values.

Language differences may occur between the adult living with HIV/AIDS and the SLP/SLT, who may be monolingual. When this is the case it is important to use interpreters and information that is clear, simple, and written in the language that the individual and family understand. SLPs/SLTs also need to spend time communicating with the interpreter before they communicate with the family to calibrate their messages and to make sure that appropriate resources have been identified as well. Low levels of literacy often exist in developing countries and impoverished communities. The literacy level of the adult living with HIV/AIDS and the family needs to be considered when preparing written information to share with them. Access to written information is important so that they can understand and review again at home when the service provider is not present.

Additionally, the SLP/SLT has a role in palliative care when the adult living with HIV/AIDS condition is deteriorating and therapy to improve functioning is not warranted. Communication and feeding are critical to the quality of life for all individuals and the SLP/SLT can provide guidance, consultation and counseling to families and other members of the team in their areas of expertise, thereby enhancing the patient's functional communication skills. There are implications for SLPs/SLTs who work with adults living with HIV/AIDS that require support and explanation regarding their communication and feeding disabilities in the absence of direct speech-language therapy. The SLP/SLT needs to consider the time required to schedule these individuals living with HIV/AIDS and their families for consultations in addition to those on their active caseloads. Providing this type of information empowers individuals and their families affected by HIV/AIDS and is an important professional function of the SLP/SLT.

SUMMARY

Clinical research and medical advances are significant contributors to the increased longevity of individuals, especially those living with HIV/AIDS in developed countries. There are great needs in developing and impoverished communities across the globe for ARV treatment. Factual information on ARV treatment, the course of HIV/AIDS, treatment, and considerations to enhance the quality of life for persons living with HIV/AIDS are critical elements that SLPs/SLTs and other health care professionals need to have knowledge of. As the number of SLPs/SLTs who have a significant amount of knowledge and experience of HIV/AIDS is inadequate to treat the number of individuals affected by HIV/AIDS, it is incumbent on all SLPs/SLTs to gain knowledge and increase their competence in treating individuals who are affected by HIV/AIDS and exhibit communication disorders. Some individuals with HIV/AIDS are living longer lives with fewer symptoms and they may have communication disorders that were present prior to their HIV/AIDS status. These adults may acquire communication disorders that are not associated with HIV/AIDS and they may develop communication disorders as a result of central nervous system damage caused by the progression of HIV/AIDS. It is important for SLPs/SLTs to remember that many individuals in impoverished communities may not have access to ARV treatment and they become terminally ill and die from the disease (Olusanya et al., 2006). SLPs/SLTs need to devise culturally appropriate intervention plans that enhance the communication skills of these individuals as well.

SLPs/SLTs who are competent to treat communication disorders in adults that are HIV negative should also acquire knowledge to effectively assess and treat those who are infected with HIV/AIDS. If SLPs/SLTs are competent to treat adults with dysphagia, then they should also be competent to treat an individual that is also living with HIV/AIDS. It is critical for SLPs/SLTs to develop cultural competence, to work collaboratively with other members of the assessment/treatment teams regarding the care and treatment of adults living with HIV/AIDS. SLPs/SLTs need to be familiar with and apply guidelines developed by the WHO, the CDC, or other governmental agencies as they are updated with respect to best practices in HIV/AIDS care as well as best practices in speech-language pathology intervention for adults in order to contribute to the quality of life of adults living with HIV/AIDS.

REFERENCES

American Speech-Language-Hearing Association. (1989). *AIDS/HIV: Implications for speech-language pathologists and audiologists* [Technical report]. Retrieved August 28, 2008, from http://www.asha.org/policy

Bell, J. E. (2004). An update on the neuropathology of HIV in the HAART era. *Histopathology*, 45(6),549–559. Neuropathology Unit, University of Edinburgh, Edinburgh, UK. Retrieved online November 29, 2004, from http://dx.doi.org/10.1111/j.1365-2559.2004.02004.x

Centers for Disease Control Antiretroviral Therapy. *A guide to primary care for people with HIV/AIDS* (Chap. 5). Available at http://www.hab.hrsa.gov/tools/primarycareguide/PCGchap5.htm

Chlebowski R. T., Grosvenor M. B., Bernhard N. H., Morales L. S., & Bulcavage L. M. (1989). Nutritional status, gastrointestinal dysfunction, and survival in patients with AIDS. *American Journal of Gastroenterology*, *84*(10), 1288-1293.

DHHS, Panel on Antiretroviral Guidelines for Adults and Adolescents. (2008, January). *Guidelines for the use of antiretroviral agents in HIV-1-infected adults and adolescents*. Pp. 1-128. Retrieved August 27, 2008, from http://www.aidsinfo.nih.gov/ContentFiles/AdultandAdolescentGL.pdf

Flower, W. M., & Sooy, C. D. (1987). AIDS: An introduction for speech-language pathologists and audiologists. *ASHA*, *29*(11), 25-30.

Hinkin, C. H., Castellon, S. A., Durvasula, R. S., Hardy, D. J., Lam, M. N., Mason, K. I., . . . Stefanski, M.. (2002). Medication adherence among HIV+ adults. Effects of cognitive dysfunction and regimen complexity. *Neurology*, *59*, 1944-1950.

Insel, K., Morrow, D., Brewer, B., & Figueredo, A. (2006). Executive function, working memory, and medication adherence among older adults. *Journals of Gerontology Series B: Psychological Sciences and Social Sciences*, *61*, 102-107.

Mathew, M., & Bhat, J. (2008). Profile of communication disorders in HIV-Infected individuals: A preliminary study. *Journal of the International Association of Physicians in AIDS Care*, *7*, 223-227.

McNeilly, L. G. (2005). HIV and communication. *Journal of Communication Disorders*, *38*(4), 303-310.

National Institute of Neurological Disorders and Stroke. National Institutes of Health. (2008, July). *Neurological complications of AIDS fact sheet*. Retrieved August 26, 2008, from http://www.ninds.nih.gov/disorders/aids/detail_aids.htm

Olusanya, B. O., Ruben, R. J., & Parving, A. (2006, July). Reducing the burden of communication disorders in the developing world. *Journal of the American Medical Association*, *296*(4), 441-444.

Panos, G., Samonis, G., Alexiou, V. G., Kavarnou, G. A., Charatsis, G., & Falagas, M. E. (2008, May). Mortality and morbidity of HIV infected patients receiving HAART: A cohort study current HIV research. *Current HIV Research*, *6*(3), 257-260.

Scaravilli, F., Bazille, C., & Gray, F. (2007). Neuropathologic contributions to understanding AIDS and the central nervous system. *Brain Pathology*, *17*(2), 197-208.

Symes, S., Suarez, P., & Eisdorfer, C. (2003). Cognitive functioning in younger and older HIV-1-infected adults. *JAIDS Journal of Acquired Immune Deficiency Syndromes*, *33*, S93-S105.

Tirwomwe, J., Rwenyonyi, C., Muwazi, L., Besigye, B., & Mboli, F. (2007). Oral manifestations of HIV/AIDS in clients attending TASO clinics in Uganda. *Clinical Oral Investigations, 11*(3), 289–292.

Wilkie, F. L., Goodkin K., Khamis, I., van Zuilen, M. H., Lee, D., Lecusay, R., & Concha, M., (1999). Cognitive functioning in younger and older HIV-1 infected adults. *Journal of Acquired Immune Deficiency Syndromes, 33*(2) S93–S105.

Zuniga, J. (1999). Communication disorders and HIV disease. *Journal of the International Associations of Physicians in AIDS Care, 5*(4), 16–23.

CHAPTER 9

External and Middle Ear Disorders Associated With HIV/AIDS

Ivan Dieb Miziara
Ali Mahmoud
Raimar Weber
Fernanda Alves Sanjar
Bárbara Elvina Ulisses Parente Queiroz

INTRODUCTION

Since the beginning of the global epidemic of human immunodeficiency virus (HIV) infection in the early 1980s, many of the initial signs and symptoms of the disease have been otorhinolaryngologic in nature (Weber, Pinheiro-Neto, Miziara, & Araújo-Filho, 2006). Ear infections are common in HIV-infected patients, especially in children, and its complications (mastoiditis and central nervous system involvement) are more common in these patients.

Despite the variation in prevalence, some studies showed otologic involvement in about 18 to 30% of patients with HIV/AIDS.

Acute otitis media and chronic suppurative otitis media are the most common otologic diseases reported, followed by external otitis (EO), otomycosis, recurrent otitis media, and otitis media with effusion (Chaloryoo, Chotpitayasunondh, & Chiengmai, 1998; Chandrasekhar et al., 2000; Prasad, Bhojwani, Shenoy, & Prasad, 2006). Some authors have even reported prevalence figures as high as 46% for otitis media in a cohort of 107 children with HIV/AIDS (Singh, Georgacalas, Patel, & Patesch, 2003). In addition, opportunistic diseases also often affect both the outer ear and the middle ear; for example, malignant (necrotizing) external otitis, chronic otitis media due to *Pneumocystis* spp., and Kaposi's sarcoma.

In this chapter we review the diseases that affect both the external ear and the middle ear of HIV-infected patients. HIV/AIDS associated pathologies of the external ear are considered first, followed by the HIV/AIDS associated pathologies of the middle ear. The prevalence, nature, clinical findings, and current treatments for each specific condition are considered.

EXTERNAL EAR DISORDERS ASSOCIATED WITH HIV/AIDS

The diseases that affect the external ear of patients with HIV/AIDS are the same as those affecting seronegative patients. The difference is that in HIV-positive patients, who have compromized immune systems, these diseases tend to be more aggressive with more serious consequences. Thus, the usual mode of therapy used in seronegative patients may be inefficient in immunosuppressed patients and require appropriate adjustments. Below, we discuss some of these diseases, from the simple external otitis to potentially more serious ones such as necrotizing malignant external otitis.

Acute External Otitis

Nature and Etiology

External otitis (EO) is an inflammation of the external auditory canal or the auricle, caused by an infectious, allergic, or dermal disorder. The annual incidence of acute EO is between 1:100 and 1:250 of the general population, and this incidence was not found to be necessarily increased in HIV-infected patients but the secondary effects may be more severe and the treatment may need to be more aggressive (Guthrie, 1999; Miziara & Valentini-Junior, 1999; Raza; Denholm, & Wong, 1995; Rowlands, Devalia, Smith, Hubbard, & Dean, 2001).

Acute EO is unilateral in 90% of the patients. It is often associated with high humidity, warm temperatures, swimming, local trauma, hearing aid or hearing protector use, and excessive cleaning or aggressive scratching of the ear canal (Agius, Pickles, & Burch, 1992; Beers & Abramo, 2004; Miziara & Valentini-Junior, 1999). Even without exposure to water, the use of objects such as cotton swabs or other small objects to clear the ear canal is enough to cause breaks in the skin and allow the condition to develop. Once the skin of the ear canal is inflamed, EO can be drastically enhanced either by scratching the ear canal with an object or by allowing water to remain in the ear canal for any prolonged period of time.

The ear canal normal flora contains a number of aerobic and anaerobic bacteria. Coagulase-negative staphylococci and coryneforms are also frequent (Brook, 1980; Stenfors & Räisänen, 2002). *Pseudomonas aeruginosa* account for the majority of the gram-negative organisms recovered from specimen swabs of acute EO, but for only about 40% of the total number of isolates. The gram-positive staphylococci were the second most common organisms recovered, accounting for 25% of total isolates, followed by members of the coryneform (diphtheroid) bacterial family (9.3%) and species of *Enterobacteriaceae* and *Vibronaceae* (*Enterobacter, Klebsiella, Serratia, Proteus*, and *Escherichia coli*—8.5%). *Aspergillus* and *Candida* were recovered from only 2 to 8% of the isolates (Roland & Stroman, 2002; Russel, Donnelly, & McShane, 1993). Roland and Stroman (2002) found a significantly lower incidence of *Staphylococcus* as a pathogen in children under 18 years old (4–8%) compared with that in adults (11–29%).

Symptoms

Symptoms of acute EO include ear pain (70%), itching (60%), or fullness (22%), with or without hearing loss (32%), or ear canal pain on chewing. The physical examination of the ear must be sensitive whenever there is earache. Signs such as pain on palpation of the tragus are suggestive of EO. The introduction of the speculum of the otoscope in the external auditory meatus can cause severe pain, if done inadvertently, making it difficult to get children to cooperate during examination. Otoscopy will reveal diffuse ear canal edema, erythema, or both, either with or without otorrhea or material in the ear canal as illustrated in Figure 9-1. A hallmark of diffuse acute EO is tenderness of the tragus (when pushed), pinna (when pulled up and back), or both. The tenderness is often intense and disproportionate to what might be expected based on visual inspection. In the severe stage, pain is intense, the lumen of the canal obstructed, and extra-canal signs such as auricular cellulitis, parotitis, or adenopathy, are likely (Agius et al., 1992; Beers & Abramo, 2004; Rosenfeld et al., 2006).

Diagnosis

The diagnosis of acute EO is done clinically. Table 9-1 shows elements proposed by Rosenfeld et al. (2006) for the diagnosis of acute EO. Laboratory tests on cultures of material obtained from the external ear, a CT scan, or an MRI must be made in cases that do not respond well to initial treatment or if there is suspicion of any complication. Possible complications of acute EO include cel-

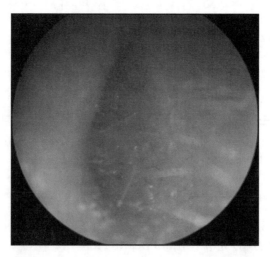

Figure 9–1. *Otoscopy of acute otitis externa with typical edema and erythema of the ear canal hindering the visibility of the tympanic membrane.*

Table 9–1. Elements of the Diagnosis of Acute External Otitis

1. Rapid onset (generally within 48 hours) in the past 3 weeks, AND
2. Symptoms of ear canal inflammation that include:
• Otalgia (often severe), itching, or fullness,
• WITH OR WITHOUT hearing loss or jaw pain*, AND
3. Signs of ear canal inflammation that include:
• Tenderness of the tragus, pinna, or both
• OR diffuse ear canal edema, erythema, or both
• WITH OR WITHOUT otorrhea, regional lymphadenitis, tympanic membrane erythema, or cellulitis of the pinna and adjacent skin

*Pain in the ear canal and temporomandibular joint region intensified by jaw motion.
Source: Reprinted from: Rosenfeld, R. M., Brown, L., Cannon, C. R., Dolor, R. J., Ganiats, T. G., Hannley, M., et al. (2006). Clinical practice guideline: Acute otitis externa. *Otolaryngology-Head and Neck Surgery, 134*(4 Suppl.), S4–S23 with permission from Elsevier.

lulite and local swelling, with or without extension to the parotid or retroauricular region, formation of abscess, osteitis, and malignant EO (Rosenfeld et al., 2006).

Management

Clinical recommendations for the treatment of acute EO are shown in Table 9-2. The initial treatment of acute EO in an HIV-positive patient is the same as that done in a patient who is HIV negative, provided no complications arise. Meanwhile, suspicion of some complications may require a more aggressive treatment approach.

Pain relief is one of the main objectives for treating acute EO. Thus, use of common analgesics such as acetoaminophen is indicated in cases of mild pain. Nonsteroidal anti-inflammatory drugs and opioids can be used in cases of moderate to severe pain. Regardless of ototopical drug selected for treatment, penetration to the epithelium is mandatory and any obstruction should be cleared (Gurney & Murr, 2003). Topical therapy allows for the administration of high concentrations of antibiotics, which can overwhelm organisms with high MICs. A solution of topical antibiotic exceeds by more than a hundredfold the tissue levels compared with what

Table 9–2. Clinical Recommendations for Treatment of Acute External Otitis

Clinical Recommendation	Evidence Rating	Comments
• Clear any obstructing debris or excess cerumen from the canal and check the integrity of the tympanic membrane and manifestations of the infection that have spread beyond the ear canal.	C	Use suction or curette/spoon device rather than irrigation until intact tympanic membrane is visualized.
• Relieve pain and discomfort with analgesics.	A	Acetaminophen or non-steroidal anti-inflammatory drugs if mild to moderate; consider opioids if severe.
• Use acidifying drops if there is mild inflammation, and consider antimicrobial drops if the disease is more advanced.	C	Select antibacterial versus antifungal agent based on clinical appearance.
• Add oral antibiotic if there is severe disease in an immunocompetent patient or if there is moderate or severe disease in those who are immunocompromised, who have diabetes or advanced age, and in patients with concomitant otitis media.	C	Consider possibility of malignant external otitis if there is severe pain, a temperature higher than 102.2° F (39°C), necrosis of canal skin, auricular chondritis, cervical adenitis, parotitis, facial paralysis, vertigo, or profound hearing loss.
• Counsel the patient about preventive measures.	C	Dry ear canals after swimming or use prophylactic acidifying drops; avoid using cotton swabs or locally sensitizing agents.

A = consistent, good-quality patient-oriented evidence; B = inconsistent or limited-quality patient-oriented evidence; C = consensus, disease-oriented evidence, usual practice, expert opinion, or case series.

Source: Adapted with permission from "Otitis Externa: Review and Clinical Update," November 1, 2006, *American Family Physician.* Copyright © 2006 American Academy of Family Physicians. All Rights Reserved.

might be expected with systemic administration (Roland & Stroman, 2002). Warming the ototopical to body temperature (e.g., by placing it in a shirt pocket or a warm room) before application helps the patient avoid the dizziness from caloric stimulation that cold liquid can incite (Osguthorpe & Nielsen, 2006). The use of oral antibiotics is reserved for cases of complications or in patients with low CD4 T-lymphocytes (Rosenfeld et al., 2006).

The widespread use of quinolones for the treatment of community-acquired infections makes the isolation of *P. aeruginosa* more difficult in HIV-infected or noninfected patients and contributes to the emergence of resistant species of *P. aeruginosa* (Bernstein, Holland, Porter, & Maw, 2007).

Malignant External Otitis

Nature and Etiology

Malignant (necrotizing) EO (also termed malignant otitis externa), as first described by Meltzer and Kelemen (1959) and Chandler (1968), is an invasive and necrotizing infection of the external auditory canal with extension to the petrous and mastoid portions of the temporal bone and skull base, which typically occurs in elderly patients with diabetes mellitus. However, several reports of malignant EO in patients with HIV/AIDS and in chemotherapy patients implicate a compromised immune system as a predisposing factor in this disease (Grandis, Branstetter, & Yu, 2004; Kielhofner, Atmar, Hamill, & Musher, 1992; Lacarte & Segura, 1990; McElroy & Marks, 1991; Muñoz & Martinez-Chamorro, 1998; Reiss, Hadderingh, Schot, & Danner, 1991; Ress, Luntz, Telischi, Balkany, & Whiteman, 1997; Rinaldo, Brandwein, Devaney, & Ferlito, 2003; Sreepada & Kwartler, 2003; Weinroth, Schessel, & Tuazon, 1994). Patients with HIV/AIDS who develop malignant external otitis tend to be younger than the typical elderly patient with this invasive ear infection, and most are not diabetic.

Pseudomonas aeruginosa is nearly always the causative organism (>98% of cases), although the administration of topical antibiotics before culture often precludes isolation of the pathogen (Ress et al., 1997; Sreepada & Kwartler, 2003). Otherwise, in patients with HIV/AIDS, as in immunocompetent individuals, there are reports of malignant EO caused by *Proteus mirabilis* (Coser, Stamm, Lobo, & Pinto, 1980) and the fungus *Aspergillus fumigates* (Cunningham, Yu, Turner, & Curtin, 1998; Hern, Almeyda, Thomas, Main, & Patel, 1996; Lyos, Malpica, Estrada, Katz, & Jenkins, 1993; Muñoz & Martinez-Chamorro, 1998; Petrak, Pottage, & Levin, 1985). Fungal etiology, also seen in people with hematologic malignancies and not so frequently in diabetes mellitus patients, makes up a significant proportion of the infections, especially in end-stage HIV/AIDS patients (Yao & Messner, 2001). Besides, there are occasional reports of malignant EO caused by other organisms, including *Staphylococcus aureus* (Bayardelle, Jolivet-Granger, & Larochelle, 1982) and *Klebsiella oxytoca* (Rodriguez, Martinez, Gonzalez, Macías, & Alburquerque, 1992), which characteristically occur in immunocompromised patients.

The infection by *P. aeruginosa* is an opportunistic one and rarely occurs in healthy people. It is a ubiquitous bacterium that is capable of growing in distilled water and is not a normal component of ear canal flora (Favero, Carson, Bond, & Petersen, 1971). This gram-negative bacterium colonizes the ear canal after small traumas or excessive exposure to water (Rubin, Yu, Kamerer, & Wagener, 1990; Sreepada & Kwartler, 2003). In the HIV/AIDS patient, some factors also contribute to the development of malignant EO with skull base osteomyelitis, for example, defects in cellular and humoral immunity, quantity and quality of lymphocytes (mainly CD4+ count <200 cells/mL), use of a higher quantity of medications, and presence of other opportunistic infections.

Symptoms

Although it is difficult to document precisely, it seems that this syndrome has been more frequently diagnosed as the index of suspicion for malignant EO and has increased among generalist physicians in the past 10 years. Although rare, pediatric cases are also being seen. In contrast to adults, children are more likely to be immunocompromised on the basis of malignancy and malnutrition. Although to our knowledge, no deaths have been reported, children tend to be more toxic with their illness, as illustrated by the development of fever, leucocytosis, and *P. aeruginosa* bacteraemia (Grandis et al., 2004; Paul, Justus, Balraj, Job, & Kirubakaran, 2001).

The clinical aspects of malignant EO are similar in HIV/AIDS patients and noninfected patients (Hern et al., 1996). Although malignant EO does not seem to be particularly prevalent in patients with HIV/AIDS, diagnosis should be considered in any patient who presents with painful otorrhea that is unresponsive to treatment regimens for simple EO (i.e., topical antibiotics and local debridement). Unlike adults, children have a more acute onset of this disease with a toxic appearance. Facial nerve paralysis is seen more frequently and rapidly but does not carry the negative prognostic significance associated with adults. Necrosis of the tympanic membrane is seen in more than half of the children and is characterized by severe otalgia and otorrhea, usually not responsive to topical drugs used to treat simple EO (Rubin & Yu, 1988; Rubin, Yu, & Stool, 1988). Pain is the remarkable symptom in malignant otitis externa: it can be associated with temporal headache, it does not improve with common analgesics, and it tends to be nocturnal. The symptom is more common in the mastoideal region and temporomandibular joint, resulting in pain with chewing. Fever is not common and otorrhea is present in the majority of patients (Hern et al., 1996; Sreepada & Kwartler, 2003). Classically, granulation tissue is frequently visible in the inferior portion of the external auditory canal at the bone-cartilage junction (at the site of Santorini's fissures). However, upon otoscopic examination of patients with HIV/AIDS, these granulations in the external auditory meatus are not so commonly found (Figure 9–2). Finding these granulations in patients with

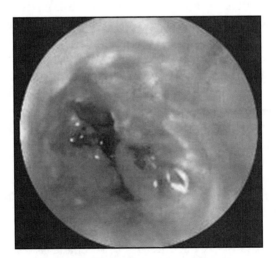

Figure 9–2. *Otoscopy of malignant otitis externa in an adult with HIV/AIDS revealing granulation in the external auditory meatus.*

HIV/AIDS is a factor of better prognosis and immunity (Ress et al., 1997; Sreepada & Kwartler, 2003). In advanced stages of the infection, osteomyelitis of the base of the skull and temporomandibular joint osteomyelitis can develop (Sreepada & Kwartler, 2003).

Osteomyelitis can be associated with the involvement of the cranial nerves (Mani, Sudhoff, Rajagopal, Moffat, & Axon, 2007). However, it may happen in any phase of the disease or in association with other central nervous system complications such as cerebral abscess, meningitis, and cavernous sinus thrombosis (Hern et al., 1996; Sreepada & Kwartler, 2003). Paralysis of the facial nerve is most common, followed (in order) by glossopharyngeal, vagal, and spinal accessory nerves at the jugular foramen, and the hypoglossal nerve as it exits the hypoglossal canal (Grandis et al., 2004).

Diagnosis

The diagnosis of malignant EO is based on a combination of clinical, laboratory, and radiographic findings. Typical signs of infection are notably absent: patients are afebrile (except children) and white blood cell count and differential are generally normal. Although nonspecific, the erythrocyte sedimentation rate (ESR) is usually markedly increased and can be used to monitor disease activity (Grandis et al., 2004; Rubin & Yu, 1988). Certain imaging modalities have proven valuable in the diagnosis and follow-up of malignant EO. Bone scans (Tc-99m methylene diphosphonate) are exquisitely sensitive because the radiotracer accumulates at sites of osteoblastic activity. However, bone scans are relatively nonspecific because they can be abnormal in the setting of simple EO. In addition, bone scans remain positive indefinitely and cannot be used to follow disease progression or resolution. There is some evidence that a quantitative bone scan can distinguish malignant EO from its more benign counterparts and can correlate with disease activity. Gallium scans (gallium citrate Ga 67) are more specific than bone scans because the radioisotope is incorporated directly into granulocytes and bacteria. Although some authors have reported that gallium scans can be used to follow disease activity, others have noted normal scans in the setting of recurrent disease (Grandis et al., 2004; Levin, Shary, Nichols, & Lucente, 1986; Sreepada & Kwartler, 2003). This kind of scan is more useful in the follow-up of patients, mainly in association with single photon emission computerized tomography

(SPECT) scanning (Stokkel, Boot, & van Eck-Smit, 1996). However, some authors have noted that normal scans can be found in patients with recurrent disease (Paramsothy, Khanijow, & Ong, 1997). Anatomic imaging studies, computed tomography, or magnetic resonance imaging are useful for detection of disease extension, progression, and resolution (Rubin, Curtin, Yu, & Kamerer, 1990). Although a CT scan is useful for identifying bone erosion, the MRI is more useful in identifying soft tissue involvement (Grandis, Curtin, & Yu, 1995). Eroded bone does not remineralize, but the regression of the soft tissue involvement is associated with the regression of the disease. Both imaging studies are also useful if there is a suspicion of skull base or central nervous system involvement (Grandis et al., 2004; Ismail, Hellier, & Batty, 2004).

Painful ear and ear discharge are also symptoms of squamous cell carcinoma of the external auditory meatus; if a patient with adequate treatment still presents these symptoms, a biopsy is required. Radiographic studies are not helpful to differentiate tumor from necrotizing infection, and histologic examination is the only definitive method to distinguish between these two entities.

Management

Oral quinolones, especially ciprofloxacin, have revolutionized the treatment of malignant EO and have replaced combination intravenous therapy. The availability of oral agents has eliminated the need for hospitalization in all but the most recalcitrant cases. With the introduction of quinolones, cure rate has increased to 90%, with few adverse effects reported. The advantages of quinolones are the low toxicity profile and excellent penetration into the bone (Barza, 1988; Wiseman & Balfour, 1994). Quinolones have not been given to children due to problems with joint development in animal models. However, ciprofloxacin has been safely administered to children with cystic fibrosis and there is a report of one child with malignant EO being effectively treated with ciprofloxacin after prolonged intravenous therapy with antipseudomonal penicillin and aminoglycoside failed (Paul et al., 2001). Therefore, ciprofloxacin may be indicated for treatment of malignant EO in rare pediatric patients (Grandis et al., 2004). Ciprofloxacin (750 mg orally twice per day) seems to be the antibiotic of choice, based on clinical experience and comparative in-vitro susceptibility studies. However, comparative trials have not been done (Levenson, Parisier, Dolitsky, & Bindra, 1991). In spite of the rapid relief of symptoms (pain and otorrhea), prolonged treatment for 6 to 8 weeks is still recommended, as indicated for an osteomyelitis. Surgical debridement may still have a role in the treatment of malignant EO in cases of abscesses and necrotic tissue. If a fungus (e.g., *Aspergillus*) is the causative organism, prolonged treatment (>12 weeks) with amphotericin B is indicated. A liposomal amphotericin preparation is recommended to keep to a minimum the incidence of nephrotoxicity (Grandis et al., 2004).

The emergence of resistant *P. aeruginosa* to ciprofloxacin is a new problem in the treatment of those patients (Berenholz, Katzenell, & Harell, 2002). In such cases, patients require hospitalization for biopsy, surgical debridement, and a prolonged course of an anti-pseudomonal β-lactam agent (ceftazidime, piperacillin, imipenem) with or without aminoglycoside. Patients with a fungal cause of malignant EO must receive prolonged treatment (>12 weeks) with an anti-fungal agent, such as anfothericin B (a less toxic liposomal form) or itraconazole (Finer et al., 2002), and surgical debridement. Hyperbaric oxygen therapy can be used as adjuvant therapy but its efficiency is still unproven (Grandis et al., 2004; Hern et al., 1996; Shupak et al., 1989; Sreepada & Kwartler, 2003).

An algorithm for diagnostic and treatment of malignant EO is presented in Figure 9–3.

Otomycosis (fungal otitis externa)

Nature and Etiology

Otomycosis or fungal otitis externa is a chronic and superficial fungal infection of the external auditory canal, with infrequent complications involving the middle ear, usually caused by *Aspergillus niger* or *Candida*, which are saprophytic microorganisms of the skin of the external meatus (Ho, Vrabec, Yoo, & Coker, 2006; Kaur, Mittal, Kakkar, Aggarwal, & Mathur, 2000; Rinaldo et al., 2003; Vennewald, Schonlebe, & Klemm, 2003).

Otomycosis may occur due to previous treatment with topical antibiotics or it may be secondary to bacterial infection (Strauss & Fine, 1991). Various other factors have been proposed as predisposing factors for otomycosis; these include a humid climate, presence

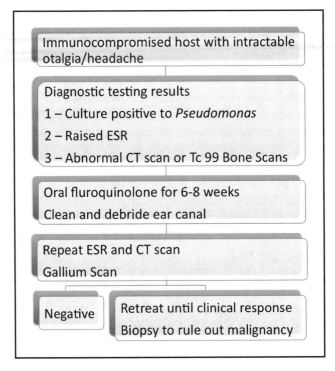

Figure 9–3. *Algorithm for malignant external otitis diagnosis and treatment. ESR = Erythrocyte Sedimentation Rate. Adapted from: Grandis, J. R., Branstetter, B. F, and Yu, V. L. (2004). The changing face of malignant (necrotizing) external otitis: Clinical, radiological, and anatomic correlations.* Lancet Infectious Diseases, 4, 34–39. *Reprinted with permission from Elsevier, Copyright 2004.*

of cerumen, instrumentation of the ear, immunocompromised host (e.g., HIV/AIDS), recently increased use of topical antibiotic/steroid preparations, wearing head clothes, presence of dermatomycoses, and swimming has also been identified (Ozcan, Ozcan, Karaarslan, & Karaarslan, 2003; Stern & Lucente, 1988). Although there has been no report of an increased incidence of otomycosis in HIV/AIDS patients, their immune-compromised state may predispose them to a higher incidence (Prasad et al., 2006). As in acute otitis externa, otomycosis is more common during summer and autumn when weather is hot and humid (Ozcan et al., 2003).

Diagnosis and Management

Clinical findings in children and adults are similar to those found in acute EO. However, the exact diagnosis of fungal otitis depends on histologic studies that show fungal invasion (Rinaldo et al., 2003). Itching of the ear is found in nearly all patients with otomycosis; hearing loss and aural fullness are also frequent symptoms as a result of accumulation of fungal debris in the canal. On otoscopic examination, we can see typical fungal colonies in the meatus as presented in Figure 9–4.

Infection with *Candida* can be more difficult to detect clinically because of its lack of characteristic appearance like *Aspergillus* and can present as otorrhea not responding to aural antimicrobials. Otomycosis attributed to *Candida* is often identified by culture data (Ho et al., 2006).

Perforation of the tympanic membrane is described as a complication due to otomycosis. The pathophysiology of the perforations may be attributed to avascular necrosis of the tympanic membrane as a result of mycotic thrombosis in the adjacent blood vessels. Most perforations heal spontaneously within a month, but about 10% of the cases may need a myringoplasty (Hurst, 2001).

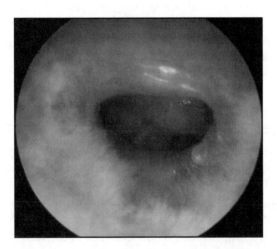

Figure 9–4. *Otoscopy (left ear) of patient with otomycosis. Typical fungal colonies are seen in ear canal. Note that the patient also presents with a perforation of the tympanic membrane.*

A standard treatment regimen for otomycosis has not yet been established. Meticulous cleaning of the ear canal may be sufficient in most of the patients. Administration of mildly acidic drops, such as boric acid and alcohol, or modified Burow's solution may be part of the initial therapy (Stern, Shah, & Lucente, 1988). If this therapy does not improve the patient's condition, we must consider invasive fungal diseases. This may require consideration of an imaging examination with computed tomography or magnetic resonance to evaluate the extension of the disease (Strauss & Fine, 1991). In cases of invasive fungal diseases, surgical debridement and systemic antifungal therapy becomes necessary (Rinaldo et al., 2003; Strauss & Fine, 1991).

MIDDLE EAR DISORDERS ASSOCIATED WITH HIV/AIDS

Studies in temporal bones of patients who had HIV/AIDS show the presence of inflammatory changes of the mucosa of the middle ear in different degrees, even in asymptomatic patients, which suggests that there is direct involvement of the middle ear with HIV/AIDS (Chandrasekhar, Siverls, & Chandrasekhar, 1992; Michaels, Soucek, & Liang, 1994).

Later, we discuss the involvement of the middle ear in patients with HIV/AIDS. The acute and chronic infections of the middle ear are probably the most frequent form of otorhinolaryngological involvement in these patients, especially among children (Miziara, Weber, Cunha-Filho, & Pinheiro-Neto, 2007; Singh, Georgacalas, Patel, & Patesch, 2003). The complications that can occur during the development of otitis media and opportunistic infections that affect the middle ear, and which are closely associated with HIV/AIDS, are considered in this section.

Acute Otitis Media

Nature and Etiology

Acute otitis media (AOM) is defined as a history of acute onset of signs and symptoms, presence of middle-ear effusion, and signs and symptoms of middle-ear inflammation. Acute otitis media is a common infection in children with and without HIV/AIDS (Newton, 2006). However, children with HIV/AIDS are more likely to suffer from otitis media than immunocompetent children (Gondim, Zonta, Fortkamp, & Schmeling, 2000; Hadfield, Birchall, Novelli, & Bailey, 1996; Shapiro & Novelli, 1998). Barnett, Kline, Pelton, and Luginbuhl (1992) observed that all HIV-infected pediatric patients developed at least one episode of AOM before the age of 3 years; in noninfected children, this prevalence was about 75%. Zuniga (1999) reported that 80% of HIV-infected children will present with three to six or more episodes of otitis media during childhood, whereas only approximately 30% of healthy children will present with three or more episodes of otitis media.

The correlation between HIV clinical stage, serum cluster of differentiation four glycoprotein (CD4+) lymphocyte count, and otitis media has been addressed by many authors. Chen, Ohlms, Stewart, and Kline (1996) observed that the incidence density of otitis media significantly increased as an HIV-infected child progressed from clinical categories A to C or moved from immunologic categories 1 to 3. Makokha et al. (2003) in Kenya demonstrated that the presence of AOM in HIV-infected children was associated with a reduction in the CD4+ lymphocyte count. However, Miziara et al. (2007) observed a higher prevalence of AOM in children receiving highly active anti-retroviral therapy (HAART) with higher CD4+ lymphocyte counts than in those receiving standard antiretroviral therapy. This may indicate that HIV-positive children with better immune status present more like HIV-negative children; that is, they are more prone to develop AOM without a chronic disease.

Children with HIV/AIDS are more susceptible to AOM than adult patients (Godofsky, Zinreich, Armstrong, Leslie, & Weickel, 1992). However, Chandrasekhar et al. (2000), in a cross-sectional study, noted that 14% of adult patients with HIV/AIDS, with an average age of 40 years, had AOM during a clinical evaluation.

Some studies confirmed that the more common bacteria responsible for the genesis of otitis media in HIV-infected children without immunosuppression are the same ones found in non-HIV-infected children: *Streptococcus pneumoniae* and *Haemophilus influenzae* (Chen et al., 1996; Marchisio, Principi, Sorella, Sala, & Tornaghi, 1996). In immunocompromised children, besides the higher number of infections (Newton, 2006), we must consider *Staphylococcus aureus* as an etiologic agent (Marchisio et al., 1996). There are reports of patients with otitis media due to *Pneumocystis carinii*, *Pseudomonas aureginosa*, and mycobacteria (Kielhofner et al., 1992; Marchisio et al., 1996; Praveen, Terry, Elmahallawy, & Horsfield, 2002).

Symptoms and Diagnosis

The clinical aspects of otitis media in HIV-infected children or in adult patients are similar to those seen in noninfected patients. Children with AOM usually present with a history of rapid onset of signs and symptoms such as otalgia (or pulling of the ear in an infant), irritability in an infant or toddler, otorrhea, and/or fever. These findings, other than otorrhea, are nonspecific and frequently overlap with those related to uncomplicated viral upper respiratory infection. Fever, earache, and excessive crying are present frequently (90%) in children with AOM; however, these symptoms are also prominent among children in acute respiratory illness without AOM (72%) (Niemela et al., 1994). In adults, the most prominent symptom is pain in the ear, following an infection of the upper airways.

Visualization of the tympanic membrane with identification of purulent middle ear effusion and inflammatory changes is necessary to establish the diagnosis of AOM with certainty. In children, to visualize the tympanic membrane adequately, it is essential that the cerumen obscuring the tympanic membrane be removed and that lighting is adequate. Appropriate restraint of the child to permit adequate examination may also be necessary. The findings on otoscopy, which suggest the diagnosis of AOM, are fullness or bulging of the tympanic membrane that may be associated with cloudiness and/or redness. Redness alone does not indicate a middle ear infection; crying or high fever may generate erythematous flush, which is usually less intense than that observed in AOM, and remits as the child quiets down. Diagnosis of AOM is certain if these three criteria are met: rapid onset, presence of middle-ear effusion, and signs and symptoms of middle-ear inflammation. Table 9–3 summarizes the elements for defining AOM.

Management

The management of pain during an episode of AOM, especially during the first 24 hours, should be addressed regardless of the use of antibacterial agents. Acetaminophen (15 mg per kg every 4–6 hours)

Table 9–3. Elements in Defining Acute Otitis Media

1. Recent, usually abrupt, onset of signs and symptoms of middle-ear inflammation and middle ear effusion

2. The presence of middle ear effusion that is indicated by any of the following:

   a. Bulging of the tympanic membrane

   b. Limited or absent mobility of the tympanic membrane

   c. Air-fluid level behind the tympanic membrane

   d. Otorrhea

3. Signs or symptoms of middle-ear inflammation as indicated by either

   a. Distinct erythema of the tympanic membrane or

   b. Distinct otalgia (discomfort clearly referable to the ear[s] that results in interference with or precludes normal activity or sleep)

Source: From American Academy of Pediatrics Subcommittee on Management of Acute Otitis Media. (2004). Diagnosis and management of acute otitis media. *Pediatrics, 113,* 1451–1465, Table 2. Reprinted with permission from The American Academy of Pediatrics, Copyright 2004.

and ibuprofen (10 mg per kg every 6 hours) provide effective analgesia for mild to moderate pain; readily available, they comprise the mainstay of pain management for AOM. Narcotic analgesia with codeine or analogs may be necessary to manage moderate or severe pain; however, its use requires prescription and there may be risks of respiratory depression or other side effects as altered mental status, gastrointestinal upset, and constipation (AAP, 2004; Bertin et al., 1996).

Currently available guidelines in English medical literature for the treatment of AOM were not developed for children with underlying conditions that may alter the natural course of AOM such as immunodeficiency in patients with HIV/AIDS. We do not recommend in AOM the observation without use of anti-bacterial agents in patients with HIV/AIDS. In the immunocompromised child with HIV infection, the physician must consider potential complications secondary to middle ear disease. Recurrent infections recalcitrant to oral antibiotic therapy, bacteremia, and meningitis are more frequently seen in children with HIV infection (Shapiro & Novelli, 1998). Based on predominant pathogens isolated from AOM, amoxicillin is the antibiotic of choice, and the dose should be 80 to 90 mg/kg per day (Piglansky et al., 2003). If no improvement in symptoms is seen within 48 to 72 hours, the patient must be reassessed to confirm the diagnosis, exclude other causes of illness, and high-dose amoxicillin-clavulanate (90 mg/kg per day of amoxicillin component, with 6.4 mg/kg per day of clavulanate in two divided doses) should be used for additional coverage for β-lactamase–positive *H. influenzae* and *M. catarrhalis* (Dagan et al., 2001). Risk factors for the presence of bacterial species likely to be resistant to amoxicillin include attendance at child care, recent receipt (less than 30 days) of anti-bacterial treatment, and age younger than 2 years. If the patient is allergic to amoxicillin and the allergic reaction was not a type I hypersensitivity reaction (urticaria or anaphylaxis), cefuroxime (30 mg/kg per day in two divided doses) can be used. In cases of type I reaction, clarithromycin (15 mg/kg per day in two divided doses) can be used in an effort to select an antibacterial agent of an entirely different class. Alternative therapy in the penicillin-allergic patient who is being treated for infection that is known or presumed to be caused by penicillin-resistant *S. pneumoniae* is clindamycin at 30–40 mg/kg per day in three divided doses. For a patient who is vomiting or cannot otherwise tolerate oral medication, a single dose of parenteral ceftriaxone (50 mg/kg) has been shown to be effective for the initial treatment of AOM (Leibovitz et al., 2000).

If symptoms persist for AOM or in cases where complications are suspected, tympanocentesis should be recommended to make a bacteriologic diagnosis (Marchisio et al., 1996). In our opinion, Gram-stain, culture, and antibacterial-agent sensitivity studies of the fluid are essential to guide additional therapy.

To prevent otitis media and other bacterial infections, exposure to viral illness in congregate living situations is not encouraged, whenever possible. However, in our experience, HIV-positive children living in homes of support have smaller chances of having a chronic disease because they receive better care (Miziara et al., 2007). Parental smoking and passive smoke exposure increase the incidence of otitis media in children; parents should therefore be asked to stop smoking. Heptavalent pneumococcal conjugate vaccine (Prevnar®) was well tolerated and immunogenic in infants with HIV infection. Reactions to the vaccine included severe induration, erythema, limited leg movement, and a fever of 103.6°F (39.8°C) after vaccination; all adverse reactions were resolved within 48 hours

(Nachman et al., 2003). However, additional studies of this vaccine are necessary to confirm long-term data on the longevity of the immune response and its benefits in terms of preventing invasive pneumococcal infection.

Recurrent Acute Otitis Media

Recurrent otitis media is defined by the occurrence of three or more episodes of AOM in a period of 6 months. These episodes are related to the level of CD4 lymphocytes; they are thus more frequent in immunocompromised patients (Chen et al., 1996; Gondim et al., 2000; Newton, 2006; Zucotti et al., 2001). In cases of recurrent otitis media, Zucotti et al. (2001) showed reduction of otitis media episodes in 100% of the children using prophylaxy with cefaclor during 6 months.

Adults make up less than 20% of patients presenting symptoms of AOM. *H. influenzae* and *S. pneumoniae* are common bacterial isolates in these patients. Compared with children, adults more often present with otalgia, ear drainage, diminished hearing, and sore throat. Opacity and redness of the tympanic membrane are equally common in children and adults. Recommended antibiotic use is the same for children and adults. Smoking should be discouraged. Nasal and oral steroids may be beneficial in patients with persistent AOM and associated allergies (Ramakrishnan, Sparks, & Berryhill, 2007).

Otitis Media with Effusion (serous or secretory otitis media)

Nature and Etiology

Otitis media with effusion (OME) is defined as the presence of fluid in the middle ear without signs or symptoms of an acute ear infection. Persistent middle-ear fluid from OME results in decreased mobility of the tympanic membrane and serves as a barrier to sound conduction. OME may occur spontaneously because of poor eustachian tube function or as an inflammatory response following AOM. Approximately 90% of children (80% of individual ears) present with OME at some time before school age, most often between the ages 6 months and 4 years. Many episodes resolve spontaneously within 3 months, but more than 30 to 40% of the children have recurrent OME, and 5 to 10% of episodes last for a year or longer (American Academy of Family Physicians [AAFP]; American Academy of Otolaryngology-Head and Neck Surgery [AAOHNS]; American Academy of Pediatrics [AAP] Subcommittee on Otitis Media with Effusion, 2004). Secretory otitis media secondary to nasopharyngeal lymphoid hyperplasia is common in children and adults with HIV/AIDS (Chen et al., 1996; Gurney & Murr, 2003; Kohan & Giacchi 1999; Prasad et al., 2006). Weber et al. (2006) and Miziara et al. (2007) also observed that 8.5% of children with HIV/AIDS had OME.

In HIV-infected adults, eustachian tube dysfunction can result from nasopharyngeal lymphoid hyperplasia, sinusitis, nasopharyngeal neoplasms, or allergies and their associated mucosal changes. Unilateral or recurrent serous otitis media in an adult warrants an evaluation of the nasopharynx to rule out large benign or malignant nasopharyngeal tumors. These lesions present as nasal obstruction, hearing loss, otitis media, and recurrent serous otitis media. Large lymphoid proliferation of the adenoids, lymphoma, and Kaposi's sarcoma occur more commonly in patients with HIV/AIDS (Moazzez & Alvi, 1998). Nasal endoscopy should be performed, with a biopsy of the nasopharynx if necessary.

Symptoms and Diagnosis

Although adults usually complain about hearing loss and ear fullness, in about half of the cases in children, neither the affected children nor their parents or caregivers describe significant complaints related to a middle ear effusion. Some children, however, may present with a sensation of ear fullness or "popping" and are often characterized by poor or inappropriate responses to environmental sounds, lack of attentiveness, behavioral changes, failure to respond to normal conversational-level speech, and the need for excessively high sound levels when using audio equipment or viewing television. Recurrent episodes of AOM with persistent OME between episodes, problems with school performance, and delayed speech or language development are also common associations of chronic OME (AAFP, AAOHNS, & AAP, 2004; Chen et al., 1996).

Diagnosis is performed with otoscopy, observing the tympanic membrane with a retracted, dull appearance with increased vascularization, without bulging, as demonstrated in Figure 9–5, and with lack of movement on pneumatic otoscopy (AAFP, AAOHNS, & AAP,

2004). Tympanometry can be used to confirm the diagnosis, which evidences a type B curve (flat sloping tympanogram with no distinct peak as illustrated in Figure 9-6; Jerger, 1970).

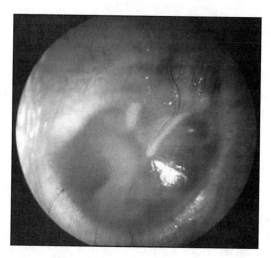

Figure 9–5. *Otoscopy (right ear) of HIV-infected children with otitis media with effusion. Tympanic membrane is dull, without bulging and presents no movement on pneumatic otoscopy, suggesting fluid in middle ear. An air bubble can be seen in the upper and anterior parts of the middle ear.*

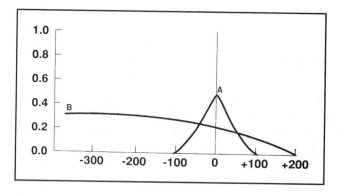

Figure 9–6. *Type A and Type B curves in tympanogram. Type A is considered normal curve; type B (flat sloping tympanogram with no distinct peak) is encountered in otitis media with effusion.*

Management

In adults, management of lymphoid proliferation on nasopharynx (adenoidectomy) usually relieves obstruction in the eustachian tube and promotes resolution of OME. In recurrences or malignant tumors such as Kaposi's sarcoma or carcinomas of the nasopharynx, which may require chemotherapy or radiotherapy, tympanostomy with insertion of ventilation tubes is indicated. Placement of ventilation tubes in adults can be performed under local anesthesia. Brody, Singh, Lee, and Sperling (2000) observed that HIV infection does not influence the indications, technique, results, or complication rate for myringotomy with placement of tubes for OME and the efficacy in relief from discomfort and improvement of hearing occurred in all cases. Recurrence of OME after tube extrusion may take place in up to 23% of the cases, especially for those who had nasopharyngeal tissue enlargement. In these patients, long-term T-tubes should be considered.

Clinicians should distinguish the child with OME who is at risk for speech, language, or learning problems from other children with OME and should evaluate hearing, speech, language, and need for intervention more promptly. Risk factors for developmental difficulties are listed in Table 9–4. Management of the child with OME

Table 9–4. Risk Factors for Developmental Difficulties in Children

Permanent hearing loss independent of OME
Suspected or diagnosed speech and language delay or disorder
Autism-spectrum disorder and other pervasive developmental disorders
Syndromes (for example, Down) or craniofacial disorders that include cognitive, speech, and language delays
Blindness or uncorrectable visual impairment
Cleft palate with or without associated syndrome
Developmental delay

Source: From American Academy of Family Physicians; American Academy of Otolaryngology-Head and Neck Surgery; American Academy of Pediatrics Subcommittee on Otitis Media with Effusion. (2004). Otitis media with effusion. *Pediatrics, 113*, 1412–1429. Reprinted with permission.

who is at increased risk for developmental delays should include a diagnostic hearing assessment, speech and language evaluation, and early tympanostomy tube insertion (Hubbard, Paradise, McWilliams, Elster, & Taylor, 1985).

After the diagnosis of OME, if the child is not at risk of having speech, language, and learning problems, treatment can be delayed by clinicians for 3 months from the date of effusion onset or diagnosis. This recommendation is based on the self-limited nature of most OME, which has been well documented in cohort studies and in control groups of randomized trials. Up to 90% of residual OME after an AOM episode resolves spontaneously by 3 months. However, only 25% of newly detected OME of unknown prior duration in children 2 to 4 years old resolves by 3 months, and documented bilateral OME of 3 months duration or longer resolves spontaneously after 6 to 12 months in only 30% of children 2 years of age or older (Rosenfeld & Kay, 2003). Clinicians should inform the parent or caregiver that the child might experience reduced hearing until the effusion resolves, especially if it is bilateral, and discuss strategies for optimizing the listening and learning environment until the effusion resolves. These strategies include speaking in close proximity to the child, facing the child and speaking clearly, repeating phrases when misunderstood, and providing preferential classroom seating (AAFP, AAOHNS, & AAP, 2004).

The treatment of OME for HIV-positive children is usually the same as used for HIV-negative children, but in our experience, resolution takes longer. OME may follow episodes of AOM. A recent meta-analysis (Koopman et al., 2008) has shown that the use of antibiotic therapy in children with AOM does not prevent the development of asymptomatic OME. However, this study did not include HIV-infected children. In the same way, no statistical or clinical benefit was found by Griffin, Flynn, Bailey, and Schultz (2006) for treating OME with antihistamines and/or decongestant in children. However, treated study subjects experienced 11% more side effects than untreated subjects (number needed to treat to harm = 9), so their use alone or in combination is not indicated. The use of antimicrobial therapy with or without steroids for OME is controversial. Although the use of oral steroids plus antimicrobial therapy show short-term benefits, the differences against control in the long term are not statistically significant (Mandel et al., 2002). The use of HAART does not seem to modify the prevalence of OME in children with HIV/AIDS (Miziara et al., 2007; Weber et. al., 2006).

When OME persists for 3 months or longer, or at any time that language delay, learning problems, or a significant hearing loss is suspected, assessment of hearing is recommended (AAFP, AAOHNS, & AAP, 2004). Hearing levels (HL) of ≤20 dB HL across the frequency range (125–8000 Hz) is considered normal hearing in children. However, if OME persists, they should be followed up with a new assessment of hearing within 3 months. Hearing levels from 21 to 39 dB can be associated with difficulties in speech, language, and academic performance, and HL ≥40 dB has been shown to have a very significant impact on speech, language, and academic performance. In these cases, tympanostomy tube insertion is indicated immediately (AAFP, AAOHNS, & AAP, 2004; Chen et al., 1996). Adenoidectomy is recommended in many cases, because it confers a 50% reduction in the need for future operations, and its benefits are independent of adenoid size (Gates, Avery, Prihoda, & Cooper, 1987). Tympanostomy tube insertion is also indicated in OME when early signs of structural damage to the tympanic membrane or middle ear are present, as retraction pockets. An algorithm for managing OME is shown in Figure 9–7.

Chronic Suppurative Otitis Media

Nature and Etiology

Chronic suppurative otitis media (CSOM) is a chronic inflammation of the middle ear and mastoid mucosa in which the tympanic membrane is not intact (perforation) and discharge (otorrhea) is present (Verhoeff, van der Veen, Rovers, Sanders, & Schilder, 2006). Bernaldez, Morales, and Hernandez (2005) observed, in a period of 10 years, a prevalence of this disease in HIV-infected children of 13.2% with an annual incidence of 3.3%. Many studies have reported CSOM among the most common ear, nose, and throat diseases in patients with HIV/AIDS, with prevalence ranging from 5 to 44% (Barnett et al., 1992; Chen et al., 1996; Gondim et al., 2000; Miziara et al., 2007; Prasad et al., 2006; Shapiro & Novelli, 1998). Weber et al. (2006) and Miziara et al. (2007) observed that children in treatment with HAART presented with a lower incidence of CSOM compared with children using other anti-retroviral therapies. This might be the result of a significant increase in the number of CD4+ lymphocytes observed in children undergoing HAART.

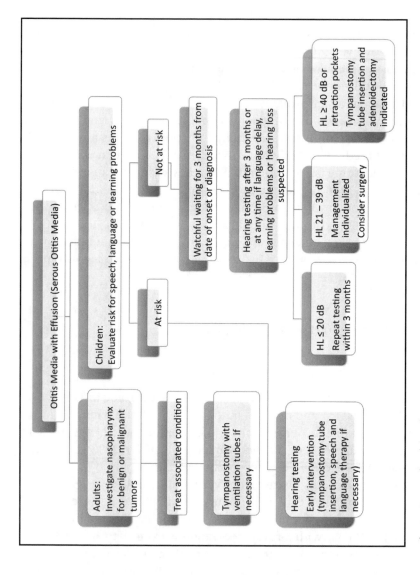

Figure 9–7. Algorithm for management of otitis media with effusion. HL = hearing level (in decibels).

The pathogenesis of CSOM is multifactorial: environmental versus genetically determined factors as well as anatomic and functional characteristics of the eustachian tube are involved. Reflux of nasopharyngeal secretions through the eustachian tube may result in contamination of the middle ear with potential respiratory pathogens. Infants and young children are especially at risk for such reflux because their eustachian tubes are short, horizontal, and "floppy" (Bluestone, 1998). Patients with HIV/AIDS more often have eustachian tube dysfunction resulting from nasopharyngeal lymphoid hyperplasia, sinusitis, nasopharyngeal neoplasms, or allergies and their associated mucosal changes. Furthermore, Recurrent acute sinusitis and chronic sinusitis are common in patients with HIV/AIDS, and the infected mucous drainage streaming into the nasopharynx from infected sinuses can cause mucosal swelling around the eustachian tube orifice and predispose patients with HIV/AIDS to CSOM. Recently, bacterial biofilms have gained attention as a source of chronic infections. A biofilm is a population of bacterial cells growing on a surface, enclosed in an exopolysaccharide matrix; as it is difficult to eradicate, this could be the source of persistent infections. Biofilms may attach to damaged tissue, such as an exposed osteitic bone and ulcerated middle-ear mucosa, or to otologic implants such as tympanostomy tubes, and are therefore thought to cause persistent infection in CSOM (Post, Stoodley, Hall-Stoodley, & Ehrlich, 2004). Kania et al. (2008) showed that adenoid tissue in children with chronic and/or recurrent otitis media contains mucosal biofilms in 54% of the cases. The bacteria encountered in CSOM in patients with HIV/AIDS are usually *Pseudomonas aeruginosa*, *Staphylococcus aureus*, gram-negative rods (*Klebsiella* spp., *Proteus* spp., and *Escherichia* spp.) and anaerobic (including *Bacteroides* spp.) and do not seem to differ from those found in noninfected patients (Bernaldez et al., 2005; Ugochukwu, Ezechukwu, Undie, & Akujobi, 2007; Verhoeff et al., 2006).

Symptoms and Diagnosis

Diagnosis of CSOM is made clinically by otoscopy, revealing otorrhea through a perforated tympanic membrane present for at least 6 weeks (Figure 9–8). Temporal CT scans are indicated in investigation of the disease. CSOM usually shows soft tissue density material in the middle ear without bone erosions (Figure 9–9). The presence of bone erosion may indicate cholesteatoma in the middle ear.

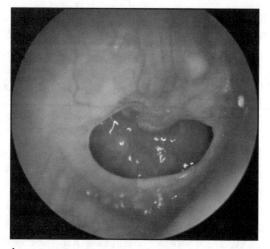

A

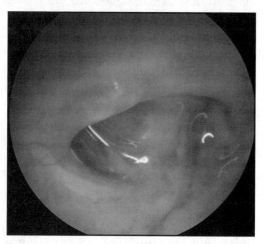

B

Figure 9–8. **A.** *Otoscopy* (right ear) *in a patient with chronic suppurative otitis media. Thickness of the mucosa in the middle ear and mild otorrhea can be seen through a perforation in the tympanic membrane.* **B.** *Otoscopy* (right ear) *in a patient with chronic suppurative otitis media. Polypoid mass and profuse otorrhea are seen in the middle ear through a wide perforation in the tympanic membrane.*

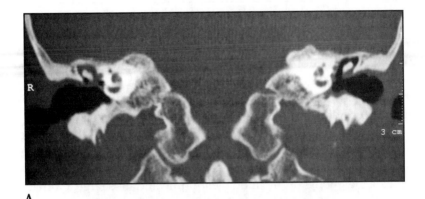

A

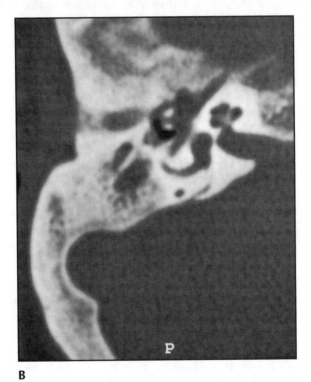

B

Figure 9–9. A. *Computed tomography scan* (coronal plane) *of a patient with HIV/AIDS revealing chronic suppurative otitis media. Soft tissue density material is seen in the middle ear, without bone erosion.* **B.** *Computed tomography scan* (axial plane) *of a patient with HIV/AIDS and chronic suppurative otitis media. Soft tissue density material is seen in the middle ear and mastoid cells, without bone erosion.*

Cholesteatoma is the presence of a destructive and expanding keratinizing squamous epithelium in the middle ear and/or mastoid process; a condition that requires surgery. Bernaldez, Morales, and Hernandez (2005) reported a 3.2% prevalence of cholesteatoma in children with HIV/AIDS and CSOM, but it does not necessarily seem that this condition is more prevalent in patients with HIV/AIDS.

The most common sequela of CSOM is hearing loss, either conductive or sensorineural, and this may affect young child's language development and school progress. Chronic infection of the middle ear, causing edema of the middle-ear lining and discharge, tympanic membrane perforation, and possibly ossicular chain disruption, results in a conductive hearing loss ranging from 20 to 60 dB (Verhoeff et al., 2006). Children who have HIV/AIDS and already face significant developmental challenges may be affected far worse by a resulting hearing loss and should be followed up as a matter of priority.

Management

Treatment of CSOM includes ear protection, aural toilet, ototopical drops, and systemic and surgical treatment. Patients, or their parents and caregivers, should be motivated to protect the infected ear with earplugs during showers and to avoid swimming or diving. Antibiotic or antiseptic eardrops, accompanied by aural toilet, are the initial recommended therapy, which can achieve dry ear in many patients. Topical quinolones (ofloxacin and ciprofloxacin) appear to be more effective than non-quinolone eardrops. Antiseptic drops, for example, aluminum acetate, boric acid, iodine powder, and povidone-iodine, commonly used for CSOM because of their low cost and availability, also are effective (Acuin, Smith, & Mackenzie, 1998). Systemic antibiotics are given both as initial therapy for CSOM and as secondary measure when topical therapy fails. Consensus is lacking as to which antibiotic to use systemically as well as about the duration of treatment in CSOM; both broad-spectrum antibiotics and culture-directed therapy have been advocated as initial oral therapy for CSOM (Verhoeff et al., 2006). When medical treatment fails to control infection in the middle ear and in those cases of CSOM with cholesteatoma, surgery is indicated. The overall success rate of surgical treatment, defined as dry ear plus an intact, mobile eardrum, may reach nearly 70%. Surgical criteria for otologic procedures should be applied to all patients, regardless of HIV status. Otolaryngologists must not withhold warranted surgical therapy because of the patient's HIV status (Kohan & Giacchi, 1999). Tympanomastoidectomy is the surgical treatment of choice in CSOM if indicated. We recommend that, in HIV-infected children, adenoidectomy should also be performed, since adenoid tissue in children with chronic and/or recurrent otitis media has been shown to contain mucosal biofilms in 54% of the cases and may contribute to inadequate functioning of eustachian tube (Kania et al., 2008).

Complications from Otitis Media

Nature and Etiology

Complications from otitis media can be classified into two major categories: intracranial (IC) and extracranial (EC). IC complications include meningitis, brain abscess (cerebral or cerebellar), extradural abscess, and sinus thrombosis; EC complications include acute mastoiditis, subperiosteal abscess, labyrinthitis, and facial paralysis.

Many authors have affirmed that otitis media complications are more common in patients with HIV/AIDS; however, it is uncertain if the immunodeficient state predisposes patients selectively to develop otitis media complications (Barnett et al., 1992; Shapiro & Novelli, 1998).

The primary ear disease underlying acute complication of OM in adult patients is more often chronic otitis media (COM) with or without cholesteatoma, and adults have more additional diseases than pediatric patients (Leskinen & Jero, 2005). Children are more likely to present with a complication to an episode of AOM in the form of mastoiditis. Complications in chronic ear disease usually follow an acute exacerbation of infection. In the progression of a middle-ear infection to an IC complication, spread may result from preformed pathways, haematogenously, and as a direct extension from the middle ear or mastoid.

The distribution of organisms in acute mastoiditis differs from that in AOM, with significantly higher rates of *S. aureus*, *S. coagulase* negative, and *S. pyogenes* and lower rates of *S. pneumoniae* and *Haemophilus influenzae*. The most common pathogens isolated from subperiosteal abscesses (SA) are *S. aureus, S. pyogenes, S. pneumoniae*, and *P. aeruginosa*. Microorganisms cultured from the external auditory canal or from the middle ear during myringotomy are not always the same pathogens isolated from the SA cavity (Luntz et al., 2001; Migirov & Kronemberg, 2004). In patients with COM and brain abscesses, multiple microorganisms are often isolated, with higher prevalence of anaerobic (including bacteroids) and gram negative as *Pseudomonas aeruginosa* and *Proteus mirabilis* (Kurien, Job, Mathew, & Chandy, 1998).

Diagnosis and Management

The wide use of available antibiotics has led to a notable decrease in the number of severe complications of otitis media and in the need for operative treatment. Petersen et al. (2007) have confirmed that the use of antibiotics reduces the risk of mastoiditis after otitis media. However, the number of episodes of AOM needed to treat to prevent one episode of mastoiditis was 4,064 (with 95% confidence interval between 2,393 and 13,456).

Complication (intra or extracranial) of otitis media should always be suspected in any HIV/AIDS patient or children with a history of chronic (more frequently) or acute otitis media presenting with high fever and signs or symptoms such as neck stiffness, severe headache, nausea and vomiting, postauricular tenderness, acute intense vertigo, facial paresis/paralysis, personality changes, as well as focal neurologic deficits. Table 9–5 summarizes some of the signs and symptoms of associated complications due to acute and chronic otitis media. A delay in the diagnosis and treatment of IC complication of otitis media can lead to increased morbidity and mortality.

If complication of otitis media is assumed as a possible diagnosis, temporal and cranial CT scans are mandatory. Brain, extradural, and subperiosteal abscesses will be evident in CT scans when enhanced by intravenous contrast. The use of contrast is also important in the diagnosis of sinus thrombosis. If IC abscesses are ruled out in patients with neck stiffness, severe headache, personality changes, or focal neurologic deficits, lumbar puncture, and CSF examination are indicated for diagnosis of meningitis. Temporal CT scans may reveal an underlying cholesteatoma that will require surgery.

Table 9–5. Signs and Symptoms Associated with
Complications of Chronic and Acute Otitis Media

High fever
Severe headache, nausea and vomiting
Postauricular tenderness
Acute intense vertigo
Facial paralysis
Personality changes
Focal neurologic deficits

Patients with complicated otitis media require hospitalization and intravenous antibiotics. Myringotomy at first examination with culturing of discharge is indicated in patients with complication of an AOM. Due to the high prevalence of *S. aureus* in mastoid subperiosteal abscesses (SA), early administration of anti-*Staphylococcus* medications in patients with SA as a complication of AOM and mastoiditis should be considered (Luntz et al., 2001; Migirov and Kronemberg, 2004). Operative treatment is recommended on patients with IC complications and abscess forming or prolonging intratemporal complications of otitis media (Leskinen & Jero, 2005). Strict surgical criteria for otologic procedures should be applied to all patients, regardless of HIV status. Otolaryngologists must not withhold warranted surgical therapy because of the patient's HIV status (Kohan & Giacchi, 1999). In suppurative otitis media with intracranial complications, craniotomy with concurrent mastoidectomy is safe and removes the source of infection at the same time that the complications are being treated. Treatment is completed with a single, short hospital stay (Kurien et al., 1998). The surgical outcome may correlate with the degree of immunocompromise in HIV/AIDS patients. Thus, a more protracted and complicated postoperative course may be expected in patients with low CD4 counts and severe ear disease. These patients may require more intensive medical therapy and monitoring (Kohan & Giacchi, 1999).

OPPORTUNISTIC INFECTIONS OF THE EXTERNAL AND MIDDLE EAR ASSOCIATED WITH HIV/AIDS

This section discusses the involvement of the external and middle ear by HIV associated opportunistic infections including otic pneumocystosis (*Pneumocystis jiroveci*), non-Hodgkin lymphoma and Kaposi's sarcoma.

Otic Pneumocystosis

Pneumocystis jiroveci (formerly *carinii*) is probably the most commonly found opportunistic agent in patients with HIV/AIDS (Madriz & Herrera, 1995). The most important site of infection by this agent is the lung, although extrapulmonary sites have been reported, such as the temporal bone (Kohan & Giacchi, 1999).

Middle ear and mastoid air cells are normally sterile. Infection at this anatomic site could develop by several routes. The area could become infected by haematogenous spread of infection, by extension of infection through lymphatic channels, by retrograde spread through the eustachian tube, or from the external auditory canal through the tympanic membrane. A hypothesis that explains ear infection by *Pneumocystis jiroveci* is the similar embryologic origin of the pulmonary alveoli and the mucosa of the tympanic membrane and middle ear epithelia (Praveen et al., 2002).

There are no reports of otic pneumocystosis in children; most reported cases are in men with average age of presentation being 33 years. Clinically, the patients present conductive hearing loss, otalgia, and otorrhea. Subcutaneous nodules and polyps in the external auditory meatus are present and the disease is uni- or bilateral. Most cases presented in the literature are primary extrapulmonary foci and pulmonary infection is not always present (Praveen et al., 2002; Rinaldo et al., 2003). Although most cases do not report destruction of the bone on CT scan imaging, there are cases where destruction of the ossicles and bony borders of the middle ear has been documented (Patel, Philpott, & McPartlin, 1999).

This opportunistic infection must be suspected in the presence of habitual treatment of external auditory meatus polyps. In these cases, a biopsy is required to exclude malignant processes from inflammatory disease and prevent a delay of early diagnosis and adequate management (Manger & Berg, 2003).

The disease responds well to established conventional therapy. Oral or intravenous trimethoprim sulfamethoxazole for at least 3 weeks is the drug of choice for otic pneumocystosis with the resultant resolution of polyps, cure of the mastoiditis, and tympanic membrane healing with minimal scarring. Other regimens include dapsone/trimethoprim and clindamycin/primaquine combinations, and atovaquone and pentamidine isethionate. Surgical excision of the otic masses or polyps may also be indicated (Mahlakwane, Ramdial, Sing, Calonje, & Biyana, 2008; Mofenson, Oleske, & Serchuck, 2004; Rinaldo et al., 2003).

Non-Hodgkin Lymphoma and Kaposi's Sarcoma

The presence of some cancers related to HIV infection, such as lymphomas and Kaposi's sarcoma have been reported in the literature with location in the middle ear or the temporal bone, but they are not as common as in other locations of the body (Michaels, Soucek, & Liang, 1994). Lymphoproliferative disease is the second most common HIV/AIDS related malignancy following Kaposi's sarcoma and is an AIDS-defining illness. Nearly one third of patients infected with HIV are expected to develop lymphoma (Kieserman & Finn, 1995; Finn, 1995). The lymphomas are mostly malignant non-Hodgkin lymphomas, and the increased risk for lymphoma in patients with HIV/AIDS appears to be related to multiple factors, including the transforming properties of the retrovirus itself, the immunosuppression and cytokine dysregulation that results from the disease, and most importantly, opportunistic infections with other lymphotrophic herpes viruses such as Epstein-Barr virus and human herpesvirus (Grogg, Miller, & Dogan, 2007; Levine, 1992).

However, the temporal bone is an extremely rare site of origin or involvement for lymphoma with a few case reports in medical literature (Goodarzi, Broberg, & Lalwani, 1998; Kieserman & Finn, 1995). Currently, following the introduction of highly active antiretroviral therapy, the risk for developing lymphoma in the context of HIV infection has decreased and the clinical outcome has improved (Grogg, Miller, & Dogan, 2007; Grulich et al., 2001).

Kaposi's sarcoma (KS) is more frequent in a temporal bone location than non-Hodgkin lymphomas. KS is an angioformative lesion characterized histologically by neoangiogenesis and proliferating spindle-shaped cells, admixed with a variable chronic inflammatory infiltrate. The development of all epidemiologic forms of KS (classic/sporadic, AIDS-associated/epidemic, and immunosuppression/iatrogenic-associated) depends largely on infection with KS herpesvirus/human herpesvirus-8 (KSHV/HHV-8). KS may occur in the ear in the form of diffuse or exophytic lesions in the ear pavilion, external auditory canal, tympanic membrane, and middle ear. When KS involves the auricles, the majority of those affected will prove to be HIV/AIDS patients (Centers for Disease Control [CDC], 1992; Rinaldo et al., 2003). Although rare, KS has been described in children with HIV/AIDS (Hadfield et al., 1996).

Persons coinfected with HIV and HHV-8 are at risk of experiencing KS, and evidence exists that progression to KS might be accelerated among persons who seroconvert to HHV-8 after being infected with HIV. Thus, preventing acquisition of HHV-8 infections among those already HIV-infected is important. Apparently, the major routes of HHV-8 transmission are oral, semen, and through blood by sharing needles. Patients should be counseled that deep kissing and sexual intercourse with persons who have high risk for being infected with HHV-8 might lead to acquisition of the agent that causes KS. HIV-infected persons should use latex condoms during every act of sexual intercourse. HIV-infected injection-drug users should be counseled not to share drug-injection equipment, even if both users are already HIV-infected, because of the chance of becoming infected with HHV-8 or other blood-borne pathogens. No recommendation can be made concerning use of drugs to prevent KS among persons coinfected with HIV and HHV-8 (CDC, 2002).

An estimated annual reduction of 39% (95% CI 35–43%) in the incidence of KS between 1994 and 2003 was seen on a large multicenter prospective study (Mocroft et al., 2004). After HAART introduction, the incidence was restricted to two cases per 1,000 persons with HIV/AIDS per year. Most individuals who developed KS while receiving HAART began treatment with low CD4 cell counts and developed KS within 6 months of the initiation of HAART. There continues to be an increased incidence of KS among homosexual men and a greatly reduced incidence of KS among patients with higher CD4 counts.

The treatment goals for KS include (1) symptom palliation; (2) shrinkage of tumor to alleviate edema, organ compromise, and psychologic stress; (3) prevention of disease progression; and (4) perhaps cure (Dezube, Pantanowitz, & Aboulafia, 2004; Di Lorenzo et al., 2007). Typical indications for systemic therapy include widespread skin involvement, extensive KS of the oral cavity, symptomatic pedal or scrotal edema, symptomatic visceral involvement, and immune reconstitution inflammatory syndrome-induced KS flare. Although several chemotherapeutic agents (e.g., bleomycin, vinblastine, vincristine, doxorubicin, and etoposide) were noted to be efficacious against KS in the past, current systemic cytotoxic therapy comprises liposomal anthracyclines (PLD and liposomal daunorubicin) and taxanes (paclitaxel) (Dezube et al., 2004; Di Lorenzo et al., 2007; Pantanowitz, 2008). A CO_2 laser may be used for lesions involving the external auditory canal, while an argon laser is preferred when the lesion involves the external auditory canal and the tympanic membrane because the tumor may be ablated without causing perforation of the eardrum (Rinaldo et al., 2003).

SUMMARY

The occurrence of disease in both the external and middle ear are relatively common in patients with HIV/AIDS, especially in children. In our experience, the incidence of such involvement may be well beyond one in every three cases. The complications due to these conditions may also be more common and severe due to the immune suppressed state of patients with HIV/AIDS and therefore require prompt detection and timely treatment. It is important to note that the advent of HAART has dramatically reduced the infection produced by opportunistic agents and decreased the incidence of complications and the possibility of chronic otitis media. But a vigilant and proactive approach to identification, diagnosis, management and follow-up of these otologic conditions in patients with HIV/AIDS is important. In this way, secondary complications that may lead to permanent or prolonged conductive hearing loss, and even increased morbidity and mortality among children and adults with HIV/AIDS, may be prevented.

REFERENCES

Acuin, J., Smith, A., & Mackenzie, I. (1998). Interventions for chronic suppurative otitis media. *Cochrane Database of Systematic Reviews, 2*, CD000473.

Agius, A. M., Pickles, J. M., & Burch, K. L. (1992). A prospective study of otitis externa. *Clinical Otolaryngology, 17*, 150.

American Academy of Family Physicians [AAFP]; American Academy of Otolaryngology-Head and Neck Surgery [AAOHNS]; American Academy of Pediatrics [AAP] Subcommittee on Otitis Media With Effusion. (2004). Otitis media with effusion. *Pediatrics, 113*, 1412-1429.

American Academy of Pediatrics [AAP] Subcommittee on Management of Acute Otitis Media. (2004). Diagnosis and management of acute otitis media. *Pediatrics, 113*, 1451-1465.

Barnett, E. D., Kline, J. O., Pelton, S. I., & Lunginbuhl, L. M. (1992). Otitis media in children born to human immunodeficiency virus-infected mothers. *Pediatric Infectious Diseases Journal, 11*, 360-364.

Barza, M. (1988). Pharmacokinetics and efficacy of the new quinolones in infections of the eye, ear, nose, and throat. *Reviews of Infectious Diseases, 10*(Suppl. 1), S241-S2477.

Bayardelle, P., Jolivet-Granger, M., & Larochelle, D. (1982). Staphylococcal malignant external otitis. *Canadian Medical Association Journal, 126*, 155.

Beers, S. L., & Abramo, T. J. (2004). Otitis externa review. *Pediatrics Emergency Care, 20*, 250-256.

Berenholz, L., Katzenell, U., & Harell, M. (2002). Evolving resistant Pseudomonas to ciprofloxacin in malignant otitis externa. *Laryngoscope, 112*, 1619.

Bernaldez, P., Morales, G., & Hernandez, C. (2005). Chronic suppurative otitis media in HIV-infected children. *Otolaryngology-Head and Neck Surgery, 133*(Suppl. 1), 243-244.

Bernstein, J. M., Holland, N. J., Porter, G. C., & Maw, A. R. (2007). Resistance of *Pseudomonas aureginosa* to ciprofloxacin: Implications for the treatment of malignant otitis externa. *Journal of Laryngology and Otology, 121*, 118-123.

Bertin, L., Pons, G., d'Athis, P., Duhamel, J. F., Maudelonde, C., Lasfargues, G., et al. (1996). A randomized, double-blind, multicentre controlled trial of ibuprofen versus acetaminophen and placebo for symptoms of acute otitis media in children. *Fundamental and Clinical Pharmacology, 10*, 387-392.

Bluestone, C. D. (1998). Epidemiology and pathogenesis of chronic suppurative otitis media: Implications for prevention and treatment. *International Journal of Pediatric Otorhinolaryngology, 42*, 207-223.

Brody, R., Singh, B., Lee, D., & Sperling, N. (2000). Management of otitis media with effusion in HIV-infected patients. *Otolaryngology-Head and Neck Surgery, 115,* 149.

Brook, I. (1980). Microbiological studies of the bacterial flora of the external auditory canal in children. *Acta Oto-laryngologica, 91,* 285.

Centers for Diseases Control. (1992). 1993 Revised classification system for HIV infection and expanded surveillance case definition for AIDS among adolescents and adults. *MMWR: Morbidity and Mortality Weekly Report, 41*(RR-17).

Centers for Diseases Control. (2002). Guidelines for preventing opportunistic infections among HIV-infected persons—2002. *MMWR: Morbidity and Mortality Weekly Report, 51* (RR-8).

Chaloryoo, S., Chotpitayasunondh, T., & Chiengmai, P. E. (1998). AIDS in ENT in children. *International Journal of Pediatric Otorhinolaryngology, 44,* 103–107.

Chandler, J. R. (1968). Malignant external otitis. *Laryngoscope, 78,* 1257.

Chandrasekhar, S. S., Conelly, P. E., Brahmbhatt, S. S., Shah, C. S., Kloser, P. C., & Baredes, S. (2000). Otologic and audilogic evaluation of human immunodeficiency virus-infected patients. *American Journal of Otolaryngology, 21,* 1–9.

Chandrasekhar, S. S., Siverls, V., & Chandrasekhar, H. K. (1992). Histopatologic and ultrastructural changes in the temporal bones of HIV-infected human adults. *American Journal of Otology, 13,* 207–214.

Chen, A. Y., Ohlms, L., Stewart, M., & Kline, M. (1996). Otolaryngologic disease progression in children with human immunodeficiency virus infection. *Archives of Otolaryngology-Head and Neck Surgery, 122,* 1360–1363.

Coser, P. L., Stamm, A. E., Lobo, R. C., & Pinto, J. A. (1980). Malignant external otitis in infants. *Laryngoscope, 90,* 312.

Cunningham, M., Yu, V. L., Turner, J., & Curtin, H. (1988). Necrotizing otitis externa due to Aspergillus in an immunocompetent patient. *Archives of Otolaryngology-Head and Neck Surgery, 114,* 554.

Dagan, R., Hoberman, A., Johnson, C., Leibovitz, E. L., Arguedas, A., Rose, F. V., et al. (2001). Bacteriologic and clinical efficacy of high dose amoxicillin/clavulanate in children with acute otitis media. *Pediatric Infectious Diseases Journal, 20,* 829–837.

Dezube, B. J., Pantanowitz, L., & Aboulafia, D. M. (2004). Management of AIDS-related Kaposi'ss sarcoma: Advances in target discovery and treatment. *AIDS Reader, 14,* 236–253.

Di Lorenzo, G., Konstantinopoulos, P. A., Pantanowitz, L., Di Trolio, R., De Placido, S., & Dezube, B. J. (2007). Management of AIDS-related Kaposi's sarcoma. *Lancet Oncology, 8,* 167–176.

Favero, M. S., Carson, L. A., Bond, W. W., & Petersen, N. J. (1971). *Pseudomonas aeruginosa*: Growth in distilled water from hospitals. *Science, 173,* 836.

Finer, G., Greenberg, D., Leibovitz, E. Leiberman, A., Shelef, I., & Kapelushnik, J. (2002). Conservative treatment of malignant (invasive) external otitis caused by Aspergillus flavus with oral itraconazole solution in a neutropenic patient. *Scandinavian Journal of Infectious Diseases, 34,* 227.

Finn, D. G. (1995). Lymphoma of the head and neck and acquired immunodeficiency syndrome: Clinical investigation and immunohistochemical study. *Laryngoscope, 105,* 1–18.

Gates, G. A., Avery, C. A., Prihoda, T. J., & Cooper J. C., Jr. (1987). Effectiveness of adenoidectomy and tympanostomy tubes in the treatment of chronic otitis media with effusion. *New England Journal of Medicine, 317,* 1444–1451.

Godofsky, E. W., Zinreich, J., Armstrong, M., Leslie, J. M., & Weickel, C. S. (1992). Sinusitis in HIV-infected patients: A clinical and radiographic review. *American Journal of Medicine, 93,* 163–170.

Gondim, L. A., Zonta, R. F., Fortkamp, E., & Schmeling, R. O. (2000). Otorhinolaryngological manifestations in children with human immunodeficiency virus infection. *International Journal of Pediatric Otorhinolaryngology, 54,* 97–102.

Goodarzi, M. O., Broberg, T. G., & Lalwani, A. K. (1998). Lymphoma of the tympanic membrane in acquired immunodeficiency syndrome. *Auris Nasus Larynx, 25,* 89–94.

Grandis, J. R., Branstetter, B. F., & Yu, V. L. (2004). The changing face of malignant (necrotising) external otitis: Clinical, radiological, and anatomic correlations. *Lancet Infectious Diseases, 4,* 34–39.

Grandis, J. R., Curtin, H. D., & Yu, V. L. (1995). Necrotizing (malignant) external otitis: Prospective comparison of CT and MR imaging in diagnosis and follow-up. *Radiology, 196,* 499.

Griffin, G. H., Flynn, C., Bailey, R. E., & Schultz, J. K. (2006). Antihistamines and/or decongestants for otitis media with effusion (OME) in children. *Cochrane Database of Systematic Reviews, 18,* CD003423.

Grogg, K. L., Miller, R. F., & Dogan, A. (2007). HIV infection and lymphoma. *Journal of Clinical Pathology, 60*(12), 1365–1372.

Grulich, A. E., Li, Y., McDonald, A. M., Correll, P. K., Law, M. G., & Kaldor, J. M. (2001). Decreasing rates of Kaposi's sarcoma and non-Hodgkin's lymphoma in the era of potent combination anti-retroviral therapy. *AIDS, 15*(5), 629–633.

Gurney, T. A., & Murr, A. (2003). Otolaryngology manifestations of human immunodeficiency virus infection. *Otolaryngology Clinics of North America, 36,* 607–624.

Guthrie, R. M. (1999). Diagnosis and treatment of acute otitis externa: An interdisciplinary update. *Annals of Otology Rhinology and Laryngology, 17,* 2–23.

Hadfield, P. J., Birchall, M. A., Novelli, V., & Bailey, C. M. (1996). The ENT manifestations of HIV infection in children. *Clinical Otolaryngology and Allied Sciences, 21,* 30–36.

Hern, J. D., Almeyda, J., Thomas, D. M., Main, J., & Patel, K. S. (1996). Malignant otitis externa in HIV and AIDS. *Journal of Laryngology and Otology, 110,* 770–775.

Ho, T., Vrabec, J. T., Yoo, D., & Coker, N. J. (2006). Otomycosis: Clinical features and treatment implications. *Otolaryngology-Head and Neck Surgery, 135,* 787–791.

Hubbard, T. W., Paradise, J. L., McWilliams, B. J., Elster, B. A., & Taylor, F. H. (1985). Consequences of unremitting middle-ear disease in early life. Otologic, audiologic, and developmental findings in children with cleft palate. *New England Journal of Medicine, 312,* 1529–1534.

Hurst, W. B. (2001). Outcome of 22 cases of perforated tympanic membrane caused by otomycosis. *Journal of Laryngology and Otology, 115,* 879–880.

Ismail, H., Hellier, W. P., & Batty, V. (2004). Use of magnetic resonance imaging as the primary imaging modality in the diagnosis and follow-up of malignant external otitis. *Journal of Laryngology and Otology, 118,* 576.

Jerger, J. (1970). Clinical experience with impedance audiometry. *Archives of Otolaryngology, 92,* 311–324.

Kaur, R., Mittal, N., Kakkar, M., Aggarwal, A. K., & Mathur, M. D. (2000). Otomycosis: A clinicomycologic study. *Ear, Nose, and Throat Journal, 79,* 606–609.

Kania, R. E., Lamers, G. E., Vonk, M. J., Dorpmans, E., Struik, J., Tran Ba Huy, P., et al. (2008). Characterization of mucosal biofilms on human adenoid tissues. *Laryngoscope, 118,* 128–134.

Kielhofner, M., Atmar, R. L., Hamill, R. J., & Musher, D. M. (1992). Life-threatening *Pseudomonas aeruginosa* infections in patients with human immunodeficiency virus infection. *Clinical Infectious Diseases, 14,* 403–411.

Kieserman S. P., & Finn, D. G. (1995). Non-Hodgkin's lymphoma of the external auditory canal in an HIV-positive patient. *Journal of Laryngology and Otology, 109,* 751–754.

Kohan, D., & Giacchi, R. J. (1999). Otologic surgery in patients with HIV-1 and AIDS. *Otolaryngology-Head and Neck Surgery, 121,* 355–360.

Koopman, L., Hoes, A. W., Glasziou, P. P., Appelman, C. L., Burke, P., McCormick, D., et al. (2008). Antibiotic therapy to prevent the development of asymptomatic middle ear effusion in children with acute otitis media: A meta-analysis of individual patient data. *Archives of Otolaryngology-Head and Neck Surgery, 134,* 128–132.

Kurien, M., Job, A., Mathew, J., & Chandy, M. (1998). Otogenic intracranial abscess concurrent craniotomy and mastoidectomy—changing trends in a developing country. *Archives of Otolaryngology-Head and Neck Surgery, 124,* 1353–1356.

Lacarte, M. P. R., & Segura, F. P. (1990). Malignant otitis externa and HIV antibodies. A case report. *Anales Otorrinolaringologicos Ibero-Americanos, 17,* 505.

Leibovitz, E., Piglansky, L., Raiz, S., Press, J., Leiberman, A., & Dagan, R. (2000). Bacteriologic and clinical efficacy of one day vs. three day intramuscular ceftriaxone for treatment of nonresponsive acute otitis media in children. *Pediatric Infectious Diseases Journal, 19,* 1040–1045.

Leskinen, K., & Jero, J. (2005). Acute complications of otitis media in adults. *Clinical Otolaryngology, 30,* 511–516.

Levenson, M. J., Parisier, S. C., Dolitsky, J., & Bindra, G. (1991). Ciprofloxacin: Drug of choice in the treatment of malignant external otitis (MEO). *Laryngoscope, 101,* 821–824.

Levin, W. J., Shary, J. H., Nichols 3rd, L. T., & Lucente, F. E. (1986). Bone scanning in severe external otitis. *Laryngoscope, 96,* 1193.

Levine, A. M. (1992). AIDS-associated malignant lymphoma. *Medical Clinics of North America, 76,* 253–268.

Luntz, M., Brodsky, A., Nusem, S., Kronenberg, J., Keren, G., Migirov, L., et al. (2001). Acute mastoiditis—the antibiotic era: A multicenter study. *International Journal of Pediatric Otorhinolaryngology, 57,* 1–9.

Lyos, A. T., Malpica, A., Estrada, R., Katz, C. D., & Jenkins, H. A. (1993). Invasive aspergillosis of the temporal bone: An unusual manifestation of acquired immunodeficiency syndrome. *American Journal of Otolaryngology, 14,* 444.

Madriz, J. J., & Herrera, G. (1995). Human immunodeficiency virus and acquired immune deficiency syndrome AIDS-related hearing disorders. *Journal of the American Academy of Audiology, 6,* 358–364.

Mahlakwane, M. S., Ramdial, P. K., Sing, Y., Calonje, E., & Biyana, S. (2008). Otic pneumocystosis in acquired immune deficiency syndrome. *American Journal of Surgical Pathology, 32,* 1038–1043.

Makokha, E. P., Ogolla, M., Orago, A. S., Koech, D. K., Mpoke, S., Esamai, F., et al. (2003). CD4 T lymphocyte subsets and disease manifestation in children with and without HIV born to HIV-infected mothers. *East African Medical Journal, 80,* 95–100.

Mandel, E. M., Casselbrant, M. L., Rockette, H. E., Fireman, P., Kurs-Lasky, M., & Bluestone, C. D. (2002). Systemic steroid for chronic otitis media with effusion in children. *Pediatrics, 110,* 1071–1080.

Manger, D. J., & Berg, R. G. (2003). *Pneumocystis carinii* infection of the middle ear and external auditory canal. Report of a case and review of the literature. *ORL Journal for Oto-Rhino-Laryngology and Its Related Specialties, 65,* 49–51.

Mani, N., Sudhoff, H., Rajagopal, S., Moffat, D., & Axon, P. R. (2007). Cranial nerve involvement in malignant external otitis: Implications for clinical outcome. *Laryngoscope, 117*, 907.

Marchisio, P., Principi, N., Sorella, S., Sala, E., & Tornaghi, R. (1996). Etiology of acute otitis media in human immunodeficiency virus-infected children. *Pediatric Infectious Diseases Journal, 15*, 58-61.

McElroy, E. A., Jr., & Marks, G. L. (1991). Fatal necrotizing otitis externa in a patient with AIDS. *Reviews of Infectious Diseases, 13*, 1246.

Meltzer, P. E., & Kelemen, G. (1959). Pyocutaneous osteomyelitis of the temporal bone, mandible, and zygoma. *Laryngoscope, 169*, 1300-1316.

Michaels, L., Soucek, S., & Liang, J. (1994). The ear in the acquired immunodeficiency syndrome: I. Temporal bone histopatologic study. *American Journal of Otology, 15*, 515-522.

Migirov, L., & Kronenberg, J. (2004). Bacteriology of mastoid subperiosteal abscess in children. *Acta Otolaryngologica, 124*, 23-25.

Miziara, I. D., & Valentini-Junior, M. (1999). Doença de causa Otorrinolaringológica em pacientes com AIDS. *Jornal Brasileiro de Medicina (Brazilian Journal of Medicine), 76*, 24-34.

Miziara, I. D., Weber, R., Cunha-Filho, B. A., & Pinheiro-Neto, C. D. (2007). Otitis media in Brazilian human immunodeficiency virus infected children undergoing antiretroviral therapy. *Journal of Laryngolology and Otology, 121*, 1048-1055.

Moazzez, A. H., & Alvi, A. (1998). Head and neck manifestations of AIDS in adults. *American Family Physician, 57*, 1813-1824.

Mocroft, A., Kirk, O., Clumeck, N. Gargalianos-Kakolyris, P. Trocha, H., Chentsova, N., et al. (2004). The changing pattern of Kaposi sarcoma in patients with HIV, 1994-2003. *Cancer, 100*, 2644-2654.

Mofenson, L. M., Oleske, J., & Serchuck, L. (2004). Treating opportunistic infections among HIV-exposed and infected children: Recommendations from CDC, the National Institutes of Health, and the Infectious Diseases Society of America. *MMWR Recommendations and Reports, 53*(RR-14), 1-92.

Muñoz, A., & Martinez-Chamorro, E. (1998). Necrotizing external otitis caused by *Aspergillus fumigatus*: Computed tomography and high-resolution magnetic resonance imaging in an AIDS patient. *Journal of Laryngology and Otology, 112*, 98.

Nachman, S., Kim, S., King, J., Abrams, E., Margolis, D., Petru, A., et al. (2003). Safety and immunogenicity of a heptavalent pneumococcal conjugate vaccine in infants with human immunodeficiency virus type 1 infection. *Pediatrics, 112*, 66-73.

Newton, J. P. (2006). The causes of hearing loss in HIV infection. *Community Ear and Hearing Health, 3*, 1-16.

Niemela, M., Uhari, M., Jounio-Ervasti, K., Luotonen, J., Alho, O. P., & Vierimaa, E. (1994). Lack of specific symptomatology in children with acute otitis media. *Pediatric Infectious Diseases Journal, 13,* 765–768.

Osguthorpe, J. D., & Nielsen, D. R. (2006). Otitis externa: Review and clinical update. *American Academy Physician, 74,* 1510–1516.

Ozcan, K. M., Ozcan, M., Karaarslan, A., & Karaarslan, F. (2003). Otomycosis in Turkey: Predisposing factors, aetiology and therapy. *Journal of Laryngology and Otology, 117,* 39–42.

Pantanowitz, L. (2008). Kaposi sarcoma: Appraisal of therapeutic agents. *Cancer, 112,* 962–965.

Paramsothy, M., Khanijow, V., & Ong, T. O. (1997). Use of gallium-67 in the assessment of response to antibiotic therapy in malignant otitis externa —a case report. *Singapore Medical Journal, 38,* 347.

Patel, S. K., Philpott, J. M., & McPartlin, D. W. (1999). An unusual case of *Pneumocystis carinii* presenting as an aural mass. *Journal of Laryngology and Otology, 113,* 555–557.

Paul, A. C., Justus, A., Balraj, A., Job, A., & Kirubakaran, C. P. (2001). Malignant otitis externa in an infant with selective IgA deficiency: A case report. *International Journal of Pediatric Otorhinolaryngology, 60,* 141–145.

Petersen, I., Johnson, A. M., Islam, A., Duckworth, G., Livermore, D. M., & Hayward A. C. (2007). Protective effect of antibiotics against serious complications of common respiratory tract infections: Retrospective cohort study with the UK General Practice Research Database. *British Medical Journal, 335,* 982–987.

Petrak, R. M., Pottage, J. C., & Levin, S. (1985). Invasive external otitis caused by Aspergillus fumigatus in an immunocompromised patient. *Journal of Infectious Diseases, 151,* 196.

Piglansky, L., Leibovitz, E., Raiz, S., Greenberg, D., Press, J., Leiberman A., & Dagan, R. (2003). Bacteriologic and clinical efficacy of high dose amoxicillin for therapy of acute otitis media in children. *Pediatric Infectious Diseases Journal, 22,* 405–413.

Post, J. C., Stoodley, P., Hall-Stoodley, L., & Ehrlich, G. D. (2004). The role of biofilms in otolaryngologic infections. *Current Opinion in Otolaryngology-Head and Neck Surgery, 12,* 185–190.

Prasad, H. K., Bhojwani, K. M., Shenoy, V., & Prasad, S. C. (2006). HIV manifestations in otolaringology. *American Journal of Otolaryngology, 27,* 179–185.

Praveen, C. V., Terry, R. M., Elmahallawy, M., & Horsfield, C. (2002). Pneumocystis carinii infection in bilateral aural polyps in a human immunodeficiency virus-positive patient. *Journal of Laryngology and Otology, 116,* 288–290.

Ramakrishnan, K., Sparks, R. A., & Berryhill, W. E. (2007). Diagnosis and treatment of otitis media. *American Academy of Family Physician, 76,* 1650–1660.

Raza, S. A., Denholm, S. W., & Wong, J. C. (1995). An audit of the management of otitis externa in an ENT casualty clinic. *Journal of Laryngology and Otology, 109*, 130–133.

Reiss, P., Hadderingh, R., Schot, L. J., & Danner, S. A. (1991). Invasive external otitis caused by Aspergillus fumigatus in two patients with AIDS. *AIDS, 5*, 605.

Ress, B. D., Luntz, M., Telischi, F., Balkany, T. J., & Whiteman, M. L. H. (1997). Necrotizing external otitis in patients with AIDS. *Laryngoscope, 107*, 456–460.

Rinaldo, A., Brandwein, M., Devaney, K., & Ferlito, A. (2003). AIDS-related otological lesions. *Acta Oto-laryngologica, 123*, 672–674.

Rodriguez, J. A. G., Martinez, I. M., Gonzalez, J. L. G., Macías, A. R., & Alburquerque, T. L. (1992). A case of malignant external otitis involving Klebsiella oxytoca. *European Journal of Clinical Microbiology and Infectious Diseases, 11*, 75.

Roland, P. S., & Stroman, D. W. (2002). Microbiology of acute otitis externa. *Laryngoscope, 112*, 1166–1177.

Rosenfeld, R. M., Brown, L., Cannon, C. R., Dolor, R. J., Ganiats, T. G., Hannley, M., et al. (2006). Clinical practice guideline: Acute otitis externa. *Otolaryngology-Head and Neck Surgery, 134*(4 Suppl.), S4–S23.

Rosenfeld, R. M., & Kay, D. (2003). Natural history of untreated otitis media. *Laryngoscope, 113*, 1645–1657.

Rowlands, S., Devalia, H., Smith, C., Hubbard, R., & Dean, A. (2001). Otitis externa in UK general practice: A survey using the UK General Practice Research Database. *British Journal of General Practice, 51*, 533–538.

Rubin, J., Curtin, H. D., Yu, V. L., & Kamerer, D. B. (1990). Malignant external otitis: Utility of CT in diagnosis and follow-up. *Radiology, 174*, 391.

Rubin, J., & Yu, V. L. (1988). Malignant external otitis: Insights into pathogenesis, clinical manifestations, diagnosis, and therapy. *American Journal of Medicine, 85*, 391.

Rubin, J., Yu, V. L., Kamerer, D. B., & Wagener, M. (1990). Aural irrigation with water: A potential pathogenic mechanism for inducing malignant external otitis? *Annals of Otology, Rhinology and Laryngology, 99*, 117.

Rubin, J., Yu, V. L., & Stool, S. E. (1988). Malignant external otitis in children. *Journal of Pediatrics, 113*, 965–970.

Russell, J. D., Donnelly, M., & McShane, D. P. (1993). What causes otitis externa? *Journal of Laryngology and Otology, 107*, 898.

Shapiro, L. N., & Novelli, V. (1998). Otitis media in children with vertically acquired HIV infection: The Great Ormond Street Hospital experience. *International Journal of Pediatric Otorhinolaryngology, 45*, 69–75.

Shupak, A., Greenberg, E., Hardoff, R., Gordon, C. Melamed, Y., & Meyer, W. S. (1989). Hyperbaric oxygenation for necrotizing (malignant) otitis externa. *Archives of Otolaryngology-Head and Neck Surgery, 115,* 1470.

Singh, A., Georgalas, C., Patel, N., & Papesch, M. (2003). ENT presentations in children with HIV infection. *Clinical Otolaryngology, 28,* 240-243.

Sreepada, G. S., & Kwartler, J. A. (2003). Skull base osteomyelitis secondary to malignant otitis externa. *Current Opinion in Otolaryngology-Head and Neck Surgery, 11,* 316.

Stenfors, L. E., & Räisänen, S. (2002). Quantity of aerobic bacteria in the bony portion of the external auditory canal of children. *International Journal of Pediatric Otorhinolaryngology, 66,* 167-173.

Stern, C. S., Shah, M. K., & Lucente, F. E. (1988). In vitro effectiveness of 13 agents in otomycosis and review of the literature. *Laryngoscope, 98,* 1173-1177.

Stern, J. C., & Lucente, F. E. (1988). Otomycosis. *Ear, Nose, and Throat Journal, 67,* 804-810.

Stokkel, M. P., Boot, C. N., & van Eck-Smit, B. L. (1996). SPECT gallium scintigraphy in malignant external otitis: Initial staging and follow-up. Case reports. *Laryngoscope, 106,* 338.

Strauss, M., & Fine, E. (1991). *Aspergillus* otomastoiditis in acquired immunodeficiency syndrome. *American Journal of Otology, 12,* 40-53.

Ugochukwu, E. F., Ezechukwu, C. C., Undie, N., & Akujobi, C. (2007). Pattern of pathogens in ear discharge of HIV-infected children in Nnewi, Southeast Nigeria. *Nigerian Journal of Clinical Practice, 10*(2), 130-136.

Vennewald, I., Schonlebe, J., & Klemm, E. (2003). Mycological and histological investigations in humans with middle ear infections. *Mycoses, 46,* 12-18.

Verhoeff, M., van der Veen, E. L., Rovers, M. M., Sanders, E. A., & Schilder, A. G. (2006). Chronic suppurative otitis media: A review. *International Journal of Pediatric Otorhinolaryngology, 70,* 1-12.

Weber, R., Pinheiro Neto, C. D., Miziara, I. D., & Araújo Filho, B. C. (2006). HAART impact on prevalence of chronic otitis media in Brazilian HIV-infected children. *Brazilian Journal of Otorrhinolayngology (Engl Ed), 72,* 509-514.

Weinroth, S. E., Schessel, D., & Tuazon, C. U. (1994). Malignant otitis externa in AIDS patients: Case report and review of the literature. *Ear, Nose, and Throat Journal, 73,* 772.

Wiseman, L. R., & Balfour, J. A. (1994). Ciprofloxacin. A review of its pharmacological profile and therapeutic use in the elderly. *Drugs and Aging, 4,* 145-173.

Yao, M., & Messner, A. (2001). Fungal malignant otitis externa due to Scedosporium apiospermum. *Annals of Otology, Rhinology and Laryngology, 110,* 377-380.

Zucotti, G., Dauria, E., Torcoletti, M., Lodi, F., Bernardo, L., & Riva, E. (2001). Clinical and pro-host effects of cefaclor in prophylaxis of recurrent otitis media in HIV-infected children. *Journal of International Medical Research, 29,* 349–354.

Zuniga, J. M. (1999) Communication disorders and HIV disease. *The Body, 17.* Retrieved November 22, 2008, from http://www.thebody.com/content/art12344.html

CHAPTER 10

Sensory and Neural Auditory Disorders Associated With HIV/AIDS

Natalie Stearn
De Wet Swanepoel

INTRODUCTION

Infection with human immunodeficiency virus (HIV) is a growing global health care concern with millions of people living with the infection. Its destructive influence on the human immune response system, which leads to acquired immune deficiency syndrome (AIDS), has a pervasive effect on the health of affected individuals. The auditory system is one of the many faculties associated with abnormalities related to HIV/AIDS, which leads to compromised auditory functioning. There are three broad categories by which HIV/AIDS can compromise auditory functioning, including pathology related to the conductive, sensory, or neural structures underlying hearing. Chapter 9 focused on the conductive auditory pathologies related to HIV/AIDS. This chapter considers the sensory and neural auditory pathologies associated with HIV/AIDS, including identification, diagnosis, and intervention for these conditions.

ANATOMY AND PHYSIOLOGY UNDERLYING
AUDITORY PATHOLOGY

The auditory system is divided into four basic systems. These include the outer ear, middle ear, inner ear, and the central auditory pathways. The outer ear funnels acoustic energy in the form of compressed air particles traveling as waves to the middle ear where the energy is changed to mechanical energy at the eardrum and ossicular chain, which in turn converts the signal to hydraulic energy in the inner ear.

The inner ear, otherwise known as the cochlea, is shaped in an upward spiral-like bony labyrinth with a membranous labyrinth on the inside. The cochlea is tonotopically organized, which means it is sensitive to specific frequencies at various intervals along its spiral-like turns. The hydraulic energy stimulates the hair cells along the tonotopically arranged cochlea at specific frequencies where action potentials are initiated by the hair cells. The cochlea is the sensory organ of the auditory system where acoustical signals are transferred to action potentials. These action potentials are representative of the frequency and temporal (time) characteristics of the auditory signal and subsequently travel through the auditory nerve (eighth cranial nerve) and enter the brainstem.

From the brainstem, the neural fibers project toward the cerebral cortex at the temporal lobe switching back and forth from each side of the brainstem with neurons multiplying in number at each nucleus along the way. Information from the right ear is directed to the left temporal lobe and from the left ear to the right temporal lobe with an additional transfer of information from one side of the brain to the other. The auditory nerves projecting from the cochlea to the brainstem constitute the peripheral auditory nervous system, and those projecting from the brainstem to the cortex constitute the central nervous system. Pathology in these structures therefore is referred to as neural based, whereas pathology in the cochlea is referred to as sensory based. In many cases of hearing loss, it is difficult to differentiate accurately whether a hearing problem is of a sensory or neural origin, and in fact it often may be both. Therefore, the term sensorineural is commonly used to specify both sensory and neural origins or merely reflect a lack of specificity in terms of site of lesion.

PREVALENCE OF AUDITORY DISORDERS ASSOCIATED WITH HIV/AIDS

As many as 75% of adults with AIDS experience some kind of auditory dysfunction as a result of the HIV infection, opportunistic coinfections, and combinations of therapies that are ototoxic (Zuniga, 1999). Exact prevalence rates for sensory and neural auditory disorders in individuals infected with HIV/AIDS, however, are difficult to establish due to significant variability between available reports. This may be attributed to the following reasons. First, the prevalence of auditory symptoms in individuals with HIV/AIDS may be underreported due to the concomitance of more overt, life-threatening conditions (Bankaitis & Keith, 1995). Prior to highly active antiretroviral therapy (HAART), many HIV-infected individuals focused on life-threatening complications of HIV, rather than quality of life issues. Hearing loss, therefore, was not accurately reported. Individuals who have benefited from HAART may now become more conscious of quality of life issues, such as hearing loss (Zuniga, 1999). Second, middle ear effusion due to otitis media, which is commonly associated with HIV, severely confounds the identification of sensory and neural hearing loss (Rinaldo, 2003). Serous otitis media and recurrent acute otitis media are the most common otologic problems in HIV-infected individuals. Otitis media, although uncommon in immunocompetent adults, may affect between 8 to 23% of the HIV-infected population (Chandrasekhar et al., 2000; Rinaldo et al., 2003; Truitt & Tami, 1999). In addition to hearing loss, as many as 46% of adults with HIV infection complain about tinnitus and 30% complain of vertigo (Marra et al. 1997).

Children infected with HIV/AIDS are particularly likely to suffer from middle ear effusion compared to immunocompetent children, and with greater severity (Hoare, 2003; Rinaldo, 2003). Reports indicate that between 18 to 50% of all children infected with HIV/AIDS may have conductive hearing loss at any given time and this probably is significantly higher for infants (Chaloryoo, Chotpitayasunondh, & Chiengmai, 1998; McNeilly, 2005; Singh et al. 2003). All children infected with HIV/AIDS will present with at least one or more episodes of otitis media, whereas only 70% of immunocompetent individuals will present with one or more episodes of otitis media during childhood. Furthermore, it is reported that 80% of HIV-infected children will present with three to six or more episodes of otitis media during childhood, whereas only approximately 30% of healthy children will present with three or more episodes of otitis media (Zuniga, 1999).

Middle ear effusion causes conductive hearing loss of a mild to moderate degree in six out of every seven children, which confounds prevalence figures of true sensory and neural hearing losses in HIV-infected individuals (Hoare, 2003). Carefully controlled studies are necessary to establish the exact prevalence of HIV-related sensory and neural hearing disorders (Bankaitis & Keith, 1995; Chandrasekhar et al., 2000).

Despite prevalence figures of sensory and neural hearing loss being confounded by middle ear effusion, the reported occurrence remains high, varying between 20 and 50% (Bankaitis & Keith, 1995; Khoza & Ross, 2002; Madriz & Herrera, 1995; Marra et al. 1997; Matas et al., 2006; Moazzez & Alvi, 1998; Roland et al., 2003). Reports do not always differentiate between sensory and neural hearing loss and they often are jointly referred to as sensorineural hearing loss. Despite the difficult task of differentiating between conductive hearing loss and sensorineural hearing loss as broad categories, it becomes even more complicated to try to differentiate between sensory and neural hearing loss. To differentiate these requires at least the use of auditory brainstem response testing (ABR) with rarefaction and condensation stimuli. In a review of available studies on prevalence data, these distinctions often are not specified.

In a study of pure-tone audiometry and ABR testing in adults with HIV/AIDS, 33% of participants presented with abnormal audiometry, whereas 56% of participants showed abnormal ABR findings (Castro et al., 2000). The increased percentage of abnormal ABR findings, in comparison to abnormal pure-tone audiometry findings, may be explained by the direct involvement of the central nervous system in HIV infection. The most direct consequence of HIV infection to the auditory system is central auditory nervous system abnormalities, which may be measured by the ABR and other auditory evoked potentials (Christensen et al., 1998). Abnormal ABR findings have been reported even in the absence of clinical manifestations of HIV/AIDS. These findings may be related to progressive encephalopathy, including abnormal neural conduction of the auditory pathways, as demonstrated by ABR testing (Reyes-Contreras et al., 2002). Findings of postmortem studies indicate that central nervous system involvement may be present in up to

90% of individuals who have HIV/AIDS (Reyes-Contreras et al., 2002). The above discussion highlights the fact that neural hearing loss or auditory disorders may have a higher prevalence in HIV-infected persons than hearing disorders of a sensory nature.

The increased prevalence of neural versus sensory auditory pathologies is particularly evident in the pediatric HIV-infected population. Children infected with HIV/AIDS are more susceptible to central nervous system involvement than adults due to their immature immune systems. HIV encephalopathy, for example, is the most common neurologic manifestation of HIV in children (Rabie et al., 2007). Neurologic involvement may result in early auditory processing disorders, which is evident by the frequent occurrence of abnormal ABR findings suggesting compromised neural integrity (Matas et al., 2006). Table 10–1 displays the prevalence rates of sensorineural hearing loss in cases of HIV/AIDS, as reported by various studies.

Table 10–1. Summary of Reports on Prevalence Rates of Sensorineural Hearing Loss in HIV-Infected Adults and Children

Authors	*Design*	*Sample*	*Prevalence*
Matas et al. (2006)	Auditory assessment	101 children (51 HIV infected children; 50 control group)	Auditory brainstem disorders in 10% of children (3–6 yrs) and in 25% of children (7–10 yrs).
Roland et al. (2003)	Retrospective design	352 HIV infected adults	27%
Khoza & Ross (2002)	Explorative design	Relationship between HIV/AIDS and auditory function in a group of adults	23%
Truitt & Tami (1999)	Literature report	Prevalence rates in adults	21–49%
Bankaitis & Keith (1995)	Literature report	Prevalence rates in adults	20–50%
Madriz & Herrera (1995)	Literature report	Prevalence rates in adults	21–49%

The onset of sensory and neural hearing loss in HIV-infected individuals may be either sudden or gradual (Chandrasekhar et al., 2000). In a study conducted on 50 HIV infected individuals between the ages of 22 and 58 years, 29% were identified with sensorineural hearing loss. Three percent reported a sudden onset of the hearing loss, 21% a gradual onset, and 6% an intermittent hearing loss (Chandrasekhar et al., 2000). Deterioration of hearing loss is related to progression of the HIV infection, and high-frequency hearing loss is expected earlier than overall hearing loss (Chandrasekhar et al., 2000).

CAUSES OF SENSORY AND NEURAL AUDITORY DISORDERS ASSOCIATED WITH HIV/AIDS

This section considers the causes of sensory and neural auditory disorders associated with HIV/AIDS. These hearing losses may occur either congenitally or be acquired after birth. There are three broad categories of etiology for sensory and neural auditory disorders, including the direct viral effect of HIV/AIDS on the auditory system, opportunistic infections, and the effects of ototoxic medication. These are presented in Table 10–2.

Direct Viral Effect of HIV/AIDS

HIV has demonstrated direct effects on the peripheral and central auditory nervous system with significant abnormalities measured by pure-tone audiometry but more commonly by auditory evoked potentials (e.g., ABR) across all age groups (Birchall et al., 1992; Matas et al., 2000; Matas et al,. 2006; Vigliano et al., 1997). Over 90% of necropsies in HIV/AIDS patients show CNS abnormalities (Koralnick et al., 1990). It is not surprising, therefore, that central auditory pathology, associated with abnormal ABR results, is one of the few audiologic manifestations directly attributable to HIV/AIDS infection (Bankaitis & Keith, 1995).

Both symptomatic and asymptomatic individuals with varying degrees of HIV infection have revealed clinical abnormalities in the ABR, indicative of neural auditory disorders (Bankaitis & Keith, 1995; Reyes-Contreras et al., 2002). Neurophysiologic studies of a

Table 10–2. Etiology of Sensory and Neural Auditory Pathology Associated with HIV/AIDS

Etiology	Effect	Type of Pathology
HIV Infection	Direct effect on nervous system	Neural auditory dysfunction and HL
Opportunistic Infections	Otitis media and cholesteatoma	CHL and SNHL
	CMV	SNHL
	Otosyphilis	SNHL
	Herpes Zoster virus	SNHL
	Meningitis	SNHL
Ototoxicity		
• *HIV treatment*	ARV regimes (zidovudine; didanosine, stavudine, lamivudine)	SNHL
• *Opportunistic infection treatment*	Antibiotics (aminoglycosides, macrolides, co-trimoxazole)	SNHL
	Antifungal agents	
	Antiviral agents	

HL = Hearing loss; CHL = Conductive hearing loss; SNHL = Sensorineural hearing loss; ARV = antiretroviral; CMV = cytomegalovirus.

21-year-old HIV-infected individual with sudden bilateral sensorineural hearing loss revealed involvement of both branches of the vestibulocochlear cranial nerves (Grimaldi et al., 1993). The ABR, which reflects the sequence of activity from the distal portion of the vestibulocochlear nerve to the level of the rostral pons of the brainstem, is a useful tool to for early detection of such effects (Bankaitis & Keith, 1995). Some of the abnormalities recorded on ABR testing in HIV-infected individuals include prolonged absolute latencies of waves III and V, and prolonged interpeak latencies of waves III to V and I to V (Bankaitis & Keith, 1995; Christensen et al., 1998; Madriz & Herrera, 1995). A more detailed discussion on abnormalities on the ABR in both adult and pediatric HIV-infected individuals is provided in the assessment section of this chapter.

The pediatric population infected with HIV is particularly susceptible to central nervous system involvement, when compared to their adult counterparts (Madriz & Herrera, 1995). HIV encephalopathy is the most common neurologic manifestation of HIV in children, affecting one in every five, and resulting in altered brain function and structure (Rabie et al., 2007). Auditory brainstem abnormality was reported in 19% of children aged 3 to 6 years, and in 8% of children aged 7 to 10 years (Matas et al., 2006). In 96% of children who died from AIDS, the CNS showed some gross or microscopic abnormalities (Kozlowski, 1992). Therefore, it is not surprising that HIV encephalopathy also may result in neural hearing disorders with a higher incidence in the pediatric population. Maternal HIV status is, however, not significantly associated with the risk of sensorineural hearing loss in infants (Olusanya, Afe, & Onyia, 2009).

The exact mechanism of CNS destruction is unclear, but it has been suggested that the virus could produce a direct effect on the brain, affecting the process of CNS maturation in the pediatric population. Alternatively, HIV may cause opportunistic infections of the CNS that generate lesions that may be primary to HIV infection or secondary to other organ involvement (e.g., hypoxic encephalopathy) (Kozlowski, 1992). In children infected with HIV, the brain continues to develop slowly, even in the absence of other clinical signs. There is no "dormant" or "latent" period for the virus. HIV is in the infected CNS cells with a low rate of duplication (Madriz & Herrera, 1995).

Furthermore, HIV may cause AIDS encephalopathy and AIDS dementia complex, which are known to result in hearing loss (Gurney & Murr, 2003). Hemorrhages and cerebrovascular events, commonly associated with HIV infection, also may result in auditory disorders. HIV-associated primary or secondary metastatic neoplasms of the central nervous system may also result in auditory disorders (Gurney & Murr, 2003).

Hearing loss in HIV-infected individuals furthermore may be caused by immune dysregulation, resultant of HIV (Sheikh et al., 2009). A single case report of Cogan's syndrome is described, in which a rare immune-mediated disorder characterized by chronic, bilateral vestibular-cochlear dysfunction and interstitial keratitis takes place. A 54-year-old, HIV-positive male is reported to have suffered from persistent vertigo, severe bilateral sensorineural hearing loss, and interstitial keratitis. No evidence of a superimposed opportunistic infection was present. Injury to the inner ear was reasoned to be caused by direct invasion by the HIV virus, or by immune dysregulation caused by the HIV virus (Sheikh et al., 2009). The subject showed dramatic improvement in vestibular and auditory symptoms in response to immunosuppressive drugs, suggesting an immunologic basis for this syndrome (Sheikh et al., 2009).

Opportunistic Infections

Opportunistic infections are the product of commonplace infections that do not produce infections in healthy individuals with intact immune systems. Auditory disorders often are a secondary manifestation of HIV infection, as a result of opportunistic infections (Bankaitis & Keith, 1995). Common opportunistic infections that may cause hearing loss include the following: otitis media, cholesteatoma, otosyphilis, cytomegalovirus, herpes zoster virus, and meningitis (Zuniga, 1999). Pathology of the sensory and neural auditory structures associated with opportunistic infections in HIV infection is commonly reported. The most frequent conditions are discussed below. It is important to note that, although the discussion of opportunistic infections includes those that are commonly associated with hearing loss, there may be several others that are less common.

Otitis Media and Cholesteatoma

Otitis media is commonly associated with HIV/AIDS, and although predoantlymin causes a conductive hearing loss, complications may lead to a permanent sensory hearing loss. Otitis media often is the first presentation of HIV infection in children, especially if it is characterized by severe disease, poor response to conventional therapies, frequent relapse, or otitis media due to an unusual organism(s) (Bernaldez, Morales, & Hernandez, 2005; Newton, 2006). Cholesteatoma is a secondary complication of chronic otitis media, which is common in patients with HIV/AIDS, due to their compromised immune system. A cholesteatoma is an epithelial pocket that may form in the tympanic membrane following a perforation or retraction of the tympanic membrane due to chronic otitis media. It is characterized by growth and resorption of adjacent bone, which ultimately may result in damage to the cochlea, in addition to significant conductive hearing loss. As many as one in every four children with HIV/AIDS, who suffer from chronic otitis media, may develop a cholesteatoma (Bernaldez, Morales, & Hernandez, 2005). Otitis media and secondary cholesteatoma, therefore, may result not only in conductive hearing loss but also in permanent sensory hearing loss in cases of HIV infection.

Cytomegalovirus

Among various opportunistic diseases, cytomegalovirus (CMV) is one of the most frequent causes of central and peripheral neurologic manifestations (Meynard et al., 1997; Vancikova & Dorak, 2001). Therefore, it also is one of the most frequent causes of sensory and neural auditory disorders resulting from opportunistic infections. CMV is documented to cause cranial nerve infection, thereby causing hearing loss if the auditory nerve is affected (Meynard et al., 1997). Sensorineural hearing loss is the most frequent symptom of congenital CMV infection. The hearing loss usually is bilateral and progressive in nature (Vallely et al., 2002). Furthermore, CMV is the leading infectious cause of brain damage and hearing loss in young children (Vancikova & Dorak, 2001). Due to its frequent occurrence in HIV-infected individuals, and its propensity to cause sensory and neural hearing loss, CMV infection should always be considered when hearing loss develops in HIV-infected individuals (Meynard, Elamrani, Meyohas, et al., 1997).

Otosyphilis

Another common opportunistic disease that frequently presents in HIV-infected individuals is syphilis. Cranial neuropathies, most commonly involving the vestibulocochlear and optic nerves, are common findings among individuals with syphilis and HIV infection (Little, Gardner, Acker, et al., 1995). Syphilis affects HIV-infected individuals at an accelerated rate when compared to non-HIV-infected individuals (Chandrasekhar et al., 2000). In persons with HIV/AIDS, the time course from the onset of syphilis infection to the presentation of otosyphilis is as short as 2 to 5 years, compared to the 15- to 30-year latency period in non-HIV-infected individuals (Truitt & Tami, 1999). Not only does syphilis affect HIV-infected individuals at an accelerated rate, but it is also more severe (Truitt

& Tami, 1999). Otosyphilis may cause a unilateral or bilateral low-frequency sensorineural hearing loss (Truitt & Tami, 1999). Hearing loss may be fluctuating, asymmetric, or sudden. Therefore, oto-syphilis should be investigated routinely in HIV-infected individuals presenting with sensory and neural auditory disorders, particularly in patients with low-frequency losses, which may be asymmetric and fluctuating.

Toxoplasmosis

Toxoplasmosis is one of the most common opportunistic infections to affect the central nervous system, and also is associated with sensory and neural hearing loss. It is a parasitic infection caused by the protozoan *Toxoplasma gondii* and is primarily associated with congenital hearing loss, although several reports of acquired hearing loss have been ascribed to the parasitic infection (Katholm et al., 1991). Cerebral toxoplasmosis is one of the characteristics of end stage AIDS with CD4 counts less than 50. The most common manifestations of toxoplasmosis include encephalitis, mental changes, fever, headaches, and confusion (Tindyebwa, Kayita, & Musoke, 2004).

Meningitis

Bacterial meningitis, an infection of the meninges surrounding the brain and spinal cord, is the most common cause of acquired infant and childhood sensorineural hearing loss (Smith, Bale, & White, 2005). Although bacterial meningitis is a life-threatening condition, the majority of individuals survive and of these at least one in every four to one in every three present with severe to profound sensorineural hearing loss, depending on the type and severity of the meningitis (Forsyth et al., 2004; Goetghebuer et al., 2000; Molyneux, 2006). Individuals with HIV/AIDS are more prone to develop meningitis due to their suppressed immune system. In South Africa, a report on pediatric hospital admissions over a 2-year period indicated that 42% of all admissions for meningitis were HIV positive (Madhi et al., 2001). The organisms causing meningitis in HIV have a different profile than in noninfected cohorts with more serious and more recurrent infection episodes (Madhi et al., 2001; Molyneux et al., 2006). Cryptococcal meningitis, *Streptococcus pneumoniae*, and tuberculosis meningitis are common in cases of HIV/AIDS-infected individuals (Madhi et al., 2001). The close association of meningitis and HIV means that permanent sensory hearing loss due to this opportunistic infection is a common symptom in surviving cases.

Herpes Zoster Virus

Herpes zoster virus infection, also known as Ramsay Hunt syndrome, occurs frequently in HIV-infected individuals. It often is associated with involvement of multiple dermatomes in shingles or the presence of disseminated disease. When the herpes zoster virus affects the auditory nerve, it is referred to as herpes zoster oticus. Herpes zoster oticus infection usually presents with unilateral ear pain and possible unilateral hearing loss. Facial palsy and impairment of the balance organs also may occur (Newton, 2006). With the increased occurrence of Ramsay Hunt syndrome in cases of HIV/AIDS, associated hearing loss must be considered routinely.

Ototoxic Medication

Ototoxicity related to HIV/AIDS is due either to the direct treatment of the condition with antiretroviral (ARV) agents or through the treatment of opportunistic infections related to the immunosuppressed condition of the individual. Reports have indicated hearing loss due to both these pathways of ototoxicity in individuals with HIV/AIDS.

Ototoxicity Related to HIV Antiretroviral Therapies

Some ARVs have been demonstrated to cause ototoxic hearing loss in case reports of adults and children (Christensen et al., 1998; Simdon et al., 2001; Vogeser et al., 1998). Although the exact mechanism is not certain, findings suggest it may be due to direct damage to the mitochondrial DNA also associated with peripheral neuropathy, pancreatitism, and lactic acidosis (Bektas et al., 2008; Newton, 2006; Shibuyama et al., 2006).

Table 10–3 provides a summary of studies investigating the ototoxicity of ARV therapies. The majority of reports are case studies of hearing loss resulting from ARV treatment. All except one report of ototoxicity have been for the class of drugs referred to as

Table 10–3. Summary of Reports on Ototoxicity Related to Antiretroviral Therapy for HIV

Studies	Design	Therapies	Outcome
Viera et al. (2008)	Retrospective (162 cases and a control cohort)	Unspecified ARV therapy	1.8% idiopathic SNHL 1.3% otosclerosis-related HL No statistically significant relationship
Schouten et al. (2006)	Prospective (8 months) observational pilot study for 33 adult subjects	Zidovudine (Group 1) Didanosine (Group 2)	No significant HL related to therapy
Poblano et al. (2004)	Prenatal effect of ARV exposed infants. Two experimental groups on different therapies and a control group assessed with auditory brainstem response.	Zidovudine (Group 1) Azidothymidine and Lamivudine (Group 2)	Infants exposed prenatally to Azidothymidine and Lamivudine showed significantly delayed wave I and I-III latencies
Rey, Heritier, and Lang (2002)	Adult case report (Prophylaxis after occupational exposure to HIV)	Stavudine Lamivudine Nevirapine	Permanent SNHL
Williams, (2002)	Adult case report	Lopinavir-ritonavir (possible interaction with azithromycin)	Reversible SNHL

continues

Table 10–3. *continued*

Studies	Design	Therapies	Outcome
Simdon et al. (2001)	Adult case reports (all older than 45 and with histories of occupational noise exposure)	Stavudine Lamivudine Didanosine Hydroxyurea	Permanent SNHL
Simdon et al. (2001) Simdon et al. (2001)		Stavudine, Lamivudine Zidovudine	
Christensen et al. (1998)	Pediatric case report	Zidovudine Didanosine	Permanent SNHL
Colebunders et al. (1998)	Adult case report	Didanosine	Reversible SNHL
Marra et al. (1997)	99 adults with HIV (43 on ARV treatment)	Zidovudine, Didanosine Zalcitabine	29% presented with SNHL. (Associated with ARV therapy for patients older than 35 years)
Monte, Fenwick, and Monteiro (1997) Martinez and French (1993) Powderly, Klebert, and Clifford (1990)	Adult case reports	Zalcitabine	Permanent and reversible SNHL

SNHL = Sensorineural hearing loss; HL = Hearing loss.

256

nucleoside reverse transcriptase inhibitors (NRTIs). There is only one report where a drug from the protease inhibitor class, lopinavir-ritanovir, was associated with hearing loss. But in this case the subject was also taking azithromycin and a possible drug interaction with ritonavir may have resulted in hearing loss. Ritonavir is a potent inhibitor of a liver enzyme (cytochrome P450) involved in metabolism of many drugs and inhibition of this enzyme may have caused increased blood levels of azithromycin (Newton, 2006).

Various NRTIs and combinations of these drugs are reported to be associated with ototoxicity in individual cases. There is a complex interaction, however, and the effects seem to be dependent on several factors including drug type, combinations of therapies, and dosages. The only study that has reported any prenatal affect on auditory functioning indicated significantly delayed auditory brainstem response (ABR) waves I and I to III for infants exposed prenatally to azidothymidine and lamivudine, whereas the group exposed only to zidovudine did not demonstrate any significant delays in latency (Poblano et al., 2004). This suggests a prenatal effect of this combination treatment on auditory functioning in infants but further studies are necessary to confirm this observation.

Interestingly, age and occupational noise exposure seem to be related to the ototoxicity of NRTIs. A significant effect of age, in subjects older than 35 years of age, on ototoxicity due to NRTIs has been reported in a group of 99 HIV-infected subjects. This has been confirmed by several case studies suggesting age as a possible contributing factor to susceptibility (Marra et al., 1997; Simdon et al., 2001). The reduction in mitochondrial DNA content induced by NRTI's, as well as mitochondrial DNA mutations associated with aging and HIV infection all may contribute to the auditory dysfunction in older subjects (Simdon et al., 2001). It is clear, however, that the ototoxic effects are not exclusively present in older subjects as illustrated by a report in a 23-year-old subject receiving a combination of therapies as a prophylaxis after occupational exposure to HIV (Rey, Heritier, & Lang, 2002).

Occupational noise exposure also has been associated with a greater susceptibility to ototoxicity of NRTI therapies and this has more recently also been confirmed in an animal study (Bektas et al., 2008; Simdon et al., 2001). The animal study indicated that mice receiving zidovudine and lamivudine and who received noise exposure showed greater auditory dysfunction, supporting the notion of a synergistic relationship between certain NRTIs and noise exposure (Bektas et al., 2008). Future studies are necessary to assess the possible pharmacogenetic, physiologic, and environmental interactions that may cause greater susceptibility in subjects receiving NRTIs.

The only study reporting no evidence of ototoxicity in NRTIs, specifically treatment with zidovudine and didanosine, was a prospective observational pilot study in 33 subjects over an 8-month period (Schouten et al., 2006). No significant changes in hearing were noted, based on pure-tone audiometry, over the 32 weeks of observation in participants taking zidovudine or didanosine (Schouten et al., 2006). This is a reasonably short period of treatment and the sample size is also limited. Use of ARV therapies for longer periods of time, different drug combinations, and dosages all may be possible factors that may contribute to ototoxicity in patients with HIV/AIDS.

The relationship between ARV therapies and ototoxicity is not straightforward and more studies certainly are warranted and necessary to isolate relationships and interactions responsible for loss of auditory functioning. What is clear, however, is that ototoxicity does occur in a subgroup of cases and is almost exclusively related to NRTIs. In addition to this, reports also suggest that older subjects, although there are clear exceptions, and subjects with a history of noise exposure may be more susceptible to ototoxicity from NRTI therapies.

Ototoxicity Related to HIV Opportunistic Infection Treatment

The second route of ototoxicity is through medications for opportunistic infections associated with HIV, which include antibiotics, antifungal, and other antiviral agents that are known to cause hearing loss (Newton, 2006). The immune-compromized condition caused by HIV predisposes these individuals to a variety of opportunistic infections, prone to recurrence, which often necessitates treatment with medications that have established ototoxic effects. For example, tuberculosis (TB) is a very common opportunistic infection associated with HIV, reportedly affecting one in every three people infected with HIV (Chan, Perez, Ben, et al., 2003). This condition, especially the multidrug resistant strains, is treated with high doses of antibiotics, including streptomycin, that are established ototoxic agents. Table 10–4 provides a list of drug classes commonly used to treat HIV complications and opportunistic infections that are associated with ototoxicity.

Table 10–4. Ototoxic Agents for HIV Complications and Associated Opportunistic Infections

Class of Medication	Examples	Organism
Antiobiotics		
Aminoglycosides	Amikacin Streptomycin	Mycobacterium tuberculosis
Macrolides	Azithromycin Clarithromycin Erythromycin	Mycobacterium avium-intercellulare complex Toxoplasma gondii
Co-trimoxazole (Trimethoprim-sulphamethoxazole		Pneumocystis jiroveci
Antifungal agents	Amphotericin	Cryptococcus
Antiviral agents Nucleotide analogue	Cidofovir	Cytomegalovirus

Source: Adapted from Newton (2006).

The ototoxicity and reversibility of ototoxic effects associated with these agents vary with age, dose, and combinations of therapies. Due to the greatly increased occurrence of opportunistic infections in children and adults infected with HIV, their risk of acquiring a drug-induced hearing loss is significantly increased compared to the general population. This is especially true because the coinfections associated with HIV/AIDS are often multiple, more serious and recur more often. Therefore, the drug therapies are prescribed more frequently and in higher dosages.

IDENTIFICATION AND ASSESSMENT OF AUDITORY DISORDERS ASSOCIATED WITH HIV/AIDS

The purpose of identification and assessment of auditory functioning for individuals infected with HIV/AIDS is to determine the presence of a disorder, and to describe the type, degree, configuration, and symmetry of the auditory disorder. This is essential for planning appropriate intervention. Early identification also may allow for the prevention or delayed progress of auditory disorders associated with HIV/AIDS. The site of the auditory disorder needs to be established so that the individual can be referred to either a medical professional, such as an ear, nose, and throat-specialist (ENT), or for appropriate auditory rehabilitation. This section discusses screening activities to identify individuals with auditory pathology, as well as a test-battery approach to assessing the auditory status of individuals infected with HIV/AIDS. The importance of a team approach and the considerations and adaptations for patients with HIV/AIDS are discussed.

Identification of Auditory Disorders

Screening for sensory and neural hearing loss should be routine practice for individuals with HIV/AIDS, due to the close association of the infection with auditory disorders. With advances in antiretroviral therapies, such as HAART, issues of quality of life, such as hearing loss, are becoming increasingly important in the holistic treatment of patients with HIV/AIDS. As many as 75% of adults living with AIDS experience some kind of auditory dysfunction due to the direct effect of HIV, opportunistic coinfections, or ototoxic combination therapies (Zuniga, 1999). Although the exact prevalence of sensory and neural hearing loss in HIV infected individuals is not known, it is estimated to be between 20 and 50% (Bankaitis & Keith, 1995; Matas et al., 2006; Roland et al., 2003). Children have a particularly high rate of central auditory abnormalities, which may impact their development detrimentally (Matas et al., 2006).

Due to the high prevalence of auditory disorders in persons with HIV/AIDS, as well as an increasing emphasis on quality of life, the need for screening for auditory disorders is clearly indicated. All health care professionals working with HIV-infected individuals should be familiar with and conduct, or refer for, a screening for auditory disorders. Table 10–5 displays screening activities for identifying hearing loss in persons with HIV/AIDS. Referral criteria, as well as relevant health care professionals to whom referrals should be made, are also included.

Table 10–5 lists a range of screening activities to conduct on HIV-infected individuals during medical evaluations. However,

Table 10–5. Procedures and Referral Criteria for Identification of Hearing Loss or Auditory Disorders Associated with HIV/AIDS

Screening Test	Description	Referral Criteria	Referral To
Case History	Questions should identify risk factors for hearing loss: • Any reported decrease in hearing sensitivity? • Any common opportunistic infections e.g. recurrent otitis media, cholesteatoma, CMV, otosyphilis, herpes zoster virus, or meningitis? • Receiving antiretroviral medication (specifically NRTIs)? • On medication for opportunistic infections, including antibiotics, antifungal, or other antiviral agents? • Any significant occupational noise exposure, which may contribute to a hearing loss? • Over the age of 35 years?	Referral if answer is "yes" to any of the case history questions. • Changes in hearing reported • If the individual presents with opportunistic infections: refer for diagnostic audiogram and medical treatment • If abnormalities on audiogram and individual is on ototoxic medication: refer for possible change in treatment regimen • If the individual has significant noise exposure and increasing age: refer for audiologic assessment, as they may be more prone to ototoxic effects	Audiologist ENT Specialist Physician (adult) Pediatrician (child)
Otoscopic Examination	The outer ear canal and tympanic membrane should be visually inspected using an otoscope.	Referral should be made if there are any of the following: • Obstructions in outer ear canal, such as cerumen, debris, etc. • If the tympanic membrane appears red, bulging or retracted, or abnormal in any way.	ENT Specialist

continues

261

Table 10–5. *continued*

Screening Test	Description	Referral Criteria	Referral To
Screening Audiogram	A baseline or screening audiogram should be conducted prior to commencing treatment with ototoxic medication.	The percentage loss of hearing (PLH) should be calculated, and referral made accordingly: • If the PLH >11.1% refer for diagnostic audiogram • If the PLH >30% refer for diagnostic audiogram & medical specialist • If there is asymmetry refer to medical specialist	Audiologist ENT Specialist
Screening Otoacoustic Emissions	Screening OAEs provide an indication of the functioning of the outer hair cells of the cochlea. An automated test should be used, with a predefined "pass" and "refer" criteria	Pass result indicates normal outer hair cell functioning of the cochlea. Refer result necessitates referral for a diagnostic audiologic assessment.	Audiologist ENT Specialist

it often is not possible to conduct all these activities, due to limited resources in terms of time and equipment. In cases where health care professionals do not have equipment for screening audiograms or screening otoacoustic emissions, they should at least conduct the case history and a thorough otoscopic examination. If any risk factors are identified from the case history, or if any abnormalities are noted on the otoscopic examination in addition to complaints by the patient, referral for diagnostic audiologic assessment should be made. The audiologist (or other hearing health care specialist) who conducts the diagnostic audiologic assessment should make appropriate referrals to ENT specialists or neurologists, as deemed necessary.

Assessment of Auditory Functioning

Individuals who meet referral criteria based on the screening procedure should undergo a comprehensive hearing assessment. The aim of the hearing assessment is to determine the type, degree, configuration, and possible etiology of a hearing loss. A test battery approach to assess the auditory status of individuals infected with HIV/AIDS is necessary to establish the site of lesion of the auditory disorder, so that appropriate intervention can be provided. Table 10-6 provides an overview of the various tests recommended for inclusion in the audiologic test battery for individuals with HIV/AIDS. Each component of the test battery is also discussed and motivated.

As seen in Table 10-6, when assessing the hearing status of individuals infected with HIV/AIDS, a complete audiologic test battery is necessary to determine the exact nature of the auditory disorder. The three main causes of sensory and neural auditory disorders in individuals infected with HIV/AIDS result in different types of auditory pathology. The direct viral effect of HIV is associated with the central nervous system, resulting in neural auditory disorders (Bankaitis & Keith, 1995). Neural auditory pathology is one of the few audiologic manifestations directly attributable to HIV infection (Bankaitis & Keith, 1995). Opportunistic infections may cause either sensory or neural auditory disorders (Bankaitis & Keith, 1995). Ototoxic medication used in the treatment of infections and neoplasms in HIV-infected individuals is the possible cochlear basis for sensory auditory disorders in these individuals (Rinaldo et al., 2003).

Table 10–6. Audiologic Test Battery for Individuals Infected with HIV/AIDS

Audiologic Test	Purpose of Auditory Test	Test Findings	
		Sensory Hearing Loss	Neural Hearing Loss
Pure-tone air- and bone-conduction audiometry	Quantifies degree, configuration, and symmetry of hearing loss. Can differentiate between conductive and sensorineural hearing loss	Loss of sensitivity, typically in high frequencies	Range of findings from no peripheral pure-tone sensitivity loss to various degrees and configurations of pure-tone loss.
Speech audiometry	Assess identification, recognition, and discrimination of words or sentences at suprathreshold and threshold levels. Measure of real-world functioning	Findings corresponds with pure-tone thresholds	Does not correspond with pure-tone thresholds. Disproportionately poor speech discrimination especially in noise.
Tympanometry	Evaluates functioning of middle ear. Describes presence and nature of middle ear disorder	May be normal or abnormal	May be normal or abnormal

Audiologic Test	Purpose of Auditory Test	Test Findings	
		Sensory Hearing Loss	Neural Hearing Loss
Acoustic reflexes	Confirms pure-tone thresholds and differentiates between sensory and neural hearing loss	Thresholds correspond with pure-tone thresholds. Absent or may be present at elevated pure-tone thresholds due to recruitment	If site-of-lesion is at VIIIth nerve or brainstem level, reflexes may be abnormal or absent. If lesion is in higher order neurons toward cortex, reflexes may be present.
Otoacoustic emissions	Objective evaluation of cochlear functioning; monitor changes resulting from ototoxic medications.	Reduced or absent depending on severity of hearing loss	OAEs may be present
Auditory brainstem responses	Differentiates between cochlear (sensory) and auditory nerve (neural) pathology.	Threshold results correspond with pure-tone thresholds. Latencies normal	VIIIth nerve or brainstem disorder, ABR abnormal or absent. Thalamic pathways of cortex, ABR may be present.
Cortical evoked responses	Identify central auditory involvement	Threshold results correspond with pure-tone thresholds. Amplitude and latency of waves (P1, N1, P2, and P3) normal.	May be abnormal amplitude and/or latency for waves (P1, N1, P2, & P3) if higher order CNS disorder

OAE = otoacoustic emission; CAEP = cortical auditory evoked potential; ABR = auditory brainstem response; CNS = central nervous system.

Table 10–6 indicates how different audiologic test results may allow the health care professional to differentiate between sensory and neural hearing loss. It is important to attempt differentiation of sensory and neural hearing loss in HIV-infected individuals as the type of loss determines intervention. Should auditory pathology be found to be sensory in nature, the cause often is either opportunistic infections or ototoxic medications. To decide whether opportunistic infections or ototoxic medication is the causal factor for the sensory hearing loss, the case history needs to be carefully analyzed.

Often, it is not possible to determine a specific cause. Multiple factors may play a role, such as a combination of opportunistic infections, ototoxic medication, as well as HIV itself. Furthermore, risk factors for auditory pathology present in HIV-negative individuals, still apply to HIV-infected individuals. These include, for example, a family history of hearing loss or presbycusis. Despite the difficulty in isolating a cause, the health care professional should attempt to identify causes to promote appropriate intervention.

Pure-Tone Audiometry

Pure-tone audiometry is a behavioral audiologic test that quantifies the degree of hearing loss and provides some information on the site of lesion. It consists of both air- and bone-conduction, and enables frequency-specific threshold determination (Chandrasekhar et al., 2000; Matas et al., 2000; Moazezz & Alvi, 1998; Vincenti et al., 2005). Chandrasekhar et al. (2000) reported deteriorating hearing loss as the HIV infection progressed based on pure-tone results, as well as earlier high-frequency hearing loss than expected due to aging. Pure-tone thresholds were significantly elevated in individuals who reported subjective hearing loss.

It is important to note that pure-tone audiometry often is normal in individuals infected with HIV/AIDS, in the presence of central/neural auditory disorders (Madriz & Herrera, 1995). Pure-tone audiometry measures only hearing sensitivity, and not hearing ability, which requires precise temporal and frequency discrimination. This does not undermine the clinical value of using pure-tone audiometry to assess individuals infected with HIV/AIDS, but rather emphasizes the importance of a test-battery approach in quantifying the exact nature and impact of the auditory disorder.

Speech Audiometry

Speech audiometry is an important component of the audiologic test battery to confirm pure-tone results but, more importantly, to provide an indication of hearing ability (Brandy, 2002; Chandrasekhar et al., 2000; Moazzez & Alvi, 1998). One of the applications of speech audiometry in the assessment of individuals infected with HIV/AIDS is to differentiate between sensory and neural auditory pathology. When the auditory disorder is sensory in nature, speech discrimination scores usually are above 90% (Truitt & Tami, 1999). Patients with HIV/AIDS, however, may show a disproportionate inability to discriminate speech in relation to their pure-tone audiometric curves due to central/neural auditory processing disorders (Madriz & Herrera, 1995). Results of speech audiometry may thus point the clinician to further testing based on the site of the auditory disorder.

Tympanometry

Tympanometry assesses middle ear functioning and is very useful to determine the presence of conductive lesions. Behavioral assessment of hearing often is confounded by middle ear effusion, which makes it difficult to differentiate between true sensory and neural auditory disorders and conductive losses (Hoare, 2003; Rinaldo, 2003). This is particularly true in individuals infected with HIV/AIDS, given the high incidence of otitis media with effusion in this population (Rinaldo, 2003). Immunocompromised children in particular are more likely to suffer from otitis media with effusion than immunocompetent children and with greater severity (Hoare, 2003; Rinaldo, 2003). Tympanometry is an essential tool in the audiologic test battery to assess middle ear functioning accurately and to assist in differential diagnosis of hearing loss or auditory pathology (Chandrasekhar et al., 2000; Fowler & Shanks, 2002; Matas et al., 2006; Moazzez & Alvi, 1998).

Acoustic Reflexes

Acoustic reflex measurements involve the presentation of sound stimuli in order to elicit the stapedial muscle reflex (Gelfand, 2002).

If acoustic reflex thresholds are elevated, it may indicate recruitment, indicative of possible cochlear pathology. Such results may be present in HIV-infected individuals with sensory hearing loss from either opportunistic infections or ototoxicity. Acoustic reflex thresholds are abnormal or absent in the case of eighth cranial nerve or brainstem dysfunction, which may be caused by the direct effect of the HIV infection on the CNS. Acoustic reflex testing is a valuable tool to assist the health care professionals in making a differential diagnosis of hearing status, and may assist in determining the site of lesion of the auditory pathology if used in a test-battery approach.

Otoacoustic Emissions

Otoacoustic emissions (OAEs) provide an objective assessment of the integrity of the outer hair cells of the cochlea. In addition to pure-tone and speech audiometry and tympanometry, otoacoustic emissions are an excellent tool to differentiate sensory from neural auditory pathology. The presence of OAEs is indicative of normal sensory or cochlear functioning (at least the outer hair cells) and, if absent, without a middle ear or ear canal obstruction, indicates the presence of sensory hearing loss. In the case of a neural hearing loss, normal OAEs may be recorded whereas other tests such as ABR and pure-tone audiometry may suggest auditory abnormalities.

Otoacoustic emissions furthermore may be used to monitor ototoxic effects of drugs administered (Garcia et al., 2001; Prieve & Fitzgerald, 2002). Antiretroviral drugs administered to individuals infected with HIV/AIDS have possible ototoxic effects (Bankaits & Keith, 1995; Gurney & Murr, 2003; Truitt & Tami, 1999). Almost all individuals with HIV/AIDS participating in an audiologic investigation conducted by Rinaldo et al. (2003) showed diminished otoacoustic emissions, suggesting cochlear dysfunction resulting from infection or ototoxicity. Ideally, individuals receiving antiretroviral therapy should receive not only a baseline audiogram but also a baseline otoacoustic emission evaluation. Subsequent follow-up evaluations with otoacoustic emissions can be used to identify any early changes in cochlear functioning before a noticeable decrease in pure-tone behavioral thresholds may be apparent. If any abnormalities are noted, these should be discussed with the treating physician to consider possible contributing factors and ultimately to investigate alternative combinations of antiretroviral therapy (Gurney & Murr, 2003).

Auditory Brainstem Response

The ABR represents synchronous neural activity in the eighth cranial nerve and brainstem pathways in response to acoustic stimuli measured with far-field electrodes on the scalp. Although otoacoustic emissions are sensitive to cochlear (sensory) pathology, the auditory brainstem response (ABR) is most sensitive to neural auditory pathology (Moazzez & Alvi, 1998; Vincenti et al., 2005). In individuals infected with HIV/AIDS, abnormal auditory brainstem responses are the most common audiologic finding, making the ABR an indispensible part of the audiologic test battery for this population (Castro et al., 2000). Central auditory nervous system abnormalities are a direct consequence of HIV infection, resulting in a high incidence of abnormal ABR results in this population (Christensen et al., 1998).

Abnormalities on ABR recordings may present during the early stages of HIV infection even before clinical symptoms are noticeable (Matas et al., 2006). Both symptomatic and asymptomatic individuals infected with HIV/AIDS have shown clinically relevant abnormalities in the ABR (Bankaitis & Keith, 1995). Structures of the auditory pathways may suffer neuropathologic changes from the HIV infection, such as subcortical demyelination and progressive encephalopathy (Bankaitis & Keith, 1995; Reyes-Contreras, 2002). This may explain why neurophysiologic studies involving ABR testing indicate abnormal findings in the early stages of HIV infection, even in the absence of clinical manifestations such as a loss in hearing sensitivity (Reyes-Contreras et al., 2002). As the HIV infection progresses, so does the frequency of ABR abnormalities (Reyes-Contreras, 2002).

Adaptations to the ABR testing protocol may be necessary in HIV-infected individuals, in order to detect subcortical demyelination as early as possible. Faster stimulus rates, which put strain on neural conduction, may reveal abnormalities in otherwise asymptomatic individuals who will only show abnormalities much later on (Bankaitis & Keith, 1995). Utilizing stimulus rates of between 21.1 per second to as high as 90 per second can unmask such subclinical abnormalities (Bankaitis & Keith, 1995).

The abnormalities reported in ABR findings for adults with HIV infection include: prolonged absolute latencies of waves III and V, as well as prolonged interpeak latencies of waves III to V and I to V (Bankaitis & Keith, 1995; Christensen et al., 1998; Madriz & Herrera, 1995). Children with HIV infection are more susceptible to central auditory pathology than adults (Matas et al., 2006). Some of the common ABR findings in children include bilaterally or unilaterally prolonged wave I to V interpeak latencies; unilaterally prolonged wave I to III and III to V interpeak latencies; and delayed onset of wave I (Christensen et al., 1998). Palacios et al. (2008) furthermore reported prolonged interpeak latencies, abnormal morphology of the ABR, and abnormal amplitude patterns in a group of 23 HIV-infected children. HIV-infected individuals also may show abnormal responses to an increased rate of stimulus presentation (Christensen et al., 1998), which is discussed in more detail under adaptations to be made to the audiologic test battery for individuals infected with HIV/AIDS.

The ABR also is very important in differentiating between neural and sensory hearing loss. If rarefaction and condensation polarity click stimuli are used, the presence of a cochlear microphonic response, representative of cochlear functioning, may be investigated. In cases of neural hearing loss, that is, auditory neuropathy, the cochlear microphonic response will be present with absent or abnormal ABR waves as opposed to conventional sensorineural hearing loss where the cochlear microphonic response will be absent. The ABR, therefore, assumes a prominent role as part of the assessment of HIV-infected individuals.

Cortical Auditory Evoked Potentials

Cortical auditory evoked potentials (CAEP) are late latency responses, measured from the scalp by far-field electrodes that occur at least 50 ms after presentation of an auditory stimulus. They are closely linked to perceptual processes, such as discrimination. Abnormal CAEPs may indicate a possible cortical lesion, whereas CAEP thresholds will correspond with behavioral thresholds if the lesion is sensory. Ragazonni et al. (1993) recorded ABR measures and CAEP measures from a group of 33 HIV-infected individuals, all of whom were neurologically asymptomatic. Although ABR results were normal, 27% of CAEP results showed longer latencies for P2,

N2, and P3 wave components, and reduced amplitude for P3 (Ragazonni et al., 1993). These findings are supported by Goodin et al. (1990), who reported similar results for CAEP measures recorded from 55 HIV-infected individuals. Delayed latencies were measured in terms of N1, P2, N2, and P3 components of the CAEP response (Goodin et al., 1990). These abnormalities were more prominent in individuals who were symptomatic from the HIV infection than in asymptomatic individuals. Seventy-eight percent of symptomatic HIV-infected individuals displayed abnormalities on CAEP indices, whereas 28% of the asymptomatic participants displayed abnormalities (Goodin et al., 1990). CAEP recordings seem to demonstrate sensitivity for detection of subclinical central nervous system involvement related to auditory processing in HIV-infected individuals. Therefore, it may prove to be a useful adjunct to the audiologic test-battery in adults infected with HIV as an early detection measure for impairments in auditory processes in the cortex. Currently, however, it is not used as a routine audiologic test procedure.

Monitoring Hearing and Auditory Functioning

Not only is it essential to utilize the above mentioned audiologic test battery to evaluate persons with HIV/AIDS, but it is just as important to regularly monitor the auditory status of these individuals. A baseline audiologic assessment is useful in individuals with HIV/AIDS from which any future changes in auditory functioning may be identified early on. This is particularly important for patients receiving ototoxic medication, before commencing treatment (Gurney & Murr, 2003). Ototoxicity of antiretroviral therapy or medications for opportunistic infections needs to be monitored to document the effects thereof and to change drug regimes if necessary (Garcia et al., 2001; Gurney & Murr, 2003). Children infected with HIV are particularly susceptible to central auditory abnormalities, more so than adults, and regular audiologic follow-up of these children is necessary if early intervention is to be a priority (Matas et al., 2006). The integrity of the peripheral and central auditory nervous system is essential to the acquisition and maintenance of speech and language, the means of communication, and plays a central role in quality of life for human beings. It is therefore of utmost priority that auditory abnormalities be identified and treated as early as possible, especially in vulnerable populations such as those infected with HIV. This necessitates proactive and timely monitoring of hearing and auditory functioning.

Adaptations for Auditory Assessment

Certain challenges must be considered when assessing the auditory status of individuals infected with HIV/AIDS in order to obtain reliable and accurate results from behavioral tests. Several HIV/AIDS-related illnesses affect the central nervous system, which may influence auditory assessment (i.e., HIV encephalopathy, subcortical dementia, cranial calcifications, cerebrovascular disease, progressive multifocal leucoencephalopathy, and meningitis (Naudé & Pretorius, 2003). Demyelination of the central nervous system associated with progressive multifocal leucoencephalopathy, subcortical dementia, and some of the other above-mentioned conditions may lead to cognitive changes that could influence the reliability of the auditory assessment. These cognitive changes may include reduced cognitive tempo or speed of thinking, attention deficits, impaired memory storage, learning difficulties, dementia, fatigue, and impaired motor activity (Naudé & Pretorius, 2003). Completing behavioral audiologic assessments that rely on active participation and the ability to concentrate on a task in the presence of such cognitive changes can be very challenging. Therefore, certain adaptations to behavioral testing procedures may be necessary to obtain reliable results. Examples of such difficulties and proposed adaptations and possible solutions are summarized in Table 10–7. It is the responsibility of the clinician to assess the individual patient, and devise solutions to each HIV-infected individual's possible cognitive difficulties.

To obtain accurate hearing thresholds, the behavioral audiologic assessment of children infected with HIV/AIDS requires additional adaptations in order to obtain accurate hearing thresholds. Children are more susceptible than adults to central nervous system involvement associated with HIV, which impacts their level of neurologic functioning (Matas et al., 2006). Therefore, these children may not be able to respond age appropriately to testing procedures. Clinicians should assess the child's developmental age prior

Table 10–7. Adaptations to Behavioral Audiologic Testing in HIV-Infected Individuals

Cognitive Deficit	Adaptation to Behavioral Audiometry
Reduced speed of thinking	• Absence of a response directly after stimulus presentations does not necessarily mean it was not heard • Provide more time for a response (press a button) • Prompt for a response repeatedly
Attention deficits and impaired memory storage	• Attention may veer from the task at hand • Repeat instructions regularly and redirect attention to task
Learning difficulties and dementia	• Difficulty understanding what is expected during behavioral testing • Repeat instructions and demonstrate appropriate responses • Ensure understanding of test instructions and repeat instructions

Source: Adapted from Naudé & Pretorius (2003).

to audiologic testing to select the most appropriate evaluation technique for each child.

The procedures for carrying out tympanometry, otoacoustic emissions, and auditory brainstem response testing should remain the same as in the adult population although it may be necessary to ensure children are sleeping either naturally or under closely supervised sedation/anesthesia. Behavioral audiologic testing, however, must be conducted either by using visual reinforcement audiometry or conditioned play audiometry. Visual reinforcement audiometry (VRA), in which an auditory stimulus is presented, and the child's response to the sound is reinforced by a bright moving animated toy, is useful in assessing peripheral hearing thresholds in young children from between approximately 7 to 36 months of age (Northern & Downs, 2002). Conditioned play audiometry is used for older children and also provides reinforcement for a correct response by praising the child (Northern & Downs, 2002). When working with children with HIV infection, the recommended ages for these procedures must be guided by developmental age as opposed to chronologic age. As neuromaturational delays and deficits are associated with HIV in children, poor or inappropriate participation may be common in assessment procedures. Neurologic or cognitive deficits are similar to those listed in Table 10–7. Children with HIV infection, for example, may have HIV encephalopathy, causing loss of memory, inattentiveness, and general apathy (Naudé & Pretorius, 2003). Adaptations may be routine practice as well as scheduling several appointments to complete an assessment.

Team Approach in Auditory Assessment

A multidisciplinary team approach is essential for assessing and treating individuals with multifaceted HIV-related disorders to ensure appropriate and comprehensive service delivery. Table 10–8 provides a list of common team members. Sensory and neural auditory disorders in individuals infected with HIV/AIDS often are only secondary to other central nervous system or neurologic complications, requiring assessment and intervention by a team of medical specialists (Meynard et al., 1997; Moazzez & Alvi, 1998). Individuals with HIV/AIDS who present with a neural auditory disorder should receive a comprehensive neurologic medical assessment, conducted by the appropriate medical personnel as a matter of priority (Truitt & Tami, 1998). Contrast-enhanced brain CT scans should be conducted, to rule out any central nervous system pathology (Rinaldo et al., 2003). It is, however, important to remember that persons with HIV/AIDS also may present with auditory pathologies found in immunocompetent individuals. Such auditory pathologies should, therefore, be kept in mind when making a diagnosis and deciding on appropriate intervention.

As discussed earlier, the diagnosis of sensory or neural auditory disorders in HIV-infected individuals may be confounded by middle ear effusion, particularly in the pediatric population (Hoare, 2003; Rinaldo, 2003). Any individual with possible middle ear effusion should promptly be referred to an ENT specialist, in order to medically manage their condition, before further audiologic diagnosis

Table 10–8. Team Members and Their Roles Regarding Sensory and Neural Auditory Disorders in HIV-Infected Individuals

Team Member	Role
General Practitioner or Primary Health Care Physician	First contact with HIV infected individual; referral source to other team members; monitoring of antiretroviral therapy regime based on audiologic results in adults
ENT	Medical assessment of auditory pathology; medical intervention for auditory complications due to HIV infection
Audiologist	Audiologic assessment, diagnosis, and monitoring; audiologic (re)habilitation
Pediatrician	Monitoring of antiretroviral therapy regime based on audiologic results in children; monitoring general development of HIV infected children; treating primary and secondary complications of HIV infection
Neurologist	Diagnosis of direct and secondary neurologic complications of HIV and recommendation of possible medical intervention

and treatment is commenced. Lastly, before starting audiologic assessment of HIV-infected individuals, it is important to consult their medication list for possible agents responsible for sensory or neural hearing loss. If ototoxic medication is suspected as a possible cause for the individual's auditory disorder, his or her physician should be consulted to discuss the possibility of an alternative regimen (Gurney & Murr, 2003).

The assessment of individuals infected with HIV/AIDS is multifaceted, and an array of medical personnel is necessary to provide the appropriate services for these individuals. Sensory and neural auditory disorders in HIV-infected individuals often are more complicated than in immunocompetent individuals. Medical personnel working with these individuals should be made aware of this to ensure that accountable services are offered to these patients with regard to the often neglected aspects of hearing and auditory functioning.

INTERVENTION FOR AUDITORY DISORDERS ASSOCIATED WITH HIV/AIDS

Treatment methods for HIV (e.g., highly active antiretroviral drugs) are rapidly advancing (Gurney & Murr, 2003). This has improved morbidity and mortality related to HIV as the virus is kept in a latent state more successfully than ever before (Gurney & Murr, 2003; Vincenti et al., 2005). Individuals with HIV infection who have access to these medications now have the prospect of longer and healthier lives with improved quality of life (Gurney & Murr, 2003). As opposed to the pressing life-threatening nature of HIV several years ago, increasingly more attention is now warranted for the more non-life-threatening quality of life issues related to HIV infection. Hearing loss is one such an issue, which has far-reaching effects on a person's quality of life, and therefore deserves special consideration in patients with HIV who are more prone to hearing loss and auditory disorders (Vincenti et al., 2005).

Prevention of HIV-Related Auditory Disorders

Prevention of HIV related auditory disorders should always be the primary goal for health care professionals working with patients infected with HIV. Various strategies for prevention of HIV-related auditory disorders are summarized in Table 10–9.

Management of HIV-Related Auditory Disorders

Many aspects of intervention for HIV-infected individuals with sensory and neural hearing loss are the same as intervention for any other individual with an auditory disorder (McNeilly, 2005). It is important, however, that the health care professional providing intervention to these individuals be knowledgeable about the progression of the disease. Hearing health care professionals, such as audiologists, should be acquainted with the HIV-infected individual's health status, as well as any factors that may impact the individual's socioemotional welfare (McNeilly, 2005). Increased flexibility in the

Table 10–9. Prevention Strategies for HIV/AIDS-Related Auditory Disorders

• Regular monitoring (every 6 months) of hearing and auditory functioning to detect disorders as early as possible
• Early identification and treatment of otitis media, to prevent secondary complications (e.g., cholesteatoma) that may cause permanent hearing loss
• Treatment of otitis media in infants and children should be particularly aggressive to avoid prolonged periods of conductive hearing loss during critical developmental periods for language, speech, and literacy
• Initiate highly active antiretroviral treatment (HAART) to prevent opportunistic infections that may lead to hearing loss
• Monitor effects of ototoxic medications with baseline audiograms at initiation and every 3 months thereafter (e.g., HAART or other ototoxic treatments for opportunistic infections)
• Review current dosages and combinations of antiretroviral drugs at first sign of ototoxicity, in order to reverse and prevent further ototoxic damage as far as possible

scheduling of appointments for intervention, for example, may be necessary as these individuals often have many diverse health care needs (Roland et al., 2003). The intervention for a hearing disorder is dependent on aspects such as the etiology, the type of disorder, and the degree and configuration of the hearing loss, and may be in the form of medical management, hearing aids, cochlear implants, or assistive listening devices, or alternative communication methods.

Medical management of HIV-related auditory disorders usually is done by ENT specialists but certain conductive hearing losses (i.e., impacted cerumen and otitis media may be treated by primary health care providers if specialist services are not available. More invasive disorders (i.e., neoplasms and cholesteatoma) require specialists for treatment, as surgery often is necessary. Often, however, medical management is not possible for these individuals, as in the case of sensory or neural hearing loss.

For persons with a sensory or neural hearing loss, it is a priority to maximize residual hearing for daily functioning by providing appropriate personal amplification. Hearing aids are electronic devices worn either behind the ear or in the ear of the individual with hearing loss to amplify sounds, specifically speech, according to the person's unique degree and configuration of hearing sensitivity. A hearing health care professional, usually an audiologist, responsible for assessing hearing status is also the professional responsible for prescribing and fitting hearing aids. The microphone of the hearing aid picks up sounds from the environment, converts the acoustic signal into an electrical signal, and sends it to the amplifier. The amplifier of the hearing aid amplifies the signal selectively according to the individual's hearing loss, which then transmits the signal to the receiver where the processed electrical signal is converted back to an acoustic signal presented to the individual's ear via tubing or an earmold (Tye-Murray, 2004). Individuals whose hearing loss is too great to benefit from amplified sound in the form of hearing aids may benefit from cochlear implants. A cochlear implant replaces the hair-cell transducer system in the cochlea by stimulating the auditory nerve directly. The nerve impulses generated by the cochlear implant travel along the neural auditory pathway and are then delivered to the brain, as if the cochlea were stimulated in a natural way (Tye-Murray, 2004).

Hearing aids and cochlear implants are communication devices worn everyday in almost all communication settings. Certain communication settings may however, require additional assistive listening devices, such as an FM system. The hearing health care professional will discuss various listening situations in the individual's daily life, and assess whether an FM system needs to be fitted. Conditions that compromise a poor listening environment include ambient noise, reverberation, and background noise. FM systems make use of radio waves to transmit sound from the source to the listener, wirelessly. The speaker may wear a wireless microphone around his or her. Their speech is frequency modulated on radio frequency carrier waves, which are transmitted to the receiver of the listener. The receiver of the FM system connects to the listener's hearing aid (Tye-Murray, 2004).

Intervention for sensory hearing loss may differ from intervention for neural hearing loss. Thus, it is important to correctly identify the type of hearing loss during audiologic assessment. Intervention for sensory and neural hearing loss are discussed below.

Management for Sensory Auditory Disorders

During intervention for sensory hearing loss, the following factors need to be taken into account: etiology of loss, degree of loss, and configuration of loss. Depending on the degree and configuration of sensory hearing loss, appropriate amplification needs to be selected and fitted. Individuals identified with a mild to severe sensory hearing loss may be fitted with hearing aids. As with immunocompetent individuals, HIV-infected individuals can benefit equally from the use of hearing aids. Hearing aid fitting and aural rehabilitation should begin as soon as the individual presents with a hearing loss significant enough to qualify for hearing aids (Madriz & Herrera, 1995; Moazzez & Alvi, 1998; Truitt & Tami, 1999). Counseling, orientation, and support should be provided for these individuals (Madriz & Herrera, 1995).

Individuals with sensory hearing loss, who have been fitted with hearing aids, may require further amplification in the form of assistive listening devices or FM systems. Certain situations, such as hearing in background noise and hearing speech at a distance, remain difficult for the hearing aid user. In such instances, an FM system may be necessary to improve the individual's hearing abilities. Children who are hearing aid users may struggle in the classroom situation, where acoustics are poor and the signal-to-noise ratio is bad. The use of an FM system enables the child to hear the speaker (teacher) clearly, while surrounding background noise is significantly reduced. Adults, who work in noisy environments with poor acoustics, also may benefit from an FM system, enabling them to overcome the challenging listening environments.

In individuals affected with bilateral profound or total sensory hearing loss, cochlear implantation may be ideal to restore a hearing level that allows them to have an acceptable quality of life (Vincenti et al., 2005). When deciding whether an individual with HIV/AIDS infection is a good candidate for a cochlear implantation, the following factors need to be taken into consideration: adherence to medication regimens; maintaining independence; and awareness of preventing HIV transmission and associated opportunistic infections (Vincenti et al., 2005).

It is essential for the individual to adhere strictly to their medication regimens to maintain their health status, and thus be able to benefit from a cochlear implant. Furthermore, it is important for them to maintain their independence, in order to be able to attend their follow-up adjustments, and maintain their cochlear implant. The medical decision to operate on an HIV-infected individual depends on the balance between the risks of the surgical procedure and the benefits of the cochlear implant for the individual (Vincenti et al., 2005). The surgical procedure can be done safely when keeping in mind that the general condition of the HIV-infected individual is the decisive factor for or against surgery (Vincenti et al., 2005).

Vincenti et al. (2005) conducted a single-case study on an HIV-infected individual who received a cochlear implant. The individual demonstrated a great increase in self-esteem, independence, and vocational prospects, following cochlear implantation (Vincenti et al., 2005). These results are supported by findings of Agwu et al. (2006), who report on a 9-year-old boy with HIV/AIDS who received a cochlear implant after developing a profound sensorineural hearing loss due to labyrinthitis ossificans. The boy experienced improved communication, as well as improved school performance and self-esteem (Agwu et al., 2006).

Roland et al. (2003) conducted a study at the New York University on seven HIV-infected individuals with profound sensorineural hearing loss, who received cochlear implants. Speech perception testing was conducted preoperatively and postoperatively. Preoperatively, the participants achieved an average word score of 1%. Postoperatively, however, the average word score was 38% (Roland et al., 2003). Furthermore, no intraoperative or postoperative surgical or medical complications were noted (Roland et al., 2003). All individuals continue to be cochlear implant users and no evidence of wound healing complications or delayed extrusion of the cochlear implant device were recorded (Roland et al., 2003). Cochlear implantation, therefore, is certainly an option for individuals who have HIV/AIDS.

In developing countries however, cochlear implantation may not always be an option due to resource constraints and very remote cochlear implant support. This field is expanding quite rapidly and in a country like South Africa cochlear implant teams and support are well established. In cases where cochlear implants are available for patients with severe to profound hearing loss, hearing aids may provide awareness of sound, but probably will not restore optimal hearing levels. Additional training in speech reading or a manual communication system, therefore, is recommended in such cases.

Whatever type of amplification the individual with sensory hearing loss receives, whether it is hearing aids, FM systems, or cochlear implants, it is essential to monitor hearing status regularly. Individuals, who have been fitted with the appropriate amplification, require follow-up audiologic assessments to accurately adjust their amplification devices and ensure that optimal amplification of speech is provided.

Management for Neural Auditory Disorders

Intervention for neural hearing loss or auditory dysfunction may be more complex and varied than that of sensory hearing loss. This is due to the range of pathologies relating to hearing and auditory functioning that may be of a neural origin. For example, an individual identified with a tumor or lesion causing a hearing loss and an individual without any evidence of a neoplasm or even a loss in hearing sensitivity but who demonstrates auditory dysfunction on a test of neural synchrony (i.e., the ABR) both may be classified as having a neural auditory disorder but their treatment will be vastly different.

In the case of a neoplasm, the ENT may provide surgical removal of the tumor, with follow-up medical and audiologic assessments. In the case where there is no evidence of loss in hearing sensitivity but there are abnormalities in neural conduction as measured on an ABR or CAEP test, as has commonly been reported in patients with HIV/AIDS, a functional approach to management should be the first course of action. The abnormalities on these tests of neural conduction should be supplemented by a detailed case history and questions about daily functioning, especially listening in noisy environments. This will provide the necessary information to decide on the use of an FM system, for example, to improve hearing ability in background noise.

As with sensory hearing loss, hearing aid fitting and aural (re)habilitation should begin as soon as the individual presents with a hearing loss significant enough to qualify for hearing aids (Madriz & Herrera, 1995; Moazzez & Alvi, 1998; Truitt & Tami, 1999). Individuals with neural hearing loss also may benefit from hearing aids, although outcomes are varied and significantly poorer than for children with sensory hearing loss. Children with neural hearing loss have dysynchronous discharge of auditory neurons, resulting in poor temporal processing. Poor temporal processing results in poor speech discrimination, especially in the presence of background noise. Amplification may make sound louder, but does not necessarily improve temporal processing abilities. A trial hearing aid fitting, therefore, is recommended for individuals with neural hearing loss until the benefit of acoustic amplification can be determined. The use of cochlear implants in individuals with neural hearing loss is becoming more widespread, and positive outcomes have been reported in many children with neural hearing loss (JCIH, 2007).

Hearing aid users with neural hearing loss may require further amplification in the form of assistive listening devices or FM systems. Certain situations, such as hearing in background noise and hearing speech at a distance, are particularly challenging for individuals with neural hearing losses (e.g., auditory neuropathy). In such instances, an FM system may be necessary to improve the individual's hearing abilities. Individuals with neural hearing loss benefit greatly from an improved signal-to-noise ratio, provided by an FM system.

Furthermore, it is essential to regularly monitor the hearing status of individuals with neural hearing loss. Amplification devices should be adjusted according to any changes in hearing status. The hearing status of individuals with neural hearing loss is expected to deteriorate with advancement of the disease. As the virus progresses, the effects on the CNS system may worsen, causing further auditory dysfunction of loss in hearing sensitivity. In the case of children with HIV encephalopathy, for example, which is degenerative, it is essential to regularly adjust their amplification devices according to their hearing status to ensure maximum speech and language development.

SUMMARY

HIV/AIDS-associated hearing loss of a sensory and neural nature is not uncommon and occurs primarily through three main etiologies. First, the direct effect of HIV on the CNS has exhibited degeneration and demyelination of auditory pathways. Second, the immune-compromized condition resulting from HIV/AIDS leads to opportunistic infections, which are common causes of hearing loss. Third, ototoxicity associated with antiretroviral medication for HIV/AIDS and medications for the secondary opportunistic infections are a real and important risk for acquired hearing loss in this population. Identification, assessment, and management strategies for hearing loss and auditory disorders associated with HIV/AIDS are formulated around these etiologies. A team approach is essential in diagnosing and managing the diverse range of symptoms that may arise. Primary and secondary prevention of hearing loss and auditory pathology through regular monitoring should be a priority in the comprehensive care of patients with HIV/AIDS.

REFERENCES

Agwu, A. G., Pasternak, R., Joyner, M., Carver, C. L., Francis, H. W. & Siberny, G. K. (2006). Nontypeable haemophilus influenzae meningitis complicated by hearing loss in a 9-year-old HIV-infected boy. *AIDS Patient Care and STDs, 20*(8), 531–535.

Bankaitis, A. E., & Keith, R. W. (1995). Audiological changes associated with HIV infection. *Ear, Nose and Throat Journal, 74*(5), 353–358.

Bektas, D., Martin, G. K., Stagner, B. B., & Lonsbury-Martin, B. L. (2008). Noise-induced hearing loss in mice treated with antiretroviral drugs. *Hearing Research, 239*(1–2), 69–78.

Bernaldez, P. C., Morales, G., & Hernandez, C. M. (2005). Chronic suppurative otitis media in HIV-infected children. *Otolaryngology–Head and Neck Surgery, 133*(2), 243–244.

Birchall, M. A., Wight, R. G., French, P. D., Cockbain, Z., & Smith, S. J. M. (1992). Auditory function in patients infected with the human immunodeficiency virus. *Clinical Otolaryngology and Allied Sciences, 17*(2), 117–121.

Brandy, W. T. (2002). Speech audiometry. In J. Katz (Ed.), *Handbook of clinical audiology* (5th ed.). Baltimore, MD: Lippincott Williams & Wilkins.

Cameron, E. (2000). The deafening silence of AIDS. *Health and Human Rights, 5*(1), 7–24.

Carvalho, M. F. P., & Tidei, R. (2001). Sudden deafness in AIDS. *Relato de Casos, 67*(2), 249–251.

Castro, N. M., Bango, M. Y., de Ureta, P. T., Garcia-Lomas, M. V., & Lopez, F. G. (2000). Hearing loss and infection with the human immunodeficiency syndrome virus. Study of 30 patients. *Revista Clinica Espanola, 200*(5), 271-274.

Chaloryoo, S., Chotpitayasunondh, T., & Chiengmai, P. N. (1998). AIDS in ENT in children. *International Journal of Pediatric Otorhinolaryngology, 44*(2), 103-107.

Chan, A., Perez, H., Ben, C., & Ochoa, C. (2003). Tuberculosis and HIV: A partnership against the most vulnerable. *Journal of the International Association of Physicians in AIDS Care, 2*(3) 106-123.

Chandrasekhar, S. S., Connelly, P. E., Brahmbhatt, S. S., Shah, C. S., Kloser, P. C., & Baredes, S. (2000). Otologic and audiologic evaluation of human immunodeficiency virus-infected patients. *American Journal of Otolaryngology, 21*, 1-9.

Christensen, L. A., Morehouse, C. R., Powell, T. W., Alchediak, T. & Silio, M. (1998). Antiviral therapy in a child with pediatric human immunodeficiency virus (HIV). Case study of audiologic findings. *Journal of American Academy of Audiology, 9*, 292-298.

Fowler, C. G., & Shanks, J. E. (2002). Tympanometry. In J. Katz (Ed.), *Handbook of clinical audiology* (5th ed.). Baltimore, MD: Lippincott Williams & Wilkins.

Garcia, V. P., Martinez, F. A., Agusti, E. B., Mencia, L. A. & Asenjo, V. P. (2001). Drug-induced ototoxicity: Current status. *Acta Otolaryngolica, 121*, 509-572.

Gelfand, S. (2002). The acoustic reflex. In J. Katz (Ed.), *Handbook of clinical audiology* (5th ed.). Baltimore, MD: Lippincott Williams & Wilkins.

Goetghebuer, T., West, T. E., Wermenbol, V., Cadbury, A. L., Milligan, P., Lloyd-Evans, N., . . . Weber, W. W. (2000). Outcome of meningitis caused by Streptococcus pneumoniae and Haemophilus influenzae type B in children in the Gambia. *Tropical Medicine and International Health, 5*(3), 207-213.

Goodarzi, M. O., Broberg, T. G., & Lalwani, A. K. (1998). Case report: Lymphoma of the tympanic membrane in acquired immunodeficiency syndrome. *Auris, Nasus, Larynx, 25*, 89-94.

Goodin, D. S., Aminoff, M. J., Chernoff, D. N., & Hollander, H. (1990). Long-latency event related potentials in patients infected with human immunodeficiency virus. *Annals of Neurology, 27*(4), 414-419.

Gurney, T. A., & Murr, A. H. (2003). Otolaryngologic manifestations of human immunodeficiency virus infection. *Otolaryngologic Clinics of North America, 36*, 607-624.

Hoare, S. (2003). HIV infection in children—impact upon ENT doctors. *Journal of Pediatric Otorhinolaryngology, 67*(Suppl. 1), S85-S90.

Joint Committee on Infant Hearing. (2007). Year 2007 position statement: Principles and guidelines for early hearing detection and intervention programs. *Journal of American Academy of Pediatrics, 120*(4), 898-921.

Katholm, M., Johnsen, N. H., Sum, C., & Willumsen, L. (1991). Bilateral sudden deafness and acute acquired toxoplasmosis. *Journal of Laryngology and Otology, 105,* 115-118.

Khoza, K., & Ross, E. (2002). Auditory function in a group of adults infected with HIV/AIDS in Gauteng, South Africa. *South African Journal of Communication Disorders, 49,* 17-27.

Koralnick, I. J., Beaumanoir, A., Hausler, R., Kholer, A., Safran, A. B., & Delacoux, R. (1990). A controlled study of early neurologic abnormalities in men with asymptomatic human immunodeficiency virus infection. *New England Journal of Medicine, 323,* 864-870.

Kozlowski, P. B. (1992). Neuropathology of HIV infection in children. In A. C. Crocker, H. J. Cohen, T. A. Kastner (Eds.), *HIV infection and developmental disabilities. A resource for service providers* (pp. 25-31). Baltimore, MD: Paul H. Brookes.

Little, J. P., Gardner, G., Acker, J. D., & Land, M. A. (1995). Otosyphilis in a patient with human immunodeficiency virus: Internal auditory canal gumma. *Otolaryngology-Head and Neck Surgery, 112,* 488-492.

Madhi, S. A., Madhi, A., Petersen, K., Khoosal, M., & Klugman, K. P. (2001). Impact of human immunodeficiency virus type 1 infection on the epidemiology and outcome of bacterial meningitis in South African children. *International Journal of Infectious Diseases, 5*(3), 119-125.

Madriz, J. J., & Herrera, G. (1995). Human immunodeficiency virus and acquired immune deficiency syndrome: AIDS-related hearing disorders. *Journal of the American Academy of Audiology, 6,* 358-364.

Marra, C. M., Wechkin, H. A., Longstreth, W. T., Rees, T. S., Syapin, C. L., & Gates, G. A. (1997). Antiretroviral therapy in patients infected with HIV-1. *Archives of Neurology, 54*(4), 407-410.

Matas, C. G., Leite, R. A., Magliaro, F. C. L., & Goncalves, I. C. (2006). Audiological and electrophysiological evaluation of children with acquired immunodeficiency syndrome (AIDS). *Brazilian Journal of Infectious Diseases, 10*(4), 264-268.

Matas, C. G., Sansone, A. P., Iorio, M. C. M., & Succi, R. C. M. (2000). Audiological evaluation in children born to HIV-positive mothers. *Revista Brasileira de Otorrinolaringologia, 66*(4), 317-324.

Mc Neilly, L. M. (2005). HIV and communication. *Journal of Communication Disorders, 38,* 303-310.

Meynard, J. L., Amrani, M. E., Meyohas, M. C., Fligny, I., Gozlan, J., Rozenbaum, W., . . . Frottier, J. (1997). Two cases of cytomegalovirus infection revealed by hearing loss in HIV-infected patients. *Biomedicine and Pharmacotherapy, 51,* 461-463.

Milazzo, L., Di Marco, A., Gervasoni, C., Rusconi, S., & Negri, C. (2000). Hearing loss as a presentation of CMV encephalitis in an HIV-1-infected patient. *Infections in Medicine, 17*(7), 495-499.

Moazzez, A. H., & Alvi, A. (1998). Head and neck manifestations of AIDS in adults. *American Family Physician, 57*(8), 1813–1822.

Molyneux, E. M. (2006). Hearing loss in Malawian children after bacterial meningitis. *Community Ear and Hearing Health, 3,* 5–6.

Molyneux, E. M., Tembo, M., Kayira, K., Bwanaisa, L., Mweneychanya, J., Njobyu, A., . . . Molyneux, M. E. (2003). The effect of HIV infection on paediatric bacterial meningitis in Blantyre, Malawi. *Archives of Disease in Childhood, 88*(12), 1112–1118.

Naudé, D. H., & Pretorius, R. E. (2003). Proposing an instructional framework for children with HIV/AIDS. *British Journal of Special Education, 30*(3), 138–143.

Newton, P. J. (2006). The causes of hearing loss in HIV infection. *Community Ear and Hearing Health, 3,* 11–14.

Northern, J. L., & Downs, M. P. (2002). *Hearing in children* (5th ed.). Baltimore, MD: Lippincott Williams & Wilkins.

Olusanya, B. O., Afe, A. J., & Onyia, N. O. (2009). Infants with HIV-infected mothers in a universal newborn hearing screening programme in Lagos, Nigeria. *Journal Compilation. Foundation Acta Pædiatrica, 98*(8), 1288–1293.

Palacios, G. C., Montalvo, M. S., Fraire, M. I., Leon, E., Alvarez, M. T., & Solorzano, F. (2008). Audiologic and vestibular findings in a sample of human immunodeficiency virus type-1-infected Mexican children under highly active antiretroviral therapy. *International Journal of Pediatric Otorhinolaryngology, 72,* 1671–1681.

Pappas, D. G., Roland, J. T., Lim, J., Lai, A., & Hillman, D. E. (1995). Ultrastructural findings in the vestibular end-organs of AIDS cases. *American Journal of Otology, 16*(2), 140–145.

Poblano, A. Figueroa, L. Figueroa-Damian, R., & Schnaas L. (2004). Effects of prenatal exposure to Zidovudine and Lamivudine on brainstem auditory evoked potentials in infants from HIV-infected women. *Proceedings of the Western Pharmacology Society, 47,* 46–49.

Rabie, H., Marais, B. J., Van Toorn, R., Nourse, P., Nel, E. D., Goussard, P., . . . Cotton, M. F. (2007). Important HIV-associated conditions in HIV-infected infants and children. *South African Family Practice, 49*(4), 19–23.

Ragazzoni, A., Grippo, A., Ghidini, P., Schiavone, V., Lolli, F., Mazzota, F., . . . Pinto, F. (1993). Electrophysiological study of neurologically asymptomatic HIV1 seropositive patients. *Acta Neurologica Scandinavica, 87*(1), 47–51.

Rey, D., L'Heritier, A., & Lang, J. M. (2002). Severe ototoxicity in a health care worker who received postexposure prophylaxis with stavudine, lamivudine and nevirapine after occupational exposure to HIV [Correspondence]. *CID, 34,* 418–419.

Reyes-Contreras, L., Silva-Rojas, A., Ysunza-Rivera, A., Jimenez-Ruiz, G., Berruecos-Villalobos, P., & Romo-Gutierrez, G. (2002). Brainstem auditory evoked response in HIV-infected patients with and without AIDS. *Archives of Medical Research, 33,* 25-28.

Rinaldo, A., Brandwein, M. S., Devaney, K. O., & Ferlito, A. (2003). AIDS-related otological lesions [Guest editorial]. *Acta Otolaryngology, 123,* 672-674.

Roland, J. T., Alexiades, G., Jackman, A. H., Hillman, D., & Shapiro, W. (2003). Cochlear implantation in human immunodeficiency virus-infected patients. *Otology and Neurology, 24,* 892-895.

Schouten, J. T., Lockhart, D. W., Rees, T. S., Collier, A. C., & Marra, C. M. (2006). A prospective study of hearing changes after beginning zidovudine or didanosine in HIV-1 treatment-naïve people. *BMC Infectious Diseases, 6,* 28-33.

Sheikh, S. I., Nijhawan, A., Basgoz, N., & Venna, N. (2009). Reversible Cogan's syndrome in a patient with human immunodeficiency virus (HIV) infection. *Journal of Clinical Neuroscience, 16,* 154-156.

Shibuyama, S., Gevorkyan, A., Yoo, U., Tim, S., Dzhangiryan, K., & Scott, J. D. (2006). Understanding and avoiding antiretroviral adverse effects. *Current Pharmaceutical Design, 12*(9), 1075-1090.

Simdon, J., Watters, D., Bartlett, S., & Connick, E. (2001). Ototoxicity associated with use of nucleoside analog reverse transcriptase inhibitors: A report of 3 possible cases and review of the literature. *HIV/AIDS, 32,* 1623-1627.

Singh, A., Georgalas, C., Patel, N., & Papesch, M. (2003). ENT presentations in children with HIV infection. *Clinical Otolaryngology, 28,* 240-243.

Smith, R. J., Bale, J. F., & White, K. R. (2005). Sensorineural hearing loss in children. *Lancet, 365,* 879-890.

Stach, B. A., Westerberg, B. D., & Roberson, J. B. (1998). Auditory disorder in central nervous system miliary tuberculosis: Case report. *Journal of American Academy of Audiology, 9,* 305-310.

Tindyebwa, D., Kayita, J., Musoke, P., Eley, B., Nduati, R., Coovadia, H., . . . African Network for the Care of Children Affected by AIDS (ANECCA). (2004). *Handbook on paediatric AIDS in Africa.* Downloadable from http://www.rcqhc.org

Truitt, T. O., & Tami, T. A. (1999). Otolaryngologic manifestations of human immunodeficiency virus infection. *Otolaryngology for the Internist, 83*(1), 303-315.

Tye-Murray, N. (2004). *Foundations of aural rehabilitation: Children, adults, and their family members.* Clifton Park, NY: Delmar Learning.

Vallely, P. (2006). Congenital infections and hearing impairment. *Community Ear and Hearing Health, 3,* 2-4.

Vancikova, Z., & Dvorak, P. (2001). Cytomegalovirus infection in immunocompetent and immunocompromised individuals—A review. *Current Drug Targets—Immune, Endocrine and Metabolic Disorder, 1*(2), 179–187.

Vigliano, P., Russo, R., Arfelli, P., Boffi, P., Bonassi, E., Gandione, M., . . . Rigardetto, R. (1997). Diagnostic value of multimodal evoked potentials in HIV-1 infected children. *Clinical Neurophysiology, 27*(4), 283–292.

Vincenti, V., Pasanisi, E., Bacciu, A., Giordano, D., Di Lella, F., Guida, M. & Bacciu, S. (2005). Cochlear implantation in a human immunodeficiency virus-infected patient. *Laryngoscope, 115*, 1079–1081.

Vogeser, M., Colebunders, R., Depraetere, K., Van Wanzeele, P., & Gehuchten, S. (1998). Deafness caused by didanosine. *European Journal of Clinical Microbiology and Infectious Diseases, 17*, 214–215.

Zuniga J. (1999). Communication disorders and HIV disease. *Journal of the International Association of Physicians in AIDS Care, 5*(4), 16–23.

CHAPTER 11

Balance Disorders Associated with HIV/AIDS

Louis Hofmeyr
Malcolm Baker

INTRODUCTION

Postural balance is a complex bodily function, essential for normal spatial orientation and movement, dependent on multiple sensory inputs, including vestibular, visual, and proprioceptive, various motor outflows, and their continuous, harmonious integration. The human immunodeficiency virus (HIV), both by direct disruption of these systems and through associated infections, neoplasms, and treatments has the potential to cause balance disturbances, with attendant functional impairment.

Although the development of antiretroviral (ARV) treatments has radically altered the picture of HIV/AIDS, many challenges remain, such as poor access to ARVs in parts of the world and the development of drug resistances, for example, by *Mycobacterium tuberculosis*. The nervous system is frequently affected by HIV/AIDS at multiple levels, including vestibular structures, and one of the more troublesome manifestations is disturbance of balance. However, detailed population-based studies on this associated manifestation are lacking.

NEUROLOGICAL AND VESTIBULAR EPIDEMIOLOGY OF HIV/AIDS

HIV infection and acquired immunodeficiency syndrome (AIDS) are currently of the major public health concerns. An estimated 38 million people are infected worldwide (UNAIDS, 2007) and through 2004, more than 20 million deaths have occurred due to the illness (UNAIDS, 2004). By far the highest prevalence of HIV infection exists in Sub-Saharan Africa, with at least 22.5 million cases and an adult prevalence of at least 5% (UNAIDS, 2007). In Sub-Saharan Africa, 57% of affected adults are women with the predominant mode of transmission being heterosexual contact. In other parts of the world, homosexual male to male and injection drug use may be more common modes of transmission. In children, most infection results from mother to infant transmission in the perinatal period (Centers for Disease Control, 2003).

After infection, the HIV virus can be detected as early as 2 weeks and HIV antibodies within 4 to 6 weeks (Allain, Laurian, Paul, & Senn, 1986). With seroconversion, a number of symptoms including fevers, sweats, malaise, lethargy, anorexia, myalgia, arthralgia, headaches, diarrhoea, lymphadenopathy, and a macular skin rash may occur (Cooper et al., 1985). Acute inflammatory demyelinating polyneuropathy (AIDP) resembling Guillain-Barré syndrome also may occur with infection (Thornton, Latif, & Emmanuel, 1991; Verma, 2001; Wulff, Wang, & Simpson, 2000).

Manifestations that may occur at various stages of HIV infection are indicated in Chapter 2 (clinical categories of the CDC classification system in HIV-infected persons). The 1993 revised CDC criteria included in the "AIDS" group a CD4-T cell count greater than 200 cells/μl or a leucocyte count consisting of more than 14% lymphocytes even in the absence of the listed conditions (Centers for Disease Control, 1992).

Neurologic system involvement is extremely common with HIV infection. An autopsy series in Tanzania (Kibayashi et al., 1999) indicated that 80% of HIV-positive cases had central nervous system (CNS) pathology including tuberculosis (TB), meningitis, and other meningitides. Modi and Modi (2004) assessed 32 HIV-positive patients with focal brain lesions by imaging, serological tests, and biopsy and found 53% to have CNS TB, 19% neurocysticercosis

(NCC), 6% to have TB and NCC, 6% to have multiple infarcts, 3% to have toxoplasmosis, 3% to have TB and cryptococcal meningitis, 3% progressive multifocal leukoencephalopathy, and 3% primary CNS lymphoma. CNS lymphoma also may mimic vestibular schwannoma (Wenzel, Götz, Lenarz, & Stöver, 2008).

HIV may affect any or multiple parts of the nervous system. Bhigjee et al. (1993) reported 33 patients with HIV and myelopathy in South Africa; of these, 36% had HTLV-1 coinfection, 18% spinal TB, 9% zoster myelitis, 6% syphilitic disease, 6% bilharzia, 3% vascular myelopathy, and 1% were attributed to seroconversion.

In adults, peripheral neuropathy may be the most common neurologic complication associated with HIV (Barohn, Gronseth, & Le Force, 1993). The most common form of neuropathy seen is distal symmetric polyneuropathy (DSP) characterized by distal pain, paresthesias, numbness, decreased or absent ankle jerks, and a protracted clinical course. Other forms of neuropathy include AIDP, CIDP (acute and chronic inflammatory demyelinating polyneuropathy), progressive polyradiculopathy, sometimes associated with cytomegalovirus infection, mononeuropathy multiplex, diffuse infiltrative lymphocytosis syndrome neuropathy, and medication-associated neuropathy.

Use of antiretroviral agents has led to a decrease in mortality rates and neurologic opportunistic infections, but possibly not DSP (Baumann & Espinosa, 2007). Muscle disorders are also well described and may arise due to HIV infection and related conditions, antiretroviral therapy, opportunistic infections, or infiltrative tumors (Francois-Jérôme Authier, 2005). Johnson, Williams, Kazi, Dimachkie, and Reveille (2003) reported on using immunomodulatory therapy for HIV-associated polymyositis, with five to eight patients treated with prednisone achieving remission and three others treated with azathioprine or methotrexate combined with intravenous immunoglobulin regaining normal strength.

Likewise, vestibular dysfunction appears to occur frequently and may occur in the early phase of HIV due to direct viral damage (Teggi, Ceserani, Lira Luce, Lazzarin & Bussi, 2008). The incidence of vertigo in HIV/AIDS patients probably is underestimated and underreported, and also may be submerged in the multitude of symptoms seen in terminally ill patients (Lalwani & Sooy, 1992). Ultrastructural analysis of vestibular end organs obtained from HIV autopsy cases revealed pathologic changes in the labyrinth wall, epithelial lining, and receptor maculae and cristae (Pappas, Roland,

Lim, Lai, & Hillman, 1995). Cytologic changes in hair cells included inclusion bodies, viral-like particles, and hair bundle formations. Epithelial lining cells, supporting cells, and connective tissue cells were also involved. Teggi, Giordano, Pistorio, and Bussi (2006) found 5 of 14 (35,7%) clinical CDC category A patients to have pure peripheral vestibular dysfunction, 3 of 11 (27,3%) in category B had both peripheral and central dysfunction, another 3 had purely central vestibular damage, and in category C, 2 of 5 had peripheral and central signs. The remaining 3 of 5 patients in category C had only central vestibular signs. On the contrary, some investigators failed to prove a higher incidence of damage to inner ear structures in patients in whom cytomegalovirus and adenovirus were isolated from the inner ear at autopsy. The lack of vestibular signs and normal inner ear histology in patients with clinical and histologic evidence of HIV dementia supported the theory that these viruses are either nonpathogenic or that viral infection occurs terminally and elicits no inflammation because of the immunosuppression from HIV/AIDS (Davis, Rarey, & Mclaren, 1995).

Essentially, HIV-associated dysfunction of any part (or multiple parts) of the vestibular and/or neurologic systems, may lead to balance disturbances and dizziness, although detailed population-based studies are lacking. In a study on hearing loss and antiretroviral therapy in patients infected with HIV-1, Marra et al. (1997) reported that 30% of 99 patients complained about vertigo related to their hearing loss. On the other hand, Khoza and Ross (2002) investigating the auditory function in a group of adults infected with HIV/AIDS in Gauteng, South Africa reported that only 9% out of 150 patients complained of vertigo. The variance of reported prevalence may relate to different diagnostic criteria.

OVERVIEW OF THE BALANCE MECHANISM: ANATOMY AND PHYSIOLOGY

The balance system in humans has evolved into a highly specialized and integrated system. Different sensory functions are utilized to supply the brain with as much information as possible to integrate and respond to specific balance and postural needs with appropriate actions. These actions aim to maintain balance function with different body positions and movements, help to orientate the body regarding its position in space, and ensure that the visual picture stays stable during head movements. Figure 11-1 illustrates the essential components of the balance system. These are discussed in the following sections as background to the ways in which HIV may disturb this complex interaction of various systems directly or indirectly.

Definitions

1. *Balance:* Balance is the means by which postural equilibrium is maintained. Disturbances may lead to dizziness, unsteadiness, incoordination, oscillopsia, ataxia, and a propensity to falls, with added morbidity. The risk of falling may be compounded by weakness, visual deficits, medication effects, arthritis, frailty, and fear.

2. *Oscillopsia:* This is a perceived sensation of oscillatory motion of the visual surround when it is not actually moving.

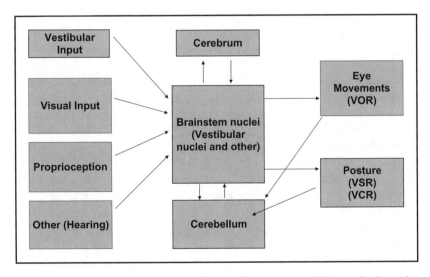

Figure 11–1. Essential components of the balance system: VOR: vestibulo-ocular reflex; VSR: vestibulospinal reflex; VCR: vestibulocollic reflex.

3. *Dizziness:* Dizziness is any sensation of disturbed or impaired spatial orientation and movement, being nonvertiginous in the absence of a false sense of rotation.

4. *Vertigo:* Traditionally derived from the Latin term *vertere* referring to rotation vertigo is a false sensation of rotation. If a patient experiences any other form of linear motion (such as bobbing or bouncing), it correctly should not be referred to as vertigo but rather described as an illusion of self-motion.

The Vestibular System

Input from the Vestibular System

The peripheral vestibular system is situated bilaterally in hard and dense bony capsules in the temporal bones on either side of the skull. This bony capsule or inner ear is divided into a part for hearing (cochlea) and a part for balance function (semicircular canals and otolithic organs). Inside these bony spaces is a membranous system filled with fluid (endo- and perilymph) (Figure 11-2).

There are three semicircular canals in each bony inner ear. They are referred to as the superior (anterior), horizontal (lateral), and posterior (inferior) semicircular canals. The semicircular canals are oriented in such a manner that they form near right angles to each other. They are involved in sensing head rotational acceleration. The horizontal canal senses the movement of the head in a horizontal plane whereas the superior and posterior canals sense movement of the head in a vertical plane. The latter two also are sometimes referred to as the vertical canals. The mechanical stimulation of angular or rotational acceleration is translated into electric neural impulses by means of the neuroepithelium in dilated portions of the membranous duct, namely, the ampullae. The ampulla consists of a gel-like organ, the cupula, which rests upon a crestlike structure, the crista. The crista supports hair cells, which serve as the receptor cells for motion. The cupula stretches across the whole ampulla and as the head rotates is moved to one or the other side causing stimulation or suppression.

The bony inner ear is divided into the cochlea, which serves as the receptor organ for hearing and the vestibular portion (semicircular canals and otolithic organs), which serves as the receptor

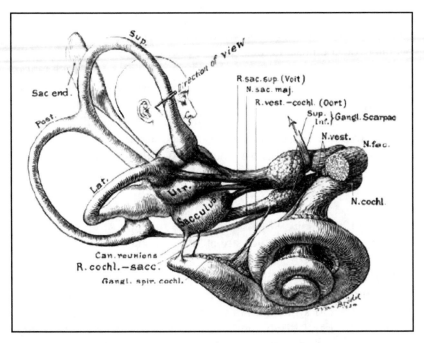

Figure 11–2. *Anatomy of the vestibular labyrinth. Structures include the utricle (Utr.), sacculus, anterior (or superior) semicircular canal (Sup.), posterior semicircular canal (Post.), and the lateral (or horizontal) semicircular canal (Lat.). Note the superior vestibular nerve innervating the anterior and lateral semicircular canals as well as the utricle. The inferior vestibular nerve innervates the posterior semicircular canal and the saccule. The cell bodies of the vestibular nerves are located in Scarpa's ganglion (Gangl. Scarpae). Drawing from original art in the Max Brodel Archives (No. 933), Department of Art as Applied to Medicine, The Johns Hopkins University School of Medicine.*

organ for balance. Both inner ears work in tandem. The vestibular functions of the inner ear include:

1. Maintaining balance.
2. Assisting with spatial orientation.
3. Keeping the retina fixed on a target during head motion.

Inside the bony inner ears a membranous system of tubes, containing fluid (endolymph), exists. The fluid in the surrounding perimembranous space is known as the perilymph. Peri- and endolymph differ in ionic content. There are two otolithic organs in each bony inner ear (i.e., the saccule and utricle). These are contained in the vestibule, which is the central portion of the inner ear. The anterior portion contains the cochlea and the posterior portion the semicircular canals. The saccule and the utricle sense gravity and linear head acceleration. The neuroepithelium that is stimulated by movement is situated in an area called the macula. The hair cells of the macula protrude into a gel-like layer covered by the otolithic membrane. The otolithic membrane is made up of calcium carbonate crystals. During motion these crystals lag the head movement, causing deflection of the cilia of the hair cells.

There are two types of hair cells, which function as receptor cells:

1. Type I hair cells, which are bulbous in shape.
2. Type II hair cells, which are slender in shape.

The hair cells contain numerous stereocilia but only one longer kinocilium. The kinocilium is semiflexible and the direction of the movement of the kinocilium in relation to the stereocilia determines whether the basal discharge is increased or decreased. This then stimulates or inhibits the neural discharge. Even at rest, there is always a resting discharge potential from the hair cells. Stimulation or an increase in the output of one semicircular canal, usually leads to an inhibition or decrease in the output of another canal on the opposite side, as they function in tandem.

The receptor cells send information to the brain via the vestibular portion of the eighth cranial nerve. Information from the superior canal, horizontal canal, utricle, and a portion of the saccule is transmitted through the superior vestibular nerve. Information from the rest of the saccule and the posterior semicircular canal is transmitted through the inferior vestibular nerve. The cell bodies of these two nerves are located in Scarpa's ganglion within the internal auditory canal of the temporal bone. In the internal auditory canal, the two vestibular portions run concurrently with fibers from the cochlea becoming the eighth cranial nerve at the entry into the pons of the brainstem.

Central Integration, Connections, and Output

The first synapse of the bipolar vestibular eighth cranial nerve axons is in the vestibular nucleus in the brainstem. The vestibular nuclei are situated bilaterally in the lower brainstem and consist of medial, lateral, superior, and inferior parts. The majority of afferents from the semicircular canals synapse in the medial and superior vestibular nuclei. The saccule and the utricle nerve fibres synapse mainly on the lateral and medial vestibular nuclei.

From the vestibular nuclei, the following pathways play a role in balance control, image stabilization and spatial orientation:

1. From the medial and superior vestibular nuclei, second-order neurons project ipsilaterally and contralaterally in the medial longitudinal fasciculus to supply the IIIrd, IVth, and VIth eye movement nuclei. Conjugated movements of the eye muscles then produce eye movements that attempt to stabilize the visual image on the retina. This is the so-called vestibulo-ocular reflex (VOR) for image stabilization during head movements.

2. From the medial and lateral vestibular nuclei, other second-order neurons supply the anterior horn cells of the cervical cord (medial vesitibulospinal tract) and the rest of the spinal cord (lateral vestibulospinal tract). The muscular movements produced by these inputs create the vestibulocollic reflex (VCR) and the vestibulospinal reflex (VSR) for static and dynamic balance control. A few of the fibers also synapse with the eye movement nuclei, which assists in producing rotational and vertical ocular adjustments during head tilt.

3. From the vestibular nuclei pathways, information is transmitted via the thalamus to the superior sylvian gyrus and inferior intraparietal sulcus region. Information from the vestibular, visual, and proprioceptive systems is integrated to create an awareness of body orientation and to form memories regarding motion and balance control.

4. The midline cerebellum is very important in the finer control of motor functions. The VOR, VCR, and VSR are influenced by the cerebellum in order to create smooth, fine, and precise movements. Pathways between the vestibular nuclei and midline cerebellum underlie this function.

5. Some of the more unpleasant symptoms, which occur with vestibular stimulation such as nausea, vomiting, excessive perspiration, and changes in heartbeat are believed to arise from connected circuitry between the vestibular nuclei and certain brainstem vegetative nuclei.

Vision

The visual system aids the patient in maintaining balance during static and moving conditions and also helps the patient with spatial orientation. Light impulses penetrate the eyes via the cornea, anterior chamber, pupil, lens, and vitreous fluid to activate the receptors on the retina.

There are two types of retinal receptor cells:

1. The rods, which are extremely sensitive to light and are the principal receptors for low light vision.
2. The cones, which have a higher acuity and are responsible for vision in bright light and color vision.

The fovea, a small part of the retina where visual acuity is the greatest, contains only cones. The optic disk is where the optic nerve originates. This area has no receptor cells and constitutes the "blind spot" in the visual field.

Bodies of ganglion cells are located in the retina and their axons pass within the optic nerve, optic chiasm, and optic tract to synapse in the lateral geniculate body of the thalamus. From the lateral geniculate body, fibers from the nasal half of one retina and the temporal half of the contralateral retina course in the geniculocalcarine tract to the primary visual receiving area in the occipital cortex. Some axons leave the optic tract to synapse in the pretectal region of the midbrain and the superior colliculus where connections are formed that mediate eye pupillary reactions and eye movements. Other axons pass from the optic chiasm to the suprachiasmatic nuclei in the hypothalamus where certain endocrine and circadic rhythms are modulated. Voluntary and involuntary (reflexive) correction of posture is possible through processing of visual inputs. Systems utilized include the saccadic, smooth pursuit, and optokinetic systems.

Saccades

Saccadic eye movements are rapid conjugate eye movements generated to fix gaze on a new target. These movements can be voluntarily or involuntarily (reflexively) generated. When voluntary, impulses are generated in the frontal eye fields of the frontal lobes of the brain. Stimulation of this area causes a contralateral conjugate lateral shift of gaze, mediated by the eye movement nuclei in the upper brainstem. Involuntary saccades are triggered by vestibular or optokinetic stimulation. When this is generated by the vestibular system, it forms part of the VOR. Involuntary saccades usually attempt to return the eye to the neutral position in the orbits. Lesions of the frontal eye fields, midline cerebellum, brainstem, and eyes may cause abnormal saccades.

Saccadic eye movements can be tested and display the following characteristics:

1. Conjugate eye deviation.
2. Short latency.
3. Accuracy with no under- or overshoots.
4. Rapidity.

Smooth Pursuit

Smooth pursuit eye movements are slow conjugated eye movements used to track slowly moving well-defined objects in the visual field. The object is registered by the fovea of the retina from where the information is transferred to the visual cortex in the occipital lobe. After interpretation, the smooth pursuit center then transfers the command for eye movement to the vestibular nuclei via the accessory optic tract and superior colliculi. In the vestibular nuclei, the eye movement is matched with the head movement and the final command for execution is given by the eye movement nuclei in the upper brainstem. Lesions of the visual system, cerebellum, and brainstem can cause abnormal smooth pursuit. Age, inattention, sedative medication, and the speed of the moving target may influence results.

Smooth pursuit can be tested and displays the following characteristics:

1. Conjugate eye deviation.
2. It is smooth in character.
3. It is symmetric.

Optokinetic Eye Movements

The optokinetic system differs from the smooth pursuit system as it is more of a reflexive eye movement. It also is generated by full-field peripheral stimulation of the retina. An example of optokinetic eye movements can be observed in the jerking eye movements of a passenger in a vehicle as he looks outside at the changing land-scape. As the features traverse the field of vision with the motion of the vehicle, the eyes demonstrate optokinetic nystagmus. The optokinetic system utilizes the same neural pathways as the smooth pursuit system. To evaluate the optokinetic response, the whole visual field should be stimulated. Asymmetric or absent responses may be indicative of pathology.

Proprioceptive and Somatosensory System

The aim of the balance system is to maintain the body's position centered over its base of support. The smaller the base, the more difficult this is. This is the reason why it is more difficult to balance on one leg than on both. In the standing position, the base of support is the feet. If the center of gravity (COG) is displaced eccentrically, three strategies are utilized to maintain balance and prevent falling. The three strategies in order of magnitude are:

1. The *ankle strategy* where small displacements of the COG produce small movements about the ankles.
2. The *hip strategy* for larger displacements of the COG where movements around the hips are mobilized to maintain balance.
3. The *step strategy* where the displacement of the COG is so large that a step is needed to increase the base of support to maintain balance.

Somatosensory information is supplied mainly by the skin touch receptors in the soles of the feet. The information gathered is transmitted in both the lemniscal and anterolateral pathways and only very extensive lesions completely interrupt touch sensation.

Proprioceptive information is supplied via the myotatic reflex arc, where stretch of a muscle leads to contraction of the muscle at a joint. Information is further supplied by the Golgi tendon organs and Pacini receptors in and around joints. The proprioceptive information is transmitted up the spinal cord in the dorsal columns. A lesion of the dorsal columns produces ataxia so that the patient walks with a broad base. Some of the axons terminate in the cerebellum but other pass via the medial lemnisci to the thalamus, cortex, and elsewhere.

Information from the somatosensory and proprioceptive pathways is utilized by the cortex of the brain to create a conscious picture of the position of the body in space.

SPECTRUM OF BALANCE DISTURBING PATHOLOGY IN HIV/AIDS

As mentioned at the outset of this chapter, there is a lack of comprehensive data on what may lead to balance disturbances in association with HIV. Anecdotal evidence, small series, and experience suggest that balance disturbances are common in HIV infection (Hausler, Vibert, Koralnik, & Hirschel, 1991; Palacios et al., 2008; Salami et al, 1991). Conditions that have been etiologically implicated are included in Table 11–1.

Detailed descriptions of the pathologies involved are beyond the scope of this chapter and may be found elsewhere. What needs to be emphasized is that neurologic pathology is frequent in HIV/ AIDS. Patients with HIV/AIDS presenting with balance disturbances may have any of the pathologies listed in Table 11–1 and sometimes multiple pathologies.

Tuberculosis is an especially prevalent co-occurring condition and may lead to meningitis, tuberculous cerebral infarction, abscesses, and other myelitis. Syphilis is another disease that should be ruled out in all patients with otologic complaints. Symptoms related to the different stages of HIV/AIDS and infections influencing fluid and electrolyte balance, cardiovascular, and respiratory function may cause nonspecific dizziness.

Treating clinicians need to be vigilant as to the multitude of possible causes and pathologies involved. More extensive investigation, than otherwise might be the case, including imaging of the nervous system and spinal tap, may therefore be warranted.

Table 11–1. Spectrum of Balance Disturbing Pathology in HIV/AIDS

HIV labyrinthitis/ vestibulitis		
Neurologic sequelae directly attributable to HIV	Encephalopathy	
	Myelopathy	
	Neuropathy (including cranial nerves)	
	Myopathy/ Motor neuronopathy	
Opportunistic and concomitant infections	Bacteria	*Mycobacterium tuberculosis* (MTB) complex
		Other mycobacteria
		Syphilis (Smith & Canalis, 1989; Morris & Prasad, 1990)
		Atypical mycobacteriosis (MAC)
		Salmonella septicemia
		Nocardia
		Listeria
	Fungi	Extrapulmonary *Pneumocystis jiroveci* (now considered to be a fungus)
		Candida species
		Cryptococcus neoformans
		Aspergillus species
		Histoplasma capsulatum
		Coccidioides immitis
		Blastomycosis
	Viruses	Cytomegalovirus
		Herpes simplex
		Herpes zoster and the Ramsay Hunt syndrome
		progressive multifocal

Table 11–1. *continued*

	Viruses *continued*	leukoencephalopathy HTLV-1
	Parasites	Neurocysticercosis
		Cerebral toxoplasma gondii
		Trypanosomiasis
		Malaria
		Strongyloides
	Rickettsia	
Neoplasms associated with HIV/AIDS	Metastatic Kaposi sarcoma of the CNS and inner ear (Michaels, Soucek, Liang,1994)	
	Lymphoma	
	Glioma	
Leukoencephalopathy of undetermined origin		
Strokes		
Antiretroviral agent complications	Abacavir associated vertigo (Fantry & Staecker, 2002)	
	Immune reconstitution inflammatory syndrome (IRIS)	
Other medication effects (side effects, interactions and ototoxicty)		
Systemic and other organ pathologies (wasting syndrome, cardiomyopathy. etc.)		
Clinical disorders not proven to be directly associated with HIV/AIDS		

CLINICAL APPROACH TO THE DIZZY PATIENT

The Case History

The history obtained from a patient with imbalance is of vital importance. "Dizziness" is a term often used by patients to describe balance disturbances but the term has different meanings to different people and symptoms caused by different pathologies may be described in the same way. Therefore, it imperative that a proper history is taken. Some clinicians may have the insight to formulate and pinpoint a problem by focusing on a few specific questions. It is more dependable, however, to utilize a dizziness questionnaire. Many such standard questionnaires exist. A dizziness questionnaire, as presented in Figure 11–3 is a simple, yet efficient, example that can be utilized.

Most patients need to be guided when answering some of these questions and it is often necessary to ask leading questions. The nature and the characteristics of the spell or balance problem, need to be defined. Second, associated medical problems, habits, and the use of medications need to be enquired about, which can help to delineate the etiology of the problem. Once the basic nature of the

---

DIZZINESS QUESTIONNAIRE

1. Describe what you are experiencing?

Spinning   Lightheaded   Passing out

Drunk feeling   Other _____

2. How long does your dizziness last?_____

Few seconds   Seconds to Minutes   Minutes to several hours

Hours to days   Continuous   Other: _____

3. How often do you get dizzy?

Only Once   More than Once   Frequency_____

Figure 11–3. Dizziness Questionnaire. From: Jacobson, G. P., & Shepard, N. T. (2008). Balance function assessment and management. *San Diego, CA: Plural Publishing, Inc. Reprinted with permission. All rights reserved.* continues

4. When do your attacks occur?

Standing up	Head Movements	Loud sounds
Sneezing	Straining	Rolling over in bed
Stress	Diet	Other _____

5. Do any of the following occur with your typical attacks?

Hearing loss	Tinnitus	Headaches
Facial Numbness	Anxiety	Change in Vision
Pain	Other _____	

6. I have the following medical problems.

Diabetes	Coronary artery disease
Stroke	Visual difficulty
Hypertension	Seizures
Migraine	Psychiatric Disease _____

7. What medications are you currently taking?

_____

_____

_____

8. Have you ever had any of the following?

Intravenous Antibiotics	Radiation Therapy	Ear Surgery
Chemotherapy	Syphilis	Noise Exposure

9. The level of my disability from dizziness is best described as:

☐ I am able to work, drive, and feel no ill effects from my dizziness.

☐ I can continue to function with my dizziness but not optimally.

☐ I need to stop when dizzy, but can return to work soon thereafter.

☐ I am incapacitated for extended periods of times because of the dizziness.

☐ I am unable to leave the house

☐ I am disabled

10. Does anyone in the family have:

Migraine	Ménière's Disease	Neurological disorder
Anxiety/Depression	Hearing loss	

11. Has the dizziness changed since the first episode?   Yes   No

If Yes :   Better   --   Worse   Shorter   --   Longer

Figure 11–3. continued

balance disturbance is ascertained (vertigo, light-headedness, ataxia, etc.), it is necessary to characterize the experience as being either episodic (spells) or an ongoing phenomenon. Replies to the following questions are instructive:

1. When did the problem first occur?
2. Did it come on suddenly?
3. Does it occur in recurrent attacks (spells)?
4. How long do they last?
5. How often do they occur?
6. Is balance normal between attacks?
7. When was the last attack?
8. Are there any warning signs that an attack is about to commence?
9. Are the attacks induced by changing of head and body position and to what extent?
10. Does closing the eyes improve or worsen the condition?

The general balance function of the patient should be noted. Determine whether there is a tendency to veer off or fall to a specific side and if this is related to the attacks. Ask if walking in the dark or on uneven surfaces or climbing stairs aggravates the condition. Other aspects to note are whether nausea, sweating, and diarrhea accompany the attacks and whether spatial disorientation is present. It should also be noted if motion sickness occurs. Ask the patient what he or she thinks might be the cause and what improves and what aggravates symptoms, if any.

Ask about any associated medical problems, habits, and medication that may contribute to or cause the problem. Vertigo may be a side effect of various pharmaceutical agents commonly used in treating HIV and associated opportunistic infections. Potentially ototoxic medications include abacavir, acyclovir, aminoglycosides, amphotericin B, azidothymidine, ddI, d4T, flucytocine, pentamidine, tetramycin, and trimethoprim-sulfamethoxasole. As the peripheral vestibular organ is situated in the inner ear, a proper history regarding ear problems and hearing loss also should be taken. Otalgia, otorrhea, tinnitus, hearing loss, fullness, and pressure in the ear and a history of ear surgery should be noted. Dizziness provoked by loud noise (Tulio phenomenon) also should be documented.

To exclude central or neurologic causes for dizziness and balance impairment a thorough history for neurologic symptoms should be taken. This is especially important in the HIV/AIDS population due to the high risk of neurologic involvement and central neurological diseases. Regarding direct HIV-1 central nervous infection, it is believed that the prefrontal cortex and parieto-occipital junction are mostly affected, followed by the vestibular cortex. The frontal eye field and supplementary eye field are minimally affected (Johnston, Miller, & Nath, 1996).

Neurologic symptoms that should be asked about are:

1. Diplopia, scotomas, photophobia.
2. Paresthesias and weakness.
3. Difficulty with speech, swallowing, and facial weakness.
4. Headaches.
5. Facial pain.
6. Tremors.
7. Loss of consciousness and presyncope.
8. Previous head and neck trauma.
9. Memory loss.
10. Risk factors of cerebrovascular disease.
11. Gait difficulty.
12. Seizures.

Eye function and adequate vision contribute significantly to balance control. Ask about loss of vision, eye movement impairment and the usage of corrective lenses. Multifocal lenses may impair visual cues for balance maintenance in the geriatric population. In the HIV/AIDS patient, possible cytomegalovirus retinal involvement should be asked about.

Cerebral hypoperfusion, with a reduction in oxygenation, can be a cause for "dizziness" or lightheadedness. Cardiovascular and especially pulmonary and hematologic causes are common in the later stages of HIV/AIDS. Postural hypotension should be ruled out.

It is known that the prevalence of psychological problems in patients with chronic dizziness can be very high. The psychological problems can be the cause, but also the result, of dizziness. Psychiatric manifestations are common in patients with HIV/AIDS. Symptoms relating to anxiety, depression, irritability, and avoidance behavior should be noted.

Previous illnesses and surgeries, medication use, allergies, family history, habits (including dietary, smoking and alcohol use), and participation in various activities such as diving and flying should be asked about. Specific emphasis also needs to be placed on symptoms relating to manifestations occurring at different stages of HIV/AIDS.

Balance disturbances are common in the general population, especially in the elderly. With the immune-compromized state associated with HIV/AIDS, concomitant diseases, opportunistic infections, and the effects of antiretroviral and other drugs, a multitude of factors may lead to imbalance. Awareness of the multitude of potentially contributing conditions is important and greater diagnostic zeal is warranted.

The Clinical Examination

The greatest burden of disease of HIV/AIDS occurs in developing countries, where funding and infrastructure often are lacking. For the purpose of this chapter, emphasis therefore is placed on the clinical examination, which provides significant information and does not require extensive infrastructure and resources.

The clinical examination prudently begins with first impressions when the patient enters the consulting area. Observing the patient's gait and movements, whether support is required, and if the patient displays obvious bruising and injuries indicative of falls may help to determine testing priorities and to verify test results later obtained. The clinical examination, as with the history taking, should be performed in a systematic manner. It is unlikely that a single finding will yield the final diagnosis and the pattern of findings of the entire clinical examination should be considered.

It is recommended that the basic general physical, neurologic, ear nose and throat (ENT) and head and neck examinations be performed before proceeding to the directed neuro-otologic examination. The focus of the examination will partly be influenced by the history; for example, patients with symptoms suggestive of lightheadedness or syncope need particular attention to be paid to the cardiovascular system, including having blood pressure and pulse checked lying and standing.

In the case of episodic vertigo, the visual and neurologic examination usually reveals no abnormalities. These are found only with the directed neuro-otologic examination (Troost, 2004). When symptoms are vaguer and include unsteadiness or disequilibrium, examination of sensation, the motor system, tendon reflexes, and cerebellar function is more likely to be abnormal. Where oscillopsia accompanies gait imbalance, bilateral-symmetric vestibular dysfunction may be present, such as may occur with meningitis, certain tumors, and toxicity (e.g., gentamycin) (Baloh, Fife, Furman, & Zee, 1996). Caloric, rotational, vestibular testing, and other directed neuro-otologic tests are especially likely to provide further findings here. Nevertheless, all patients with undiagnosed balance disturbances require a complete neurologic examination. Components of the neurologic examination are described here only briefly, as there are many detailed reference works on this topic (e.g., Mayo Clinic, 1997).

Basic Neurologic Examination

Level of Consciousness

A decreased level of consciousness may be associated with metabolic encephalopathy, medication side effects, meningitis, malignancy, extensive cerebral infarction, extensive intracranial multifocal lesions, and others.

Cognitive Impairments

These may be assessed by basic mental status examinations and more extensive psychometric evaluations. Abnormalities range from subtle apraxias to frank dementia, which may be seen with multifocal infarcts, infections, tumors, and other conditions.

Cranial Nerve Examination

Examination of visual acuity and visual fields may reveal a visual component of balance disturbance. Papilledema or absent venous pulsations on fundoscopy should raise concern regarding raised intracranial pressure (and may contraindicate the performing of a spinal tap). Decreased corneal sensation may indicate cerebello-pontine angle pathology. Bedside hearing tests (tuning fork acuity, Rinne and Weber) may point to audiologic disease, which would warrant further audiologic assessment. Cranial nerves IX to XII abnormalities may indicate skull base or nasopharyngeal pathology such as might be seen with certain neoplasms or meningitis.

Ocular Movement Examination

Strabismus should be checked for as this may be a relatively nonspecific cause of disequilibrium. Asymmetrical slowing of the adducting eye may indicate brainstem infarction or infection or a mass lesion of the posterior fossa. Finding spontaneous or induced nystagmus is crucially important in diagnosing peripheral, central, or systemic causes of imbalance.

Sensory Examination

Distal sensory changes may indicate peripheral neuropathy. A sensory level may be seen with myelopathy, whereas hemisensory loss is likely associated with central nervous system pathology. Selective loss of vibration sense and proprioception may be seen with neurosyphilitic tabes dorsalis or vitamin B deficiency. Typically, these patients rapidly lose balance and fall in any direction when closing eyes with the Romberg test but may be relatively steady with eyes open. Peripheral vestibulopathy tends to cause the patient to fall to the side of abnormality with eye closure.

Motor System Examination

Diffuse or focal weakness may indicate CNS (including spinal) or neuromuscular disorders. Hyporeflexia typically occurs with peripheral disorders, whereas hyper-reflexia may indicate spinal or cerebral dysfunction.

Cerebellar System Examination

Definite limb or truncal ataxia or incoordination strongly suggests a CNS disorder, most likely involving the cerebellum or its connections. Lesions of the vermis may selectively affect the trunk, whereas cerebellar hemisphere lesions tend to affect limb coordination.

Unsteadiness with Romberg testing with eyes open and only slightly worsening with eye closure strongly suggests a cerebellar dysfunction. Gait also is frequently abnormal. In the HIV setting, tumors, abscesses, infarcts, and granulomas may involve the cerebellum.

Symptoms and signs indicating the likely diagnoses and useful special investigations are indicated in the algorithm in Figure 11–4.

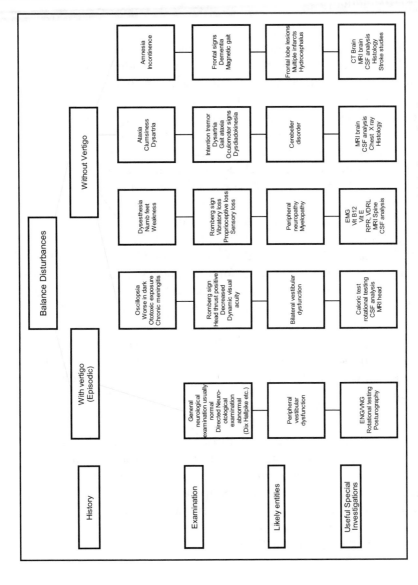

Figure 11–4. *Algorithm for the investigation of HIV/AIDS patients with balance disorders.*

311

Basic Ear, Nose, and Throat Examination

Ear Examination

The ear can be involved in various ways in patients with HIV/AIDS. Otologic diagnoses include otitis externa, otitis media, conductive hearing loss, sensorineural hearing loss, and mastoiditis (Rarey, 1990). Histopathologic changes in 49 temporal bones from 25 patients with HIV included severe otitis media in 5 patients (20%), low-grade otitis media in 15 (60%), labyrinthine cryptococcosis in 2, Kaposi sarcoma in the eighth nerve in 1, and CMV inclusion-bearing cells in the inner and middle ear of 6 (24%) (Michaels, Soucek, & Liang, 1994).

Ear evaluation should include examination of the external ear, ear canal, and tympanic membrane. Congenital abnormalities should be noted. Wax needs to be removed before the tympanic membrane can be assessed and before caloric testing is performed.

A tympanic membrane perforation, infection, and cholesteatoma can cause dizziness and these are contraindications for caloric testing using water. If the ear is infected and especially if discharging, a representative swab should be taken for microscopy, culture, and sensitivity. Tissue samples, where indicated, should be sent for histologic analysis.

Tuning fork tests (including Weber and Rinne) may be performed before formal audiologic testing is requested. The findings can dictate whether specific imaging studies (e.g., CT or MRI) are required.

The Nose, Throat, Mouth, and General Head and Neck Examination

In cases of HIV/AIDS, the nose, throat, mouth and head and neck areas often are involved and should be part of the standard basic evaluation of all patients with balance disturbances. Some of the examinations performed will overlap those performed as part of the neurologic examination. An overview of nose, throat, mouth and general head and neck conditions to look for in patients with HIV/AIDS is highlighted in Table 11-2.

Directed Neuro-Otologic Examination

The following section discusses some of the clinical tests that can be performed on patients with dizziness and balance-related disorders.

Table 11–2. An Overview of Nose, Throat, Mouth and General Head and Neck Conditions in Patients with HIV/AIDS

Nasal manifestations	Nonspecific Nasal Obstruction
	Allergic and Nonallergic Rhinitis
	Rhinosinusitis
	Herpes Simplex
	Herpes Zoster
	Seborrheic Dermatitis
	Kaposi's Sarcoma
	Non-Hodgkin Lymphoma
Throat manifestations	Recurrent Aphthous Ulcers
	Benign Lymphoid Hyperplasia (also Adenoids)
	Epiglottitis
	Herpes Simplex
	Cytomegalovirus
	Kaposi's Sarcoma
	Non-Hodgkin Lymphoma
Oral manifestations	Candida
	Herpes Simplex
	Herpes Zoster
	Hairy Leucoplakia
	Recurrent Aphthous Ulceration
	Xerostomia
	Gingivitis and Periodontitis
	Kaposi's Sarcoma
	Non-Hodgkin Lymphoma
	Squamous Carcinoma
General Head and Neck manifestations	Salivary Gland Involvement
	Mycobacterial Infections
	Herpes Zoster
	HIV Lymphadenopathy
	Seborrheic Dermatitis
	Bell Palsy
	Kaposi's Sarcoma
	Non-Hodgkin Lymphoma
	Other Infections

These are all clinical tests and no sophisticated equipment is needed to perform them. The sensitivity is high but the specificity (maybe excluding the Dix Hallpike test for benign paroxysmal positional vertigo) is usually lower. Therefore, it should be noted that the tests do not stand alone and should always be interpreted as part of a test battery.

The Romberg Test

The Romberg test is a useful clinical test to evaluate static balance function. It is discussed here as part of the directed neuro-otologic examination but is actually dependent on the integration of information from three sensory systems in maintaining truncal balance, namely, the visual, vestibular, and proprioceptive systems. These three systems supply information to the cerebellum, which is utilized to coordinate and maintain balance by its influence on the motor control system.

The examiner needs to be close to the patient at all times to give support and prevent falling and injury. The patient is asked to remove his or her shoes and stand upright on a firm surface for 30 seconds. The arms are crossed in front and the eyes kept open. Swaying or losing balance at this stage is difficult to interpret and may be due to more than one system being involved. Severe proprioceptive problems, acute vestibular dysfunction, and midline cerebellar lesions can be the cause. Weakness also may cause instability and performing other tests to rule out certain neurological disorders is required. Age also plays a role and should be taken into account when interpreting results. Older patients more often suffer with musculoskeletal problems and decreased general strength. The patient is then asked to close the eyes in order to remove the visual system input. At this point, only the vestibular and proprioceptive systems will contribute to maintaining balance and patients with acute vestibular loss and proprioceptive problems will lose their balance.

The Romberg test also is considered positive when the patient needs to open the eyes, unfold the arms, or take a step. With acute vestibular loss, the patient usually will fall toward the involved side. It should also be noted if the patient sways abnormally without losing balance, as this may indicate a functional problem or malingering.

The modified version of the Romberg test is performed with the patient standing heel to toe. This decreases the base of support and makes it more difficult to maintain balance. Any test scenario that decreases the proprioceptive input (for instance standing on a foam cushion) also will make the test more sensitive for vestibular deficits. However, if tests are not standardized and age-related norms are not taken into account, one should be cautious in interpreting results.

The Fukuda Stepping Test

Ask the patient to march on the spot, with arms extended 90 degrees forward and eyes closed, for 50 steps. If the patient sways to either side by more than 45 degrees, the test is considered positive, as illustrated in Figure 11-5. This can be indicative of a unilateral vestibular loss. When bilateral vestibular loss is suspected, care should be taken to prevent the patient from falling. An example of this is seen with tuberculosis (commonly occurring in patients with HIV/AIDS) which has been treated with aminoglycosides or other ototoxic drugs.

Gait Testing

Gait should be assessed by asking the patient to walk on a straight line, first with the eyes open, and then with eyes closed. Observe if the patient veers off to one side, displays abnormal swaying of the arms, and also note, when the patient turns around, whether there is a corrective step or sway to a specific side. The patient can then be asked to walk heel to toe, with eyes open and closed to increase the demand on the vestibular system. Once again, the possibility of falling and injury exists and care should always be taken to prevent this.

Spontaneous and Gaze-Evoked Nystagmus

Nystagmus is the involuntary, oscillatory movement of the eyes in a horizontal, vertical, rotational, or multiple directions. Movement usually consists of a slow phase and a fast corrective saccade. The direction of saccadic nystagmus as described, is the direction toward which the fast component of the eye movement is beating. In the case where the movement is primarily rotational, the direction is described as being either clockwise or counterclockwise, once again depending on the fast component. Pure rotational nystagmus strongly suggests a central nervous system disorder. Sometimes, when originating in the visual system, it may consist only of two slow

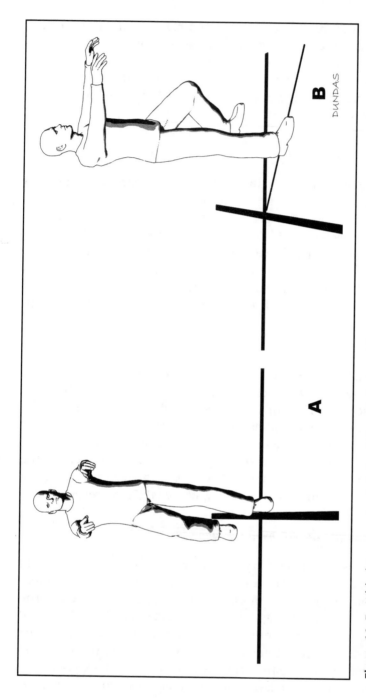

Figure 11–5. *With the arms extended at a 90° angle in front of the body, and the eyes closed, the patient marches in place for 50 steps.* **A.** *Normal Fukuda stepping test result.* **B.** *Abnormal Fukuda stepping test result with rotation greater than 45°. From: Jacobson, G. P., & Shepard, N. T. (2008). Balance function assessment and management. San Diego, CA: Plural Publishing, Inc. Reprinted with permission. All rights reserved.*

pendular phases. Other abnormal, irregular, or unequal eye movements generally require further central nervous system investigation. Nystagmus which is present only when fixating gaze off center, and does not suppress while fixating, is termed gaze-evoked nystagmus. Gaze-evoked nystagmus typically is associated with pathology of the gaze holding centers in the brainstem. The centers involved for horizontal gaze holding are situated in the neural integrator that consists of the vestibular nuclei, vestibulocerebellum and the nucleus prepositus hypoglossi (NPH). Vertical gaze nystagmus originates in the interstitial nucleus of Cajal in the upper brainstem and associated systems. Endpoint nystagmus sometimes can be mistaken for gaze nystagmus but is, in fact, a physiologic phenomenon that occurs in the extreme positions of eye fixation. It usually fatigues over time.

Before testing for spontaneous and gaze-evoked nystagmus, the range of normal eye movements including conversion should first be assessed. Abnormalities here may influence nystagmus findings. Spontaneous nystagmus occurs without any stimulation of the patient. Depending on its nature, it can indicate a peripheral or central disorder. When spontaneous nystagmus is of peripheral origin, it can be suppressed by fixating gaze and follows Alexander's law. Alexander's law states that the intensity of the nystagmus is greater when the patient looks in the direction of the fast phase of the nystagmus as indicated in Figure 11-6.

It therefore is possible that it may only be present when gazing in one direction. Ask the patient to look straight forward, while keeping the head still for at least 1 minute. The patient should then look 30° to the left, right, upward, and downward. Nystagmus due to peripheral vestibular causes will be suppressed by visual fixation. It therefore will be easier to notice when visual fixation is suppressed or eliminated. Clinically, this can be accomplished by having the patient close one eye while examining the other with an ophthalmoscope. Alternatively, the patient can be asked to look at a large white surface without visual cues. The most reliable method, however, is to use conventional Frenzel lenses or video Frenzel, if the facility is available. Nystagmus without fixation should be observed for 30 seconds. A Frenzel lens has a diopter of +20 and eliminates visual fixation. An internal light makes it easier for the examiner to observe nystagmus. Peripheral vestibular nystagmus also can be enhanced if the patient is asked to perform simple concentration-diverting exercises such as answering general questions.

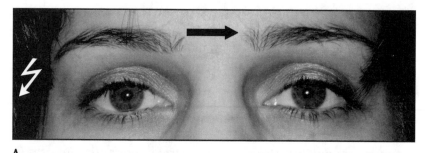

A

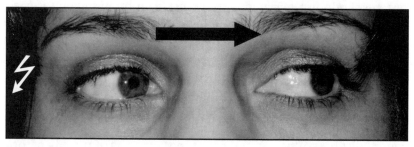

B

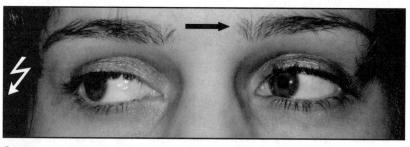

C

Figure 11–6. Alexander's law. *The fast phase of the nystagmus (black arrow) is directed away from the affected side with the acute peripheral hypofunction (white arrow) (**A**). When the direction of gaze is toward the fast phase of the nystagmus, the amplitude of the nystagmus is larger and more obvious (**B**). When the direction of gaze is toward the slow phase of the nystagmus, the amplitude of the nystagmus is smaller and less obvious (**C**). As the patient improves, the nystagmus will later only be visible with gaze in the direction of the fast phase (**B**).*

Smooth Pursuit and Saccade Testing

The head should be kept still to minimize any vestibular stimulation and to maximize visual acuity. Abnormalities in smooth pursuit and saccade testing are indicative of central disorders and unless spontaneous nystagmus is severe, it will not significantly influence test findings.

Saccades are tested in the horizontal and vertical planes. The examiner sits in front of the patient, asking him or her to fixate on the examiner's index finger held about 30 cm in front of the patient. The index finger of the other hand is held 30° off center and the patient is then asked to shift gaze to the other index finger on command of the examiner. Tests are repeated to the left and right in the horizontal plane and up and down in the vertical plane. The saccades should be rapid with no visible latency and accurate with no under- or overshoot of the eyes. Conjugate eye movements should be checked prior to this test to check for pronounced spontaneous nystagmus.

Smooth pursuit testing may be abnormal in older patients or in patients with inattention and caution must be exercised when interpreting test results. The patient is asked to fixate on the examiners index finger, which is moved in the horizontal plane and then in the vertical plane. Vertical smooth pursuit is more difficult to perform and following of a target downward may sometimes be jerky with saccades. Any irregular and asymmetric responses should be noted. Lesions of the vestibulocerebellum cause abnormal smooth pursuit.

A specific asymmetric response in the horizontal plane with the adducting eye movement being more impaired can be a sign of pathology of the medial longitudinal fasciculus in the brainstem. If bilateral, internuclear ophthalmoplegia may indicate multiple brainstem infarcts, or multiple sclerosis.

The Cover–Uncover Test

The patient is asked to fixate on a target. The examiner covers one eye and then uncovers, observing for an upward eye movement. When the tested eye moves up, the other eye usually moves down. The other eye is then also tested by covering and uncovering.

A positive test result is indicated by the ocular tilt reaction, elicited on the ipsilateral side of testing. The ocular tilt reaction consists of a lateral head tilt (toward the other side), skew deviation of the eyes (hypotropia of the undermost eye), and ocular torsion. This is seen in acute utricular lesions and pathology in the graviceptive pathways in the brainstem.

Head Shake Nystagmus

If spontaneous nystagmus is not seen, the head of the patient can be shaken in a horizontal plane to elicit nystagmus. First, rule out neck pathology that limits movement and causes pain. Ask the patient to close the eyes, tilt the head 30° forward to align the horizontal canal, and shake the head for 20 seconds. On termination of shaking, the eyes are immediately opened and observed for nystagmus. A positive response is characterized by three or more beats and indicates an abnormality in the central velocity storage system of the brainstem or an uncompensated peripheral disorder.

The Head Impulse Test

This test is used to examine the vestibulo-ocular reflex (VOR) as illustrated in Figure 11-7. Neck pathology, which impairs movement and causes pain, should be ruled out. The head of the patient is held firmly between the hands of the examiner and while the

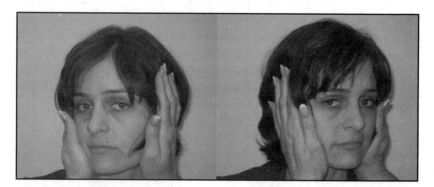

Figure 11–7. *The head impulse test. An intact bilateral vestibulo-ocular reflex (VOR) of the horizontal semicircular canals. With the head impulse test (head thrust test) the patient is able to maintain visual fixation on a stationary object in front during rapid head movements.*

patient is asked to fixate on a target, the head is suddenly and unpredictably thrust either to the left or right. The amplitude of the movements need not be large and emphasis should be on the acceleration. A catch-up saccade at the end of the head movement constitutes a positive result and is indicative of a defective VOR involving the horizontal semicircular canal with head movement toward the involved side as indicated in Figure 11–8.

Although slightly more difficult to perform and to interpret, it can also be used to test the vertical canals. For this, the head is turned 45° toward the side being tested and head thrusts are performed in the vertical plan. A catch-up saccade with the head thrust in the backward direction indicates a defect in VOR of the posterior semicircular canal on the side the head is tilted toward. A catch-up saccade with the head movement forward indicates a defective VOR of the superior semicircular canal on the side the head is tilted toward.

Hyperventilation-Induced Nystagmus

In some cases, nystagmus can be induced by means of hyperventilation. The occurrence of nystagmus after a period of hyperventilation for 90 seconds may implicate a demyelinating disorder such as multiple sclerosis, acoustic neuroma, or microvascular compression of the eighth cranial nerve. Other conditions such as migraine and anxiety also may yield positive results.

Positional and Positioning Testing

Positional nystagmus refers to nystagmus that occurs when the patient is in a specific position and the nystagmus usually persists. Positioning nystagmus is short lasting and is elicited only when the patient changes head position.

With the patient seated, observe whether nystagmus is present. The patient should then be asked to lie back so that any nystagmus or change in nystagmus in the supine position can be observed. If nystagmus is seen, it is important to determine whether the nystagmus subsequently disappears. After 1 minute, the patient is turned on the side and again observed for nystagmus. After 1 minute the patient should turn back and completely around to the other side.

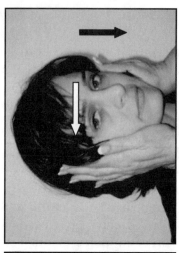

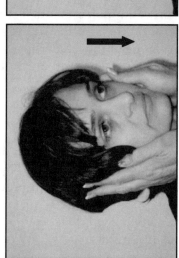

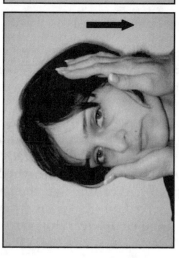

Figure 11–8. *A positive head impulse test. The patient will display a catch-up saccade (white arrow) to the stationary visual target in front with the head impulse test (head thrust test) toward the affected side. This is indicative of a defective vestibulo-ocular reflex (VOR) of the left horizontal semicircular canal (black arrow).*

In this sequence of positioning, it is important to document the latency of nystagmus, the direction, and whether it disappears. Benign paroxysmal positional vertigo (BPPV) is a very common form of positioning vertigo (with nystagmus) where the direction of the nystagmus changes with different head positions. It is common to have a delay or latency before the nystagmus commences and then it usually disappears within 1 minute.

BPPV is a condition in which loose particles or degenerated otoconia float in the semicircular canals. When the patient is lying on the side and the fast component is beating towards the ground, the nystagmus is called geotropic. When it is beating upward, it is called ageotropic. Positional nystagmus lasting longer than 1 minute also can be caused by conditions such as vestibular migraine, microvascular compression, perilymph fistulas, Ménière's disease, alcohol intoxication, and latent spontaneous nystagmus due to vestibular neuronitis. To be able to distinguish among these conditions is difficult and history and clinical findings should be correlated with the specific nystagmus.

BPPV involving the posterior semicircular canals probably is the most common form of peripheral vertigo (with nystagmus) seen. The Dix Hallpike test (Dix & Hallpike, 1952) is performed to assess this condition. The patient is asked to turn the head 45° toward the examiner while seated. After excluding back and neck pathology, the patient is moved backward to the supine position with the head hanging down by about 20° (Figure 11-9).

A positive response indicating BPPV would be that the patient develops, after a latency of a few seconds, a typical upbeating torsional nystagmus with the direction toward the lower ear. The nystagmus usually is accompanied by a sensation of vertigo and not infrequently by nausea. It usually terminates within a minute. In some cases, a sensation of vertigo is experienced without accompanying nystagmus. In other cases, nystagmus can be observed without the patient experiencing vertigo. In these cases, it is more likely that the pathology is central. Vertigo of peripheral origin usually is accompanied by nystagmus.

Pressure-Induced Nystagmus

With pressure-induced tests, the aim is to look for inner ear conditions that are influenced by changing of intracranial pressure or

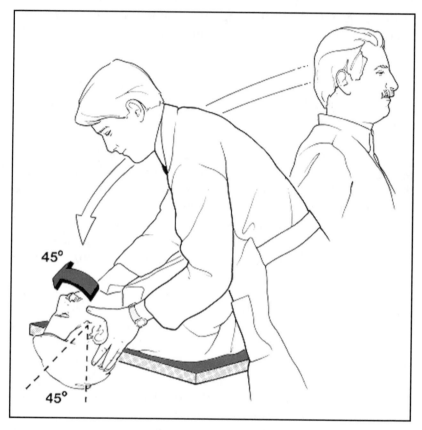

Figure 11–9. *The Dix Hallpike test for benign paroxysmal positional vertigo (BPPV) affecting the left ear. Figure reprinted with permission from Troost, B. T., & Patton, J. M. (1992). Exercise therapy for positional vertigo.* Neurology, 42, 1441–1444.

middle ear pressure. Perilymph fistulas and dehiscence of the semicircular canals can present with nystagmus when the patient is asked to perform a Valsalva maneuver or perform a squatting position to increase intracranial pressure. The Valsalva maneuver is performed by asking the patient to exhale against a closed mouth and nose in order to force air through the eustachian tubes and into the middle ear spaces. This will increase the pressure in the middle ears, causing the tympanic membranes and ossicles to move outward, and will elict vertigo in patients with fistulae. Alternatively, the pressure increase in the middle ears also can exert pressure directly on a fistula causing inward movement of the inner ear fluid resulting in vertigo. Although a negative response does not exclude pathology, provoking nystagmus in response to increased pressure may indicate fistulas, a mobile footplate, or a semicircular canal dehiscence.

The Dynamic Visual Acuity Test (DVA)

This is a useful test to evaluate the VOR. The principle involved is that the patient needs an intact vestibular system to stabilize the eyes during head movements greater than 2 Hz (2 oscillations per second). At slower head movements, the patient utilizes the visual system and the vestibular system is not tested. It is advisable to have an assistant when performing this test. The patient is seated and the static visual acuity obtained by using a standard visual acuity chart. The row with the smallest letters or figures that the patient is able to read is documented. The head of the patient is then shaken from left to right at a frequency of 2 Hz at small amplitudes of no more than 10 degrees. While this is performed, the dynamic visual acuity is tested. It is normal to lose up to two rows of acuity during movements but if the patient loses three or more rows an uncompensated unilateral vestibular lesion or bilateral vestibular loss should be suspected. It is recommended to use more than one chart to prevent the patient learning the sequence. In this way, the horizontal VOR is tested. This test also can be performed for the vertical VOR if the head is shaken up and down.

Caloric Testing

For many years, the caloric test has been one of the fundamental tests performed in the assessment of dizzy patients. It is one of the most important methods of investigation of the equilibrial sense organ as it allows the separate examination of each labyrinth (Hamersma, 1957). The basic caloric test is straightforward and can easily be performed in any outpatient setting.

It is based on the principle that, when water that differs in temperature from body temperature is injected into the ear canal, it elicits nystagmus. The temperature current that is created in this way is transferred via the tympanic membrane, temporal bone, and middle ear space to the inner ear. A water stimulus colder than body temperature inhibits the inner ear and, when the patient is supine with the head raised 30° on a pillow, it causes a nystagmus beating away from the ear being tested. A water stimulus warmer than body temperature stimulates the inner ear and causes a nystagmus beating toward the injected ear. The greater the difference in temperature between injected fluid and the body, the greater the response of nystagmus (and vertigo sensation).

The standard bithermal caloric test is performed with cold water at 30°C and warm water at 44°C. In cases of tympanic membrane perforation, water irrigation is not advisable and air injection into the ear canal should be used. Besides giving an unreliable result, water in the middle ear injected through a perforation can cause severe vertigo and infection.

Responses are recorded for both ears using cold and warm water and the caloric difference and directional preponderance calculated. To perform the caloric test accurately, the temperature of water should be closely controlled and the resulting nystagmus recorded. Unfortunately, this can only be accomplished accurately with specific equipment.

However, it is possible to perform a caloric test as part of the clinical examination and cold tap water may simply be used. The idea is to compare the two sides and see if responses can be elicited and how these compare regarding latency, intensity, and duration. Intensity can be classified as 0 to 4 with 0 being no response and 4 being a maximal response. The minimum ice water caloric test (MIWCT) is a standardized test where three ice cubes are added to tap water to lower the temperature to 4°C within approximately 13 minutes before irrigation. Irrigation with 0.5, 1, or 2 ml can be performed and appears to be a suitable bedside investigation of vestibular function (Schmäl, Lübben, Weiberg, & Stoll, 2005).

The reaction in caloric testing is based on a reflex and the results can demonstrate hyperfunction (with central pathology), hypofunction, asymmetry (usually a difference of 20–25%), or total loss of function. The caloric test, however, stimulates the horizontal canal and superior vestibular nerve segment preferentially and may not detect pathology involving the inferior vestibular nerve. Unfortunately, the frequency of the stimulus of the caloric test is very low (0.002–0.004 Hz) and actually nonphysiologic. A loss of caloric response does not imply a nonfunctioning labyrinth. Other tests stimulating at higher frequencies such as rotational testing may still be normal. Therefore, results obtained with the caloric test should be interpreted with caution.

Clinical Rotation Chair Testing

It is known that stimulating the peripheral vestibular apparatus by means of a caloric test is a nonphysiologic stimulus equivalent to a frequency between 0.002 and 0.004 Hz and accelerations of less than 10 degrees/s^2. The VOR usually functions at much higher frequencies physiologically; therefore, the fact that a patient does not have function on caloric testing does not imply absent peripheral vestibular function. Rotation stimuli use higher stimulation rates and are a more physiologic way of testing the VOR. This augments information obtained by the caloric test.

The patient is placed on a rotatable office chair with armrests for support. The patient is then asked to tilt the head forward by 30° to position the horizontal canal so it is selectively tested. The patient should then close the eyes before being rotated to one side at the rate of 0.5 Hz or one turn per 2 seconds. After the 10th rotation the patient is immediately asked to open the eyes, and is observed, preferably using Frenzel lenses or a videonystagmoscope. Nystagmus normally is observed and the time it takes to stop is recorded. The time it takes to stop is related to the time decay constant used in computerized rotation chair testing and a value of less than 10 seconds indicates possible peripheral vestibular dysfunction. After 3 minutes, the test can be repeated to the other side. In such a manner, an asymmetry in the two vestibular systems can be elicited, which may indicate a peripheral lesion with an incomplete dynamic compensation in the central nervous system. The major limitation of this test is that it cannot be used to isolate one peripheral system from the other because each stimulus affects both sides simultaneously.

Advanced Laboratory Vestibular Testing

With advanced vestibular testing, equipment is utilized to accurately measure findings evident by clinical testing but also to obtain information that cannot be seen clinically. The equipment is, however, expensive and not readily available in developing countries. The cost/benefit ratio of utilizing such equipment is debatable. Many vestibular laboratories also utilize experimental devices and much experimental work is being performed to learn more about the balance function in humans. A brief description of advanced measures is provided in this section.

Computerized Dynamic Posturography

This test examines the balance system of a patient, integrating visual, vestibular, and proprioceptive functions. It can test a patient's balance function in challenging visual and supportive (proprioceptive) environments. The test can mimic certain experiences of daily life. Although this test cannot usually be used in isolation, it can coordinate findings obtained with standard vestibular (e.g., the caloric) tests in some vestibular conditions. It is helpful in the rehabilitative management of patients and also can be used to identify patients with functional problems and malingering. In some cases of central vestibular and extravestibular central nervous system pathology, posturography may be the only helpful test. Different apparatus may offer several testing protocols (Figure 11–10).

Static and dynamic posturography in patients with asymptomatic HIV/AIDS indicated that the entire vestibular system tends to be involved from the early stages of HIV infection. In HIV-positive subjects, a variable dysfunction in the reflex control of long latency is observed, which correlates with alteration of the central dopaminergic system; in HIV/AIDS patients, the central nervous system damage appears more important, globally distributed and correlates with immunosuppression (Dellepiane, Medicina, Mora, & Salami, 2005).

Vestibular-Evoked Myogenic Potentials (VEMP)

Vestibular-evoked myogenic potential (VEMP) testing is a test of the descending vestibulocollic system and vestibulocollic reflex (VCR). The evoked potentials refer to the modulation of the tonic electromyogram (EMG) activity of the neck muscles induced by vestibular activation. As with conventional evoked potentials, these responses need averaging for their detection. The VEMP response consists of an initial positivity (P13) followed by a negativity (N23).

The saccule is slightly sensitive to sound and this fact underlies the basis of the test. A stimulus (usually click sounds) is presented to the ear, which then relays through the saccule to the inferior vestibular nerve to the medial and lateral vestibular nuclei in the brainstem. From there, the medial vestibulospinal tract (MVST) and the lateral vestibulospinal tract (LVST) relay impulses to the neck and the leg muscles, respectively. In cervical or cVEMP testing, one

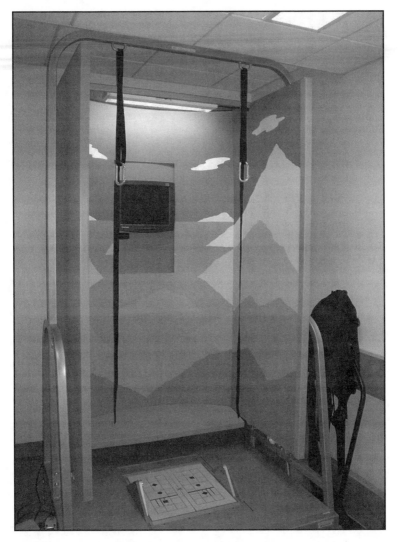

Figure 11–10. *A computerized dynamic posturography system.*

measures the response in the sternocleidomastoid muscle, which is most commonly used.

The VEMP test can be used to examine numerous conditions such as Ménière's disease, acoustic neuroma, and the superior semicircular canal dehiscence syndrome. In the lower tracing in Figure 11-11, no VEMP could be elicited on the right side. The patient

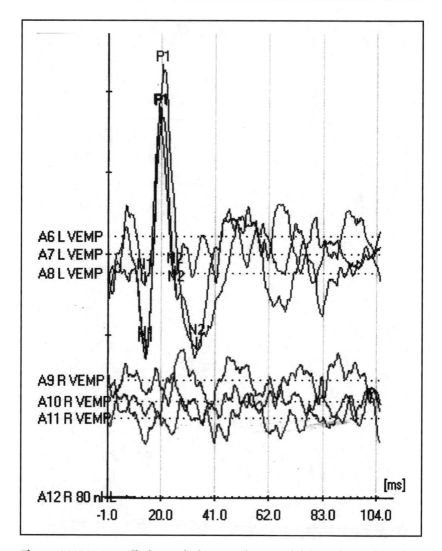

Figure 11–11. *A vestibular evoked myogenic potential (VEMP) waveform in a patient with a right-sided acoustic neuroma of the inferior vestibular nerve. In the lower tracing no VEMP could be elicited on the right side.*

was later diagnosed with a right-sided acoustic neuroma of the inferior vestibular nerve.

As more research evidence accumulates, VEMP testing is expected to assume an increasingly important role in the battery of tests. Unlike The equipment is less expensive than that for other specialized procedures.

Electronystagmography (ENG) and Videonystagmography(VNG)

Nystagmography is a technique for recording nystagmus and is considered to be the gold standard for vestibular assessment. Electronystagmography (ENG) utilizes electrodes affixed to the face of the patient in such a way that the corneoretinal electric potentials generated by the movement of the eyes, can be recorded.

In videonystagmography (VNG) either goggles fitted with a small video camera or goggles fitted with an infrared camera are placed on the patient's eyes. The camera records the patient's eye movements and displays them on a video/computer screen as seen in Figure 11-12. Usually, the eyes as well as the nystagmus tracing are displayed. The software used in the systems enables the examiner to record even very minor nystagmus and the video playback facility is handy to study and reassess the nystagmus.

The four main components of ENG/VNG are:

1. Tracking tests of a visual object (ocular motor testing)
2. Nystagmus testing (spontaneous, hyperventilation, Valsalva induced, etc.)
3. Positional and positioning (Dix Hallpike) testing
4. Caloric testing (illustrated in Figure 11-13)

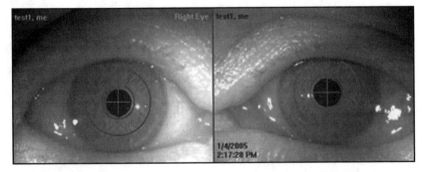

Figure 11–12. *Photograph showing how software in a video eye-movement recording system permits the identification of the pupil and iris. From: Jacobson, G. P., & Shepard, N. T. (2008).* Balance function assessment and management. *San Diego, CA: Plural Publishing, Inc. Reprinted with permission. All rights reserved.*

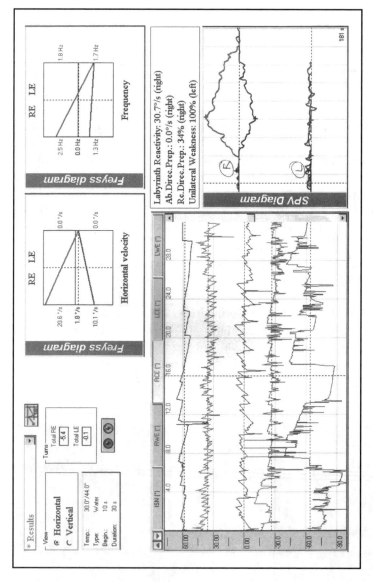

Figure 11–13. *Bithermal caloric response in an HIV patient with left-sided vestibular neuronitis. Note the slight spontaneous nystagmus to the right in the upper black tracing. Spontaneous nystagmus needs to be considered when interpreting the result of a caloric test. The caloric responses are absent on the left side.*

In patients with HIV-1 infection, abnormalities in vertical eye movements and relative asymmetries in smooth pursuit gains, both horizontally and vertically, are more sensitive and consistent indicators of CNS dysfunction than are horizontal eye movement abnormalities or measurements of absolute smooth pursuit gain and phase (Johnston, Miller, & Nath, 1996).

Electronystagmographic anomalies were noted in 57% of patients with HIV/AIDS and ARC who also had abnormal audiologic test results (Hausler et al., 1991). Spontaneous and positional nystagmus, often vertical or rotatory, asymmetric rotatory pendular tests, incomplete visual fixation suppression, saccadic ocular pursuit, abnormal optokinetic nystagmus, and hyporeflexia or areflexia on caloric examination were observed. The proportion of abnormal results was significantly higher in symptomatic and asymptomatic HIV-seropositive patients than in the seronegative control group. It also should be noted that, in patients with HIV/AIDS without neurologic symptoms, subclinical disturbances do exist and necessitate specialized testing (Salami et al., 1991).

In some conditions, for instance, BPPV, the VNG is very helpful in determining the involved canal but in the majority of cases the VNG findings must be correlated with the history and clinical examination to make a diagnosis.

Rotation Testing

Rotation systems should be used in conjunction with conventional ENG or VNG testing. The systems are usually expensive, however, and the information obtained may be of limited practical value. However, rotation chair testing is helpful in diagnosing bilateral vestibular loss, picking up abnormalities missed by conventional testing, and for assessing children in whom caloric testing is difficult (Shepard & Telian, 1996). An asymmetry in testing can indicate an uncompensated, peripheral vestibular lesion. Rotation chair testing is not aimed at isolating one peripheral side as the site of pathology because when rotated the stimulus affects both sides simultaneously.

There are two forms of rotation test. In one, the patient is seated on a chair and the whole body rotated, as illustrated in Figure 11-14. In the other, the patient moves his or her own head from left to right at a predetermined rate. In both forms of testing,

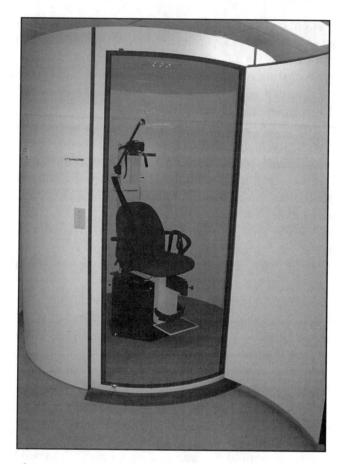

Figure 11–14. *A rotation system where the whole body can be rotated.*

the nystagmus response of the eyes is recorded and then compared with the patient's body or head movement. The results are expressed by using parameters such as gain, phase, and asymmetry.

With the whole body rotation testing system, different protocols exist. In addition, optokinetic nystagmus, optokinetic after nystagmus, and visual-vestibular suppression can be tested. Off-vertical axis testing (OVAR) is performed by tilting the axis of the rotation chair with respect to the gravitational axis and is used to assess otolith function.

Other Investigations

Depending on the disorder suspected or diagnosed, the following other investigations may be requested:

1. *Diagnostic audiometry* (pure tone, speech reception and speech discrimination)
2. *Immittance testing* (tympanometry and acoustic reflex testing)
3. *Otoacoustic emissions (OAEs):* Diminished otoacoustic emissions are very common and may indicate cochlear dysfunction resulting from infections or ototoxicity. Emissions also may be diminished due to subclincal otitis media with effusion (Soucek & Michaels, 1996).
4. *Electrocochleography (ECochG) and auditory brainstem responses (ABR):* Abnormal results obtained by ECochG may also indicate cochlear dysfunction as with OAE's and is useful in diagnosing Ménière's disease. Abnormal ABR responses are indicative of retrocochlear pathology such as acoustic neuroma and neuropathy.
5. *Plain x-rays, computerized tomography (CT), and magnetic resonance imaging (MRI of the head and spine):* Plain x-rays have been replaced in general by CT and MRI but are still useful to detect gross pathology if the latter two are not available. CT is preferred in cases where bony definition is important, such as in examination of the temporal bones. MRI gives superior information regarding soft tissue (Figure 11–15).
6. *Blood tests* (CD4 count, viral load, liver functions, Vitamin B12, lactate, serology, autoimmune screen, WR, VDRL)
7. *CSF analysis* (in particular for tuberculosis, bacteria, fungi, and cytology)

CLINICAL DISORDERS CAUSING BALANCE DISTURBANCE NOT NECESSARILY ASSOCIATED WITH HIV/AIDS

Numerous disorders, not necessarily related to HIV/AIDS, can cause dizziness and imbalance. At this time, insufficient population-based studies have been performed to know the incidence and preva-

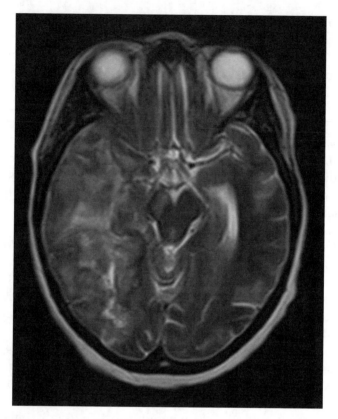

Figure 11–15. *T2-weighted MRI of the brain of a patient presenting with a balance disturbance showing extensive vasculitic pathology also involving the brainstem. The patient had HIV with pulmonary tuberculosis.*

lence of the majority of disorders causing dizziness and imbalance in patients with HIV/AIDS. It is beyond the scope of this chapter to discuss all the possible causes for dizziness and imbalance in the general population. There are many textbooks in neurology, neurotology and otorhinolaryngology that discuss these conditions in detail as well as Web sites with relevant topics (Brandt, 2000; Goebel, 2001; Hain, 2008.).

In health systems in developed countries, these disorders may be managed by specialists in major centers with state of the art facilities. In developing countries, such management frequently is not feasible. Nevertheless, with advances in telemedicine, allowing access to outreach liaison programs and specialist consultation, applying world-class approaches may be possible.

Table 11-3 lists some of the more frequently seen conditions that can cause dizziness, imbalance, and falls which are not necessarily directly associated with HIV/AIDS. The pervasive effects of HIV, however, may result in an increased occurrence of some of these conditions as initial research reports seem to indicate.

Table 11–3. Causes of Dizziness, Imbalance, and Falls That Are Not Necessarily Associated with HIV/AIDS

Ear Problems	
Wax	Labyrinthine concussion
Acute and chronic middle ear disease	Infective labyrinthitis
	Acoustic neuroma
Cholesteatoma	Bilateral vestibular damage (including ototoxic drugs)
Benign paroxysmal positional vertigo (BPPV)	
	Microvascular compression syndrome
Ménière's disease	
Otosclerosis	Otolithic dysfunction
Vestibular neuronitis	Glomus tumors
Perilymph fistula	Auto immune inner ear disease (AIED) e.g., Cogan syndrome
Temporal bone fractures	
Neurologic Problems	
Vertiginous migraine	Enchephalitis
Demyelination	Cervical vertigo
Transient ischemic attacks (TIAs) and stroke	Whiplash injury
	Chiari malformation
Structural brain lesions (trauma, hematomas, neoplasms, infections)	Basilar invagination
	Parkinsonism
Epilepsy	Toxins, (e.g., Lithium, carbon monoxide)
Cerebellar degeneration	
Meningitis	Vitamin B12 deficiency

continues

Table 11–3. *continued*

Visual Problems	
Diplopia	Inappropriate corrective lenses
Ocular pathology	Visual illusions

Hematologic Problems	
Anemia	Syncope
Hyperviscosity syndromes	Cardiac dysrhythmia
Antiphospholipid syndrome	Cardiac failure
Hemodynamic problems	Subclavian steal syndrome
Hypotension	Carotid sinus syndrome
Vertobrobasilar insufficiency	Cardiac vegetations
Postural hypotension	

Skeletal Problems	
Cervical spine problems	Hip and knee replacement surgery
Osteoarthritis and other arthritides	

Metabolic and Endocrine Problems	
Hypoglycemia	
Hypothyrodism	

Psychological and Psychiatric Problems	
Anxiety	Functional problems
Depression	Malingering
Phobic postural vertigo (BPV)	

Other	
Motion sickness	
Mal de debarquement (MDD)	
Alcohol	
Medication side effects and interactions (Including certain ARVs)	

TREATMENT

Treatment of Dizziness and Balance-Related Disorders Caused by HIV/AIDS

Treatment of HIV-associated balance disturbances needs to be directed primarily at identifiable causes. For this reason alone, proper clinical evaluation and subsequent special investigations are vital. With regard to special investigations, more aggressive workup is often warranted including CNS imaging (MRI and other), spinal tap, nystagmography, and histologic analyses. Central to treatment is the use of combination highly active antiretroviral therapeutic agents (HAART). This is a rapidly developing and constantly changing field. Detailed description is beyond the scope of this review (see Chapter 3). It is sufficient to say that currently there are five major classes of ARVs, (Hoffmann & Mulcahy, 2007), namely:

1. Nucleoside and nucleotide reverse transcriptase inhibitors (NRTIs)
2. Non-nucleoside reserve transcriptase inhibitors (NNRTIs)
3. Protease inhibitors (PIs)
4. Fusion inhibitors
5. Entry inhibitors

Medications are used in various combination regimens. What combinations of ARVs and at what point administration should be instituted (e.g., with CD4 counts below certain levels) is a field that is continuously changing (see Chapter 3). It also should be emphasized that certain medications, used in the treatment of HIV/AIDS may lead to balance disturbances, such as the NRTIs abacavir, didanosine (ddI), and stavudine (d4T). The development of a balance disturbance may require their cessation, usually with change to a different regimen. Use of ARVs may not significantly lower the prevalence of certain neurologic conditions such as distal sensory neuropathy and myopathy but it certainly does reduce the incidence of opportunistic infections, which may affect systems related to balance control.

Treatment of Opportunistic and Concomitant Infections and Neoplasms

Opportunistic infections and neoplasms warrant specific treatment regimens; for example, tuberculosis requires a multidrug antimycobacterial regimen with adaptations in the event of drug resistances. These patients occasionally develop bilateral vestibular paresis as a consequence of the vestibulo- and ototoxic effects of certain drugs. Balance impairment in these patients is permanent and difficult to manage. Oscillopsia and difficulty walking in the dark and on uneven surfaces are problematic. Vestibular rehabilitation often is the only option. Concomitant infections such as syphilis should be aggressively treated with appropriate antibiotic regimens. Neoplasms may require surgical intervention, radiotherapy, and chemotherapy. As with tuberculosis, some of the chemotherapeutic drugs are oto- and vestibulotoxic and surgery near the brain and vestibular apparatus as well as radiation-induced neuritis can permanently affect balance function.

Therapy for Clinical Disorders Not Necessarily Related to HIV/AIDS

Pharmaceutical Therapy for Dizziness

Medication can be used as symptomatic relief for vertigo and nausea. In Table 11–4, some of the treatment options for acute vertigo and nausea in adults are illustrated. In the majority of cases, medications are only for short-term use as long-term treatment with drugs causing central depression can be detrimental to a patient's balance and cognitive function. Medication also is used in the treatment of specific conditions (Table 11–5).

Surgical Interventions for Dizziness

The majority of useful surgical procedures are offered by otolaryngologists and neurotologists and to a lesser extent neurosurgeons. Strict surgical criteria for otologic surgery should be applied to all patients, regardless of HIV status. Warranted surgical therapy should not be withheld because of the patient's HIV status. Surgical outcomes, however, do correlate with the patient's degree of

Table 11–4. Treatment of Acute Vertigo and Nausea in Adults

Name	Dosage	Use	Side Effects
Anticholinergic			
Glycopyrrolate	1–2 mg q12h po	Vs ae	Anticholinergic side-effects
Antihistamines			
Cyclizine	50 mg q8h po or 100 mg q8h sup or 1 ml q8h im	VS	Sedation, moderate anticholinergic
Cinnarizine	25 mg q8h po	VS	Sedation
Promethazine	25–50 mg q4–6h po or q4–6h im or q4–6h sup	VS AE	Sedation
Benzodiazepines			
Diazepam	5–10 mg q6–12h po or q4–6h im or q4–6h iv	**VS**	Sedation, tolerance, addiction
Lorazepam	1–2 mg q8–12h po	VS	Sedation, tolerance, addiction
Clonazepam	0.5 mg q8h po	VS	Sedation, tolerance, addiction
Alprazolam	0.5 mg q8h po	VS	Sedation, tolerance, addiction
Butyrophenone			
Droperidol	2.5–5 mg q12h im	**VS AE**	Sedation, respiratory depression, extrapyramidal reaction
Phenothiazine			
Prochlorperazine	5–10 mg q4–6h po or q6h im or 25 mg q12h sup	AE	Extrapyramidal reaction
Seretonin Antagonists			
Odansetron	8 mg q12h po or 8–32 mg iv slowly	**AE**	Headaches

Vs = mild vestibular suppressant, VS = moderate vestibular suppressant, **VS** = strong vestibular suppressant, ae = mild anti-emetic, AE = moderate anti-emetic, **AE** = strong anti-emetic

Source: Bhansali, S. A. (2001). Therapy: Medical alternatives. In J. Goebel (Ed.), *Practical management of the dizzy patient.* (1st ed., p. 307). Philadelphia, PA: Lippincott Williams & Wilkins.

Table 11–5. Pharmacologic Management of Dizziness Not Necessarily Related to HIV/AIDS

Treatment	Condition
Betahistine	Ménière's disease
Aminoglycosides	Ménière's disease
Diuretics	Ménière's disease
Migraine treatment	Vestibular migraine
Antiepileptic drugs	Vestibular epilepsy
	Microvascular compression
Corticosteroids	Vestibular neuronitis
	Autoimmune inner ear disease
Antibiotics	Ear infections
Psychiatric drugs	Anxiety, phobias, etc.
Vitamin B12	Vitamin B12 deficiency

immunocompromise. A more protracted and complicated postoperative course may be expected in patients with low CD4 counts (Kohan & Giacchi, 1999). Surgical procedures are divided into nondestructive (e.g., patching of an inner ear fistula), selectively destructive (e.g., selective vestibular nerve section), and destructive (e.g., transcanal or transmastoid labyrinthectomy) (Figure 11–16).

Intratympanic gentamycin is often used in treating Ménière's disease and can be regarded as a staged destructive procedure. It should be emphasized that, with destructive procedures, the balance system as a whole is weakened. No destructive surgical procedure should ever be performed unless proper appropriate diagnostic methods have been utilized and unless a structured vestibular rehabilitation program can be offered (Hofmeyr, 2006). The risk/benefit ratio should also be assessed and the patient thoroughly informed. Vestibular rehabilitation should be utilized after surgery.

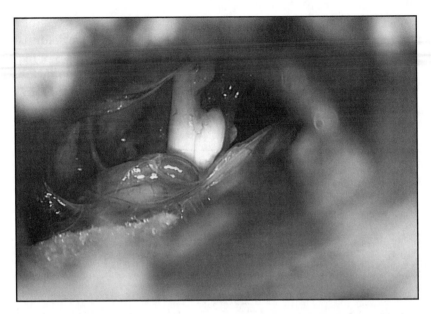

Figure 11–16. *A selective vestibular nerve section performed by the author in a patient with Ménière's disease on the left side. The sparing of the cochlear division on the left side (inferior side) of the eighth cranial nerve can be visualized. The retrosigmoid approach was utilized.*

Physical Therapy

Vestibular rehabilitation is extremely important in the management of patients with dizziness and balance-related disorders and should be a multidisciplinary approach (Herdman, 1999). Patients with stable unilateral vestibular deficiency and those with bilateral vestibular dysfunction (e.g., due to tuberculosis treatment with ototoxic drugs) will benefit most. It also is helpful in the rehabilitation of patients with central pathology of a stable nature. Patients with fluctuating disease, however, tend to respond poorly because of CNS adaptability difficulty. Techniques are based on adaptation, substitution, and habituation. Adaptation exercise programs are used primarily in unilateral vestibular loss where recovery results from adaptive capabilities of the vestibular system. The vestibular system learns to function with different vestibular neural inputs. Substitution exercise programs are used for patients with severe bilateral vestibular loss and attempt to replace vestibular function. Visual and somatosensory inputs are optimized. No mechanism, however, fully compensates for the loss of vestibular function. Vestibular habituation is used in patients with motion sickness and utilizes gradual central adaptation or conditioning to an environmental stimulus.

Vestibular maneuvers such as the Epley maneuver (Figure 11-17) are used as primary treatment for BPPV and work on the principle

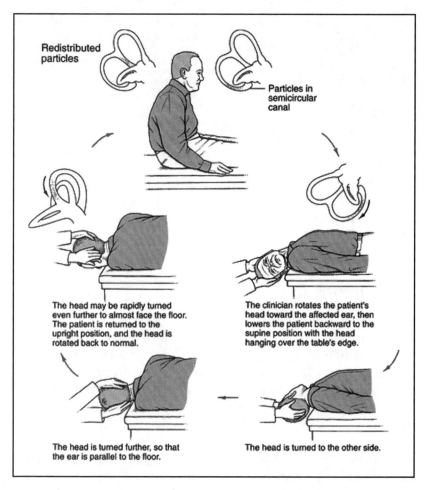

Figure 11–17. *The Epley maneuver performed for posterior canal benign paroxysmal positional vertigo (BPPV) affecting the right ear. From:* The Merck Manual of Diagnosis and Therapy, *18th ed., p. 792, edited by Robert Porter. Copyright 2007 by Merck & Co., Inc., Whitehouse Station, NJ. Retrieved February 4, 2009 from: http://www.merck.com/mmpe*

that otoconia and debris are displaced from the semicircular canals, where they cause inappropriate stimulation and symptoms (Epley, 1992). Physical therapy also includes devices such as neck collars used for cervical vertigo. Supportive devices such as canes, walking frames and wheelchairs may need to be offered for some patients where physical therapy fails.

SUMMARY

Balance disturbances are frequent and troublesome in the HIV population and may be associated with viral infection, associated conditions and treatments or occur independently. Awareness of the many possible causes, with appropriate investigations and targeted and symptomatic therapies, offers the best chance of meaningful improvement for the majority of patients.

REFERENCES

Allain, J. P., Laurian, Y., Paul D. A., & Senn, D. (1986). Serological markers in early stages of human immunodeficiency virus infection in haemophiliacs. *Lancet, 2*(8518), 1233-1236.

Baloh, R. W., Fife, T. D., Furman, J. M., & Zee, D. S. (1996, March). Chronic disequilibrium without vertigo. In *Continuum, 2*(2).

Barohn, R. J., Gronseth, G. S., & Le Force, B. R. (1993). Peripheral nervous system involvement in a large cohort of human immunodeficiency virus-infected individuals *Archives of Neurology, 50*(2), 167-171.

Barré-Sinoussi, F., Chermann, J. C., Rey, F., Nugeyre, M., Chamaret, S., Gruest, J., . . . Montagnier, L. (1983). Isolation of a T-lymphotropic retrovirus from a patient at risk for AIDS. *Science, 220*, 868-871.

Baumann, R. J., & Espinosa, P. S. (2007). Neuroepidemiology of HIV/AIDS. In P. Portegies & J. R. Berger (Eds.), *HIV/AIDS and the nervous system, Handbook of clinical neurology* (3rd ed., pp. 3-31). Amsterdam, The Netherlands: Elsevier B.V.

Bhigjee, A. I., Vinsen, C., Windsor, I. M., Gouws, E., Bill, P. L. A., & Tait, D. (1993). Prevalance and transmission of HTLV 1 infection in Natal / Kwa Zulu. *South African Medical Journal, 83*, 665-667.

Brandt, T. (2000). *Vertigo: Its multisensory syndromes.* London, UK: Springer.

Broder, S., & Gallo, R. C. (1984). A pathogenic retrovirus (HTLV-III) linked to AIDS. *New England Journal of Medicine, 311*, 1292-1297.

Buescher, J. L., Gross, S., Gendelman, H. E., & Ikezu, T. (2007). The neuropathogenesis of HIV-1 infection. In P. Portegies & J. R. Berger (Eds.), *Handbook of clinical neurology* (Vol. 85, 3rd series). *HIV/AIDS and the nervous system* (pp. 45-67). Amsterdam, The Netherlands: Elsevier B.V.

Centers for Disease Control. (1981a). Pneumocystic pneumonia—Los Angeles. *MMWR Morbidity and Mortality Weekly Report, 30*, 250-252.

Centers for Disease Control. (1981b). Kaposi's sarcoma and Pneumocystic pneumonia among homosexual men—New York City and California. *MMWR Morbidity and Mortality Weekly Report, 30*, 305-308.

Centers for Disease Control. (1981c). Follow-up on Kaposi sarcoma and Pneumocystic pneumonia. *MMWR Morbidity and Mortality Weekly Report, 30*, 409-410.

Centers for Disease Control. (1992). 1993 revised classification system for HIV infection and expanded surveillance case definition for AIDS among adolescents and adults. *MMWR Morbidity and Mortality Weekly Report, 41*(RR17).

Centers for Disease Control. (2003). *HIV/AIDS surveillance report 2003*. Retrieved May 31, 2008, from http://www.HIVMedicine.com

Cooper, D. A., Gold, J., Maclean, P., Donovan, B., Finlayson, R., Barnes, T. G., et al. (1985). Acute AIDS retrovirus infection. Definition of a clinical illness associated with seroconversion. *Lancet, 1*(8428), 537-540.

Curthoys, I. S., Kim, J., McPhedran, S. K., & Camp, A. J. (2006). Bone conducted vibration selectively activates irregular primary otolithic vestibular neurons in the guinea pig. *Experimental Brain Research, 175*(2), 256-267.

Davis, L. E., Hjelle, B. L., Miller, V. E., Palmer, D. L., Llewellyn, A. L., Merlin, T. L., . . . Wiley, C. A. (1992). Early brain invasion in iatrogenic human immunodeficiency virus infection. *Neurology, 42*, 1736-1739.

Davis, L. E., Rarey, K. E., & McLaren, L. C. (1995). Clinical viral infections and temporal bone histologic studies of patients with AIDS. *Otolaryngology-Head and Neck Surgery, 113*, 695-701

Dellepiane, M., Medicina, M. C., Mora, R., & Salami, A. (2005) Static and dynamic posturography in patients with asymptomatic HIV-1 infection and AIDS. *Acta Otorhinolaryngologica Italica, 25*(6), 353-358.

Dix, R., & Hallpike, C. (1952). The pathology, symptomatology and diagnosis of certain common disorders of the vestibular system. *Annals of Otology, Rhinology and Laryngology, 6*, 987-1016.

Epley, J. M. (1992). The canalith repositioning procedure: for treatment of benign paroxysmal positional vertigo. *Otolaryngology Head and Neck Surgery, 107*, 399-404.

Fantry, L. E., & Staecker, H. (2002). Vertigo and abacavir. *AIDS Patient Care and STDs, 16*(1), 5–7.

Francois-Jérôme Authier, P. C. (2005). Skeletal muscle involvement in human immunodeficiency virus (HIV) infected patients in the era of highly active antiretroviral therapy (HAART). *Muscle Nerve, 32*(3), 247–260.

Gallo, R. C., Salahuddin, S. Z., Popovic, M., Shearer, G. M., Kaplan, M., Haynes, B. F., . . . Safai, B. (1984). Frequent detection and isolation of cytopathic retroviruses (HTLV-III) from patients with AIDS and at risk for AIDS. *Science, 224*(4648), 500–503.

Goebel, J. A. (2001). *Practical management of the dizzy patient.* Philadelphia, PA: Lippincott Williams & Wilkins.

Hain, T. C. (n.d). Retrieved June 15, 2008 from http://www.tchain.com/

Hamersma, H. (1957). *The caloric test. A nystagmographical study.* Thesis, University of Amsterdam.

Hausler, R., Vibert, D., Koralnik, I. J., & Hirschel, B. (1991). Neuro-otological manifestations in different stages of HIV infection. *Acta Otolaryngologica, Supplementum, 481*, 515–521.

Herdman, S. J. (1999). *Vestibular rehabilitation.* Philadelphia, PA: F. A. Davis.

Hoffmann, C., & Mulcahy, F. (2007) Overview of antiretroviral agents 2007. In C. Hoffmann, J. K. Rockstroh, & B. S. Kamps (Eds), *HIV medicine 2007* (pp. 93–126). Paris, France: Flying Publisher.

Hofmeyr, L. M. (2006). Current treatment of Ménière's disease. *Specialist Forum, 6*(9), 60–68.

Jacobson, G. P., & Shepard, N. T. (2008). *Balance function assessment and management.* San Diego, CA: Plural Publishing.

Johnson, R. W., Williams, F. M., Kazi, S., Dimachkie, M. M., & Reveille, J. D. (2003). Human immunodeficiency virus associated polymyositis: A longitudinal study of outcome. *Arthritis and Rheumatism, 49*(2), 172–178.

Johnston, J. L., Miller, J. D., & Nath, A. (1996). Ocular motor dysfunction in HIV-1-infected subjects: quantitative oculographic analysis. *Neurology, 46*(2), 451–457.

Khoza, K., & Ross, E. (2002). Auditory function in a group of adults infected with HIV/AIDS in Gauteng, South Africa. *South African Journal of Communication Disorders, 49*, 17–27.

Kibayashi, K., Ng'walali, P. M., Mbonde, M. P., Makata, A. M., Mwakagile, D, Harada, S., . . . Tseunenri, S. (1999). Neuropathology of human immunodeficiency virus 1 infection. Significance of studying in forensic autopsy cases at Dar es Salaam, Tanzania. *Archives of Pathology and Laboratory Medicine, 123*, 519–523.

Kohan, D., & Giacchi, R. J. (1999). Otologic surgery in patients with HIV-1 and AIDS. *Otolaryngology-Head and Neck Surgery, 121*(4), 355–360.

Lalwani, A. K., & Sooy, C. D. (1992). Otologic and neurotologic manifestations of acquired immunodeficiency syndrome. In T. A. Tami (Ed.), *Otolaryngologic Clinics of North America* (pp. 1183–1197). Philadelphia, PA: Saunders.

Lee, K. C., & Tami, T. A. (1998) Otolaryngologic manifestations of HIV. *HIV InSite knowledge base chapter* (pp. 1–23). Retrieved October 13, 2007, from http://hivinsite.ucsf.edu/InSite?page=kb-04-01-13

Mayo Clinic. (1997). *Mayo Clinic examinations in neurology.* St. Louis, MO: Mosby, Elsevier.

Marra, C. M., Wechhin, H. A., Longstreth, W. T., Rees, T. S., Syapin, C. L., & Gates, G. A. (1997). Hearing loss and antiretroviral therapy in patients infected by with HIV-1. *Archives of Neurology, 54,* 407–410.

McArthur, J. C., Brew, B. J., & Nath, A. (2005). Neurological complications of HIV infection. *Lancet Neurology, 2005, 4,* 543–545.

Michaels, L., Soucek, S., & Liang, J. (1994). The ear in the acquired immunodeficiency syndrome I. Temporal bone histopathologic study. *American Journal of Otology, 15,* 515–522.

Modi, M. M. A., & Modi, G. (2004). Management of HIV–associated focal brain lesions in developing countries. *QJM, Monthly Journal of the Association of Physicians, 97,* 413 –421.

Morris, M. S., & Prasad, S. (1990). Otologic disease in the acquired immunodeficiency syndrome. *Ear, Nose, and Throat Journal, 69,* 451–453.

Nzilambi, N., De Cook, K. M., & Forthal, D. N. (1988). The prevalence of infection with immunodeficiency virus over a 10-year period in rural Zaire. *New England Journal of Medicine, 318*(5), 276–279.

Palacios, G. C., Montalvo, M. S., Fraire, M. I., Leon, E., Alvares, M. T., & Solorzano, F. (2008). Audiologic and vestibular findings in a sample of human immunodeficiency virus type-1-infected Mexican children under highly active antiretroviral therapy. *International Journal of Pediatric Otorhinolaryngology, 72,* 1671–1681.

Pappas, D. G. Jr., Roland, J. T. Jr., Lim, J, Lai, A., & Hillman, D. E. (1995). Ultrastructural findings in the vestibular end-organs of AIDS cases. *American Journal of Otology, 16*(2), 140–145.

Rarey, K. E. (1990). Otologic pathophysiology in patients with human immunodeficiency virus. *American Journal of Otolaryngology, 11*(6), 366–369.

Rubbert, A., Behrens, G., & Ostrowski, M. (2007). Pathogeneses of HIV-1 infection. In C. Hoffmann, J. K., Rockstroh, & B. S., Kamps (Eds.), *HIV Medicine 2007* (pp. 59–86). Paris, France: Flying Publisher.

Salami, A., Cordone, G., Melagrana, A., Barbieri, M., Morandi, N., & Rizzo, F. (1991). Otoneurological abnormalities in AIDS patients. *International Conference on AIDS, 215*(7), 16–21.

Schmäl, F., Lübben, B., Weiberg, K., & Stoll, W. (2005). The minimal ice water caloric test compared with established vestibular caloric test procedures. *Journal of Vestibular Research, 15*(4), 215-224.

Shepard, N. T., & Telian, S. A. (1996). *Practical management of the balance disorder patient.* San Diego, CA: Singular Publishing Group.

Smith, M. E., & Canalis, R. F. (1989). Otologic manifestations of AIDS: The otosyphilis connection. *Laryngoscope, 99*, 365-372.

Soucek, S., & Michaels, L. (1996). The ear in the acquired immunodeficiency syndrome: II. Clinical and audiologic investigation. *American Journal of Otology, 17*(1), 35-39.

Tardieu, M., & Bautet, A. (2002). HIV-1 and the central nervous system. *Current Topics in Microbiology and Immunology, 265*, 183-195.

Teggi, R., Ceserani, N., Lira Luce, F., Lazzarin, A. & Bussi, M.(2008). Otoneurological findings in human immunodeficiency virus positive patients. *The Journal of Laryngology and Otology, 122*, 1289-1294.

Teggi, R., Giardano, L., Pistorio, V., & Bussi, M. (2006). Vestibular function in HIV patients. *Acta Otorhinolaryngologica Italica, 26*(3), 140-146.

Thornton, C. A., Latif, A. S., & Emmanuel, J. C. (1991). Guillain-Barré syndrome associated with human immunodeficiency virus infection in Zimbabwe. *Neurology, 41*(6), 812-815.

Troost, T. (2004). Dizziness and vertigo. In G. Bradley, R. B. Daroff, G. M. Fenichel, & J. Jankovic, (Eds.), *Neurology in clinical practice* (4th ed., pp. 233-245). Philadelphia, PA: Butterworth Heineman.

UNAIDS. (2004). *2004 report on the global HIV/AIDS epidemic* (4th global report). Retrieved August 17, 2009 from: http://www.unaids.org/bangkok2004/gar2004_html/GAR2004_00_en.htm

UNAIDS. (2007). *AIDS epidemic update.* Retrieved August 17, 2009, from http://data.unaids.org/pub/EPISlides/2007/2007_epiupdate_en.pdf

Verma, A. (2001) Epidemiology and clinical features of HIV 1 associated neuropathies. *Journal of the Peripheral Nervous System, 6*(1), 8-13.

Wenzel, G. I., Götz, F., Lenarz, T., & Stöver, T. (2008). HIV-associated cerebral lymphocyte infiltration mimicking vestibular schwannoma. *European Archives of Otorhinolaryngology, 265*, 1567-1571.

Wulff, E. A., Wang, A. K., & Simpson, D. M. (2000). HIV-associated peripheral neuropathy: Epidemiology, pathophysiology and treatment. *Drugs, 59*(6), 1251-1260.

CHAPTER 12

Dysphagia and Related Assessment and Management in Children with HIV/AIDS

Hilda Pressman

INTRODUCTION

Children living with HIV/AIDS face numerous challenges of which feeding difficulties and nutritional issues are very prominent. The effects of these associated feeding difficulties related to HIV/AIDS are pervasive and hold far-reaching implications. In light of the new generation of improved antiretroviral (ARV) therapies which result in reduced mortality and increased life expectancy, concerns about quality of life are becoming more important. Feeding difficulties in children with HIV/AIDS certainly has a devastating impact on their quality of life apart from the risk of death. This chapter will therefore provide some background on the feeding difficulties and nutritional issues that children with HIV/AIDS may be faced with as a backdrop to a discussion on assessment and intervention for this vulnerable population.

ACQUISITION OF HIV/AIDS IN CHILDREN ASSOCIATED WITH FEEDING

Feeding issues potentially affect all babies born to mothers who are HIV+. In addition to in utero exposure through transplacental passage of the virus and perinatal exposure through infected maternal blood and vaginal secretions, breast milk can be a source of infection (vertical infection). Researchers estimate 29% HIV transmission with consistent breast feeding with the risk of transmission being highest in the early months after birth (Pressman, 1992; U.S. National Institute of Allergy and Infectious Disease, 2004).

Reducing Transmission Associated with Feeding

Prior to the availability of antiretroviral therapy, about 25% of pregnant women with HIV in the United States had been found to transmit the virus to their babies. Comparable statistics are reported in developing countries. This number is reduced to less than 2% if the woman takes the drugs before and during birth and the baby is given the drugs after birth. Even when the medication is only given to the mother during labor and delivery, the rate of perinatal transmission can still be decreased to less than 10%. Elective cesarean section has also been used to reduce the chance of exposure for the baby. In 1992, the estimated number of perinatally acquired AIDS cases in the United States was 945. In 2004, this number was decreased to an estimated 48 cases (Centers for Disease Control and Prevention [CDC], 2006). In the Ukraine, some 97 percent of HIV+ children were infected by their mothers. As of May 2004, UNICEF indicated that in the Ukraine over 90% of HIV+ pregnant women were receiving antiretroviral treatment. Their newborn babies were also receiving treatment (United Nations International Children's Emergency Fund). In the Western Cape Province in South Africa, AZT plus nevirapine is being used and the rate of mother-to-baby HIV infection has been reduced from 22% in 2004 to less than 5% in 2008 (Dugger 2008). In KwaZulu-Natal South Africa where only nevirapine was used the rate of transmission was 23% (Dugger, 2008; Rabie, Marais, & Cotton, 2008). In several states in the United States, the law allows for testing all pregnant mothers unless they opt out.

Although this is very promising, unfortunately, the medication is not readily available in many countries and the number of children with HIV/AIDS remains very high. The rate of HIV seropositivity among malnourished children was reported at 21.7% with the highest seroprevalence in underweight children at 47.4% (Angami et al., 2004). In the United States 10 to 14% of infants who acquire HIV acquire it through breast milk. In developing countries this number is one-third to one-half of all HIV infections (Fowler & Newall, 2002). Rabie, Marais and Cotton (2006) note that the risk is greatest during the first few months of life. The degree of risk varies with the mother's HIV status, that is, a high viral load or seroconversion during the period of breast feeding. Antiretroviral treatment is not fully able to suppress the secretion of HIV in breast milk.

Risk Assessment Regarding Breast Feeding

In developed countries, where formula is readily available, mothers who are HIV+ are advised not to breast feed their children. This has been problematic in countries such as South Africa, India, and China where formula is not readily available or affordable, water may not be safe, and where there is a stigma attached to the mother who is not breast feeding her child. In these situations, the benefits of breast feeding are judged to outweigh the potential risk of HIV transmission. UNAIDS/WHO/UNICEF currently recommends avoidance of all breast feeding when replacement feeding is "affordable, feasible, acceptable, sustainable, and safe" (Shankar et al., 2005; p. 961). For those who must breast feed, the recommendation is exclusive breast feeding (nothing passes baby's lips except breast milk with the exception of routine oral polio vaccinations and co-trioxazole prophylaxis) with early weaning. This is reported to pose a lower transmission risk than mixed feeding, as water, juices, or food may introduce bacteria that could lower immune response and increase the risk of transmission of HIV. Rabie, Marais, and Cotton (2006) note that exclusive breast feeding, which has this very strict definition, is difficult to enforce. Rapid weaning is recommended at around 6 months of age with purees and milk provided instead of breast milk. It is important that the breast feeding mother eat well and stay as healthy as possible. In South Africa some mothers have begun to pasteurize their breast milk. Certain hospitals have chosen to implement breast milk pasteurization programs and have trained mothers to do this at home. This reduces the infectivity of expressed breast milk (Rabie, Marais & Cotton, 2006) but still continues to be a possible source of infection for the child.

Shankar et al. (2005) studied the issue of breast feeding in India from 2000 to 2004. In the study, there were 146 HIV+ pregnant mothers and 29 HIV– pregnant mothers. After each of the mothers was tested for HIV, they had a posttest counseling session. During this session, the risks and benefits of feeding choices in the context of HIV were discussed. Four options were presented including exclusive breast feeding and early weaning (at 6 months), infant formula, modified animal milks (cow or buffalo), or heat-treated breast milk. An increase was noted in the percentage of women with HIV who breast fed from 60% (in 2000 to 2002) to 88% (in 2003 to 2004). This was thought to be due to the information given to the mothers of an increase in morbidity that had been noted in non breast-fed infants. The morbidity included pneumonia, acute gastroenteritis, and sepsis.

A recent finding reported that 3 cases in the United States, since 1993, have been reported where babies were infected with HIV through food being prechewed by an infected parent or caregiver (Gaur et al., 2009). Saliva does contain HIV, but usually in amounts too low to cause transmission. It is assumed that the infected chewers had inflammations or open sores in their mouths, which passed the virus to infants through cuts or other common teething conditions. This information is important as prechewing food is common in many cultures and in places where prepared pureed food or equipment to puree home prepared foods are not available. Additionally, it should be noted that prechewing significantly reduces the food value that the child receives.

DYSPHAGIA

Dysphagia is the term used to describe feeding and swallowing disorders. Difficulty may occur in sucking, eating from a spoon, chewing food, swallowing solids and or liquids, selectivity of type and texture of food, coughing or choking when eating, or food sticking in the throat or chest. In addition to eating and drinking, difficulty with swallowing may affect the control of saliva, taking oral medications, and managing tooth brushing.

The Phases of Feeding and Swallowing

There are four phases of feeding and swallowing, each of which may be affected by HIV/AIDS. Difficulty may be seen at any point from birth on. The oral preparatory phase involves taking the liquid or food into the mouth (sucking from breast, bottle, or straw, or taking food off a spoon) and includes the process of chewing when children are on whole food. In the oral initiation phase, the food is gathered together into a cohesive bolus and transmitted posteriorly to allow for a swallow. In the oral preparatory and oral initiation stages, children may have difficulty sucking, they may not manage the food or liquid in their mouths causing food to fall out of the mouth, and they may manage purees and soft solids but may lose liquid if they try to drink from a cup. Some children may not chew efficiently and may have weak and/or discoordinated tongue movements. Some children will easily gag on food that has any increased texture. We would expect to see a child move to some table foods by 10 to 12 months of age. In children with dysphagia, meals may be prolonged to an hour or more. They may also pocket food in their cheeks and can hold this food for hours, which may set them up for a choking episode. These deficits put them at risk for not being able to meet their nutritional needs. A child should follow his or her growth curve and when they begin to fall off, they are said to have failure to thrive. Children with oral stage dysphagia may drool more than typical for age.

When food or liquid is passed into the pharynx, a series of contractions moves it through the pharynx and into the esophagus. The upper esophageal sphincter opens to allow the food to pass into the pharynx and then closes to prevent refluxate from getting into the pharynx. Breathing stops at the moment of swallow to prevent the material falling into the airway. If the food or liquid falls into the airway, it is called penetration if it occurs above the vocal folds, and aspiration if the material passes below the vocal folds. This can have a significant effect on the lungs. Some individuals will cough if the bolus is misdirected and they may bring it back into the pharynx to be re-swallowed safely. Others do not cough and so there is no warning that aspiration is occurring. A very high percentage of children with developmental disabilities aspirate silently. In the pharyngeal phase, there may be a delay in triggering the swallow with material falling into the open airway. Children may have material left in the pharynx after the rest of the bolus passes into the esophagus. Both of these difficulties increase the risk of aspiration. It is said that feeding is the most complicated thing that a newborn has to do. Signs of pharyngeal phase dysphagia include coughing during or after the meal, choking or gagging, voice with wet or gurgly sounds, or a sensation of food sticking in the throat. Pharyngeal phase problems may exist without any signs and would be classified as silent aspiration. If aspiration is occurring, there may be increased upper respiratory problems (pneumonia, chronic bronchitis, or asthma that is not under control). Instrumental assessment of swallow such as modified barium swallow (MBS) or flexible endoscopic evaluation of swallowing (FEES) may be necessary.

Once in the esophagus, the bolus is again moved by a series of contractions (peristalsis) until it empties into the stomach. The lower esophageal sphincter opens to allow the bolus to pass into the stomach. It then closes to keep the material from moving back up. Food, liquid, or acid coming back up from the stomach into the esophagus is called reflux and is termed gastroesophageal reflux disease (GERD) if it is an ongoing problem. If the refluxate passes above the upper esophageal sphincter, into the pharynx, mouth, nose, and/or trachea it is called laryngopharyngeal reflux (LPR) and may affect the vocal folds. Refluxate that gets to the oropharynx may be aspirated and can be dangerous for the lungs due to the acid component in the material. Signs of esophageal phase dysphagia include frequent spitting up or vomiting, arching or stiffening when eating, a hoarse voice, and a preference for liquids over solid food. Reflux has been implicated in esophagitis, ear infections, sinusitis, and damage to the vocal folds (Arvedson & Brodsky, 2002). Understanding the complexity of the normal swallow and the difficulties that children or adults may have when eating allows the healthcare provider to be alert for evidence of difficulty with feeding and swallowing and to intervene or make an appropriate referral.

Dysphagia in Children with HIV/AIDS

There is a paucity of research regarding feeding and swallowing difficulties in children with HIV/AIDS. In a study by Pressman and Morrison (1988), of 55 children with HIV/AIDS who were followed ongoing as part of a multidisciplinary program, 25 (45%) were found to have symptoms of dysphagia at some point during their illness. Eleven of these children (44%) had mild to moderate difficulties in that they were able to be maintained on oral feeding but had difficulty with specific consistencies, had insufficient intake to meet their caloric needs, feeding time was prolonged, and they were unable to progress from bottle to purees or from purees to chewables as appropriate for age or a combination of factors. Fourteen (56%) had severe dysphagia. They had overall developmental delay (6), intermittent dysphagia secondary to *Candida* (6), progressive encephalopathy (3), and dysphagia related to a brain tumor (1). They were unable to be maintained solely on oral feedings. Many of the children were at risk for nutritional compromise. Some had muscle wasting as an effect of malnutrition, which affected the heart, respiratory muscles, ability to clear secretions and aerate the lungs, and decreased the strength and coordination of the muscles of deglutition. They also demonstrated anorexia secondary to pain during feeding and/or related to side effects of their medication. Nine children required hyperalimentation to support their nutrition and one had an NG tube.

In a study in 1992, Pressman reported on 96 children ages 4 months to 17 years and 3 months, who were seen for screening of speech, language, and feeding/swallowing skills. Only the first screening of each child was reported. Of these 96 children, 20.8% had some degree of dysphagia. Among the group there was difficulty with all phases of feeding and swallowing, including coughing on food or liquid, slow feeding (more than 30 minutes), failure to thrive, gagging on solids and chewables, inability to transition from purees to solids, and decompensation of feeding skills secondary to odynophagia (pain on swallowing). The infections associated with odynophagia were candida esophagitis, herpes gingivastomatitis, and CMV esophagitis. Three percent of the children had suffered a CVA. Developmental delay was identified in 19.8% of the children. This involved significant motor involvement and microcephaly. In many cases, this was associated with prenatal factors other than HIV/AIDS including use of drugs and alcohol during pregnancy, poor prenatal care, prematurity, and low birth weight. Progressive encephalopathy was seen in 7.3% of the children. The children with progressive encephalopathy lost feeding skills and had to revert to nonchewables. They lost the ability to self-feed and oral feeding time was notably prolonged. Four percent of the children required placement of a gastrostomy tube to supplement oral feeding.

De Lange (2003) found irregular tongue function in 5/12 children ages 6 to 36 months, who took a longer time to complete their meal. Angami et al. (2004) found that the prevalence rate of HIV+ children among malnourished children was 21.7%. Underweight children had an even higher prevalence of 47.4% and children with kwashiorkor had the lowest seroprevalence at 10.5%. No other studies were found that specifically looked at feeding and swallowing. Many of the papers published only addressed causes of dysphagia, such as those that follow.

Dysphagia and Neurologic Disease

HIV crosses the blood-brain barrier causing neurological complications in many children. Davis-McFarland (2002) notes that pediatric HIV is neurotrophic, and therefore more likely to initially affect the central rather than peripheral nervous system. Van Rie, Harrington, Dow, and Robertson (2007) note that children may be more vulnerable to neurological complications of HIV-1 infection and that this usually indicates a poor prognosis. HIV often invades the central nervous system (CNS) early in infection. The encephalopathy that develops may be static or progressive. Children with static encephalopathy demonstrate developmental delay in infancy and nonprogressive motor deficits. McNeilly (2005) reported seeing children with cerebral palsy with spastic quadriplegia and mental retardation. Children are also noted to have acquired microcephaly with a decrease in serial head circumference measurements and brain atrophy on CT. Seizure disorder is often seen. Rabie, Marais, van Toorn, Nourse, New, and Goussard (2007) noted that nasopharyngeal incoordination which can cause food or liquid to come from the nose may be an important indication of neurological disease. Some of the children with static encephalopathy may go on to develop progressive encephalopathy. Van Rie et al. (2007) report that "experience with children on antiretroviral therapy (ART) revealed a high rate of arrested HIV related encephalopathy, but also high rates of residual behavioral problems, neurologic, cognitive and scholastic impairments and risk for relapse" (Rie et al., p. 3). Communication deficits including receptive and expressive language, as well as articulation disorders and oral motor deficits are frequently seen and may be related to neurologic impairment and/or medical, social, and educational factors. See Section II (Chapters 7 and 8) of this book for further information on communication disorders associated with HIV/AIDS in children.

Children with neurologic disorders are at increased risk of dysphagia at all phases. There is a critical period from birth to 2 years of age for presenting a variety of foods and textures to typically developing children. During this period, children develop sensory tolerances as well as eating behaviors and related swallowing skills. Those who do not have the experiences during this critical period may develop hypersensitivity and difficulty in managing table foods. They may require therapeutic intervention to help them achieve this goal. Many children with HIV/AIDS do not have the opportunity to explore a variety of foods during this critical period due to illness and/or developmental delay. Rabie, Marais, van Toorn, Nourse, et al. (2007) note that "swallowing disorders may contribute significantly to morbidity in HIV-infected infants." They further note that coughing or liquid coming from the nose associated with feeding is "suggestive of poorly coordinated swallowing, which is a particular problem in children with encephalopathy."

Children with progressive encephalopathy related to HIV/AIDS show neurologic deterioration including loss or plateau of developmental milestones, progressive motor deterioration, impaired brain growth, generalized weakness, stroke, or mass lesions of the central nervous system. In some children, the neurologic condition may be the first AIDS defining illness. Van Rie et al. (2007) noted that HIV-1 enters the central nervous system (CNS) soon after infection and may persist over the course of the infection. The CNS is immature and brain growth may be impaired. This may affect motor, cognitive, and language functions. In children with progressive encephalopathy, the loss of developmental milestones may lead to decompensation and a decrease in chewing skills. Even hand to mouth coordination for self-feeding may be affected. Meningitis and toxoplasmosis also can affect the brain and cause loss of skills. Miller (2003) notes that HIV encephalopathy may be present in up to 16% of children with HIV-1 infection.

In children with neurologic impairment, the feeding complications include increased risk of aspiration while feeding (usually silent), which may lead to aspiration pneumonia or chronic lung disease, nasopharyngeal incoordination leading to food or liquid coming through the nose, poor chewing, difficulty self-feeding, and ultimately malnutrition. When children encounter difficulties with eating and swallowing they tend to take much longer at mealtimes and eat less. Prolonged mealtimes affect weight gain due to the calories that are expended during the feeding and digestive processes. Refusal of food often is seen. Mealtimes of 30 minutes are suggested as children usually eat 90% of what they will ultimately eat in the first half hour. Many children require 3 small meals and 3 snacks, all of which should be calorically dense. Some children who had previously fed themselves may need to be fed. In one study, Pressman (1992) found 3% of the children had a CVA. CNS opportunistic infections are less frequent in children compared with adults. Early identification and intervention in children with neurologic deficits associated with HIV/AIDS is critical to helping these children meet their potential.

Effect of Infectious Diseases on Oral Intake

Infectious diseases associated with HIV/AIDS often have an effect on intake of food. Most commonly there is odynophagia, or pain on swallowing caused by fungal infections. These include oral candidiasis, cryptococcus, and histoplasma. *Candida* has been reported in the oral, laryngeal, and esophageal mucosa. The appearance is of a milky pseudomembrane that may wipe off but then leave a raw bleeding surface. Oral candidiasis may be an early sign of illness or progression of disease. Rabie, Marais, van Toorn, Nel, and Cotton (2007) note that this is the most frequent oral manifestation in HIV+ children. Epiglottitis has been reported causing dysphagia, odynophagia, and hoarseness, and sometimes causing airway obstruction. Oral candidiasis is frequently readily responsive to medications, but esophageal candidiasis requires a much longer period of treatment. New species of *Candida* are emerging with some drug resistance being noted, specifically for fluconazole. Other forms of infection include herpes gingivostomatitis, viral esophagitis, and gastritis. Nausea and vomiting may be secondary to drugs, infection, or illness. Colitis and esophagitis, as well as herpes simplex, may affect the ability of the body to absorb food. Many medications used to treat HIV/AIDS may be associated with nausea, vomiting, abdominal pain, and/or diarrhea (Table 12–1).

Behardien (2006) followed 268 children over a two-year period, ages 1 month to 10 years and 8 months, with a mean age of 3½ years. All were vertically infected. The study found that 70.1% of the children had oral lesions, 38.8% had oral candidiasis, 36.6% had pseudomembranous candidiasis, 5.6% had ulceration NOS, 3.4% had periodontal conditions, 0.7% had herpes simplex virus infection, and 3.0% had xerostomia (dry mouth). Xerostomia often is a side effect of medication. Dry mouth can increase dental caries, as saliva is important in bathing the teeth throughout the day and can significantly affect the ability to manage dry food in the mouth.

Other infections that may affect children include cytomegalovirus (CMV) and toxoplasmosis. In the experience of Pressman and Morrison (1988) this may affect brain function, as both CMV and toxoplasmosis may pass the blood-brain barrier. Gastroenteritis commonly causes diarrhea. Colitis and esophagitis also are seen. Herpes simplex is seen in the mouth in the form of gingivostomatitis. If it is extensive and persists for more than 4 weeks it is considered

Table 12–1. Medications Associated with Nausea, Vomiting, Abdominal Pain, and Possibly Diarrhea

Abacivir	Erythromycin	Ritonavir
Acyclovir	Ganciclovir	Saquinavir
Amprenavir	Indinavir	Stavudine
Azithromycin	Lamivudine	Sulfonamides
Ciprofloxacin	Nelfinavir	Zidovudine
Clarithomycin	Nevirapine	
Dideozyinosine	Pentamidine	
Efavirenz	Rifampin	

an AIDS defining condition. Painful recurrences are seen. Infectious diseases are very common in children with HIV/AIDS and frequently result in decrease or refusal of feeding as well as a decline in development including communication. Ongoing clinical intervention needs to be adapted to the child's ability to participate at any given time in their illness.

Failure to Thrive

"Failure to thrive" is the term used to distinguish children who are not growing along their curve or who have fallen off their curve. Wasting is one of the principal criteria for the diagnosis of symptomatic AIDS. The CDC defines wasting in children younger than 13 as persistent weight loss of more than 10% of baseline, downward crossing of at least two percentile lines on the weight for age chart in a child age 1 or older, or less than the 5th percentile on the weight for height chart on two consecutive measurements at least 30 days apart. Butensky (2001) states that levels of specific nutrients can affect disease expression. Nutritional status can impact the quality of life and survival. Growth may be affected by a low CD4-T lymphocyte count, infections such as pneumonia, maternal drug use during pregnancy, a lower infant CD4 T-cell count, and exposure to antiretroviral therapy. Children have greater nutritional issues compared to adults as they have the added demands for growth and development. Rabie, Marais, van Toorn, Nourse, et al. (2007) note that poor food security, poor nutrition choices, and chronic diseases such as tuberculosis (TB) may be additional contributing factors. These difficulties are frequently seen in developing countries (Table 12–2).

Gastrointestinal manifestations of AIDS include diarrhea, malabsorption, nausea, and vomiting. Additionally, anorexia can be primary or a side effect of HIV. Absence of appetite may be secondary to pain from inflammation and ulcers of the upper GI tract or a side effect of medication. Anorexia is also associated with anxiety and depression. Growth in HIV-infected children remains below the growth in age-matched, gender-matched uninfected children. Children may have poor oral intake, increased metabolic needs (Oleske, Rothpletz-Puglia, & Winter, 1996), inability to obtain adequate food, poor nutritional choices, and/or gastrointestinal malabsorption. Infections may affect the gastrointestinal (GI) tract. Persistent and

Table 12–2. Factors Associated with Failure to Thrive

• Decreased nutritional intake   • Increased nutritional needs – Dysphagia   – Increased metabolic rate – Odynophagia   – Fever – Anorexia   – Infection • Gastrointestinal issues   – Cardiac requirements – Malabsorption   – Respiratory requirements – Chronic diarrhea   • Psychosocial issues – Nausea   – Inability to obtain adequate food – Vomiting   – Caregiver illness

chronic diarrhea increases caloric needs by 25%. Metabolic rate may be increased and many of the children have increased nutritional requirements due to protein wasting, fever, infections, and sepsis. Some children suffer from chronic vomiting and nausea or chronic diarrhea. Children also have been found to have resting energy expenditures that are increased. Malnutrition predisposes children to further infection and malabsorption. They may require a higher level of calories than a child without HIV. Higher intake has been associated with improvement in weight and fat mass. Malnutrition has a very significant effect on the child's ability to communicate and to learn. The weakness associated with malnutrition makes all movements effortful. Hypotonia may be seen to affect oral motor skills. The child may be lethargic and the desire to communicate may be decreased. Stimulability for therapeutic tasks also may be affected.

Psychosocial Issues

Psychosocial factors may have an effect on a child's ability to meet nutritional needs. These include poverty, limited access to health care, and illness in the biological or caregiving family members. The medical status of the direct caregivers may cause erratic caregiving. Bringing children for appointments and administering medications may be problematic. In South Africa many children are placed in residential care centers because the parents are unable to take care of them or unwanted children are abandoned (de Lange, 2003). Many of the children with HIV/AIDS need to have their food prepared to a soft or pureed consistency, which adds to the burden of food preparation. In some countries, the equipment needed to puree foods may not be available and jarred purees do not have the same caloric density as home-prepared purees. High calorie foods can be offered at meal and snack time (see Table 12–4 in section on Intervention). This is helpful for children who tend to eat small quantities. Some of the children who were previously independent feeders may need to be fed. Pressman and Morrison (1988) and Pressman (1992) encountered children who reached the phase in progressive encephalopathy where they needed assistance with feeding and/or needed to move from regular table food to soft to chew or pureed foods. Caregivers found this very disturbing as it was a major signal in the decline of the children. Children may face social isolation because of their special food needs, oral motor deficits, and possible need to be fed beyond an age when that is considered appropriate. Mealtime is often an opportunity for language stimulation as children and adults talk during the meal, but as mealtime is often distressing due to the child's special needs, this opportunity is often lost.

IDENTIFICATION AND REFERRAL

The ability to work with an HIV/AIDS team is a critical factor in the evaluation, monitoring, and management of patients. In addition to the members of the entire pediatric HIV/AIDS team, the feeding team members typically include a physician, speech-language pathologist/speech-language therapist (SLP/SLT), physical therapist (PT), occupational therapist (OT), dietician, and nurse. All of these individuals should be pediatric specialists. Additionally, the caregiver should be an integral part of the team. It is only with feedback from the caregiver that recommendations can be made which can be carried out at home. Pressman and Morrison (1988) and Pressman (1992) had the opportunity to work in an HIV/AIDS program with Dr. James Oleske and the other members of his team in Newark, NJ. Children were seen in a weekly clinic and the authors attended each of the clinics. All patients were referred to the speech-language pathologist for evaluation and follow-up. In these studies, children presented with poor weight gain, refusal to feed, inability to tolerate specific consistencies, and coughing or choking associated with eating. Additionally, children were seen as inpatients as needed. For the in patients, odynophagia was a significant reason for referral. Infants would be admitted to the hospital with sudden refusal of the bottle. When the SLP/SLT fed the child, immediate sucking was seen. This then stopped and screaming was heard. After calming, the same thing recurred. This became a recognizable pattern of *Candida*, which sometimes was not noted orally but was present in the pharynx and/or esophagus.

Children exhibiting the following difficulties should be referred to the SLP/SLT for evaluation: (1) nutritional factors including failure to thrive, which is often associated with limited intake, refusal of oral feeding, and pain associated with eating or drinking; (2) dysphagia issues including difficulty sucking from breast or bottle, decreased oral containment of food (i.e., food falls out of the mouth), inability to progress from purees to table food often accompanied by gagging, prolonged chewing, "pocketing" of food in the cheeks even after the meal is finished, inability to progress from bottle to cup, meals that last more than 30 minutes, decrease in intake often associated with progressive encephalopathy, report of coughing or choking during or after the meal, sometimes associated with aspiration pneumonia, chronic bronchitis, or asthma, wet or gurgly vocal quality after eating, food or liquid coming out of the nose during or after meals, significant drooling beyond teething or the child's report of the sensation of food being caught in their throat; and (3) respiratory issues including reactive airway disease, pneumonia, or bronchitis. The indications for referral to a SLP/SLT is summarized in Table 12-3.

Rabie, Marais, van Toorn, Nourse, et al. (2007) note that when uncoordinated swallowing occurs the SLP/SLT can provide invaluable assistance. McMeans (2005) indicates that HIV+ infants may have a weak suck, which may lead to inadequate intake of breast milk or formula and that older children may demonstrate poor chewing and feeding skills. McMeans (2005) further notes that difficulty with swallowing may lead to poor oral intake or complete refusal and that there is a risk of aspiration and pneumonia associated with swallowing problems. Additionally, children with neurologic deterioration

Table 12–3. Indications for Referral to a SLP/SLT

- Nutritional Factors
  - Failure to thrive
  - Refusal of oral feeding
  - Pain associated with eating or drinking

- Dysphagia issues
  - Difficulty sucking from breast or bottle
  - Decreased oral containment of food
    - Food falls out of mouth
  - Inability to progress from purees to table food
  - Prolonged chewing
  - "Pocketing" of food in the cheeks
  - Inability to progress from bottle to cup
  - Meals that last more than 30 minutes
  - Decrease in intake often associated with progressive encephalopathy
  - Report of coughing or choking during or after the meal
    - Sometimes associated with respiratory problems
    - Wet or gurgly vocal quality after eating
  - Food or liquid coming out of the nose during or after meals
  - Significant drooling beyond teething
  - Child's report of the sensation of food being caught in their throat

- Respiratory issues
  - Reactive airway disease
  - Asthma
  - Pneumonia
  - Chronic bronchitis

may lose feeding skills leading to inadequate intake of nutrients. The members of the feeding team must be well trained, not only in their area of specialty, but also in working with children with HIV/AIDS. This may require mentorship and supervision until the individual demonstrates the level of knowledge necessary to work independently. Even when working independently in their own area of expertise, members of the feeding team continue to rely on each other's expertise in providing the most appropriate intervention. The SLP/

SLT often serves as the coordinator of the feeding team due to their expertise in dysphagia management. Different members of the team may be called on for specific children, but the team should meet on some regular schedule to review cases together.

ASSESSMENT

Taking the History

A good history is the first and often one of the most revealing aspects of the assessment. The medical chart provides much of the information that is needed, but an interview with the caregiver and the child is critical. Important issues to address are the symptoms of the problem including the concerns of the caregiver and the concerns of the child. Concerns of the other team members may be found in the chart review or by direct contact. Identifying the onset of the problem may help to link it to changes in medication or changes in neurologic function. Nutritional status is critical and members of the feeding team should be relied on to provide necessary information. The SLP/SLT will want to determine whether the child is following a curve on the growth chart or is falling off. Body Mass Index should be calculated to look at weight for height. Questions should be asked that would identify gastrointestinal difficulties, including anorexia or decrease in appetite, as well as vomiting or diarrhea. Indications of respiratory difficulties such as pneumonia, bronchitis, or asthma should be determined. An exacerbation of asthma symptoms or inability to manage asthma as expected may be secondary to ongoing micro aspiration. A list of current medications should be obtained and assessed for side effects that may be exacerbating the problems. A history of hospitalizations should be obtained. The SLP/SLT will want to ascertain how nutritional and hydration issues are currently being addressed. What type of diet is the child on, that is, regular, soft to chew, ground, or pureed? Does the child feed independently? Are any special utensils needed? Does the child use a bottle and/or cup? What foods and feeding techniques have been most accepted? Is the child taking a supplement in order to meet nutritional needs? Does the child take a multivitamin with fluoride? A three-day recall diet is often helpful to indicate what typical meals and snacks are like. This should be filled out contemporaneously for three days, one of which should be a weekend. The support of a dietician is invaluable in assessing whether the child is meeting nutritional needs and in making suggestions as needed. History forms are available in the literature (Arvedson & Brodsky, 2002; Sheppard, 1995).

Clinical Assessment

The next aspect of the assessment is the clinical examination, which the SLP/SLT may perform independently or with other members of the feeding team. If this is done independently then the child will be referred for further evaluations as needed. The benefit of being seen by the feeding team as a whole is that fewer appointments have to be made and a consensus can be reached.

Before beginning the clinical assessment, the SLP/SLT should put on gloves and any other protective gear that is deemed necessary. Universal precautions assume that everyone is potentially a carrier of HIV/AIDS and/or other infectious diseases. For further details see Chapter 4. The SLP/SLT first will assess anatomy. Oral and thoracic structures are assessed for malformations or evidence of muscular disorders. The PT on the team will be helpful in assessing thoracic structures and function. The child may have concomitant difficulties unrelated to HIV/AIDS or may have deficits secondary to neurologic impairment. Children with HIV/AIDS often have "thrush" or *Candida*. This looks like a white milky coating of the surface of the tongue and/or gums, which can be very painful and affect intake. There may be complete refusal of oral feeding in some children, especially the young bottle or breast fed children possibly indicating *Candida* in the mouth, pharynx and/or esophagus. If the child is being breast-fed, *Candida* can be passed back and forth between mother and child and so both must be treated. If teeth have not been well cared for there may be dental caries, loose teeth, or inflamed gums, all of which can affect acceptance and management of solid food. Additionally, aspiration of saliva, which contains increased bacteria from dental caries, increases the chances of respiratory compromise. Bleeding gums present a special problem for caregivers due to concerns regarding transmission. Drooling or pooling of oral secretions should be noted. This may be indicative of problematic swallowing. The voice should be noted to determine if it has a wet or gurgly vocal quality, which may indicate pooling of secretions in the pharynx. Hoarseness may be indicative of ongoing laryngopharyngeal reflux or *Candida* on the vocal folds.

The child's postural stability for trunk, head, and neck is critical for safe and efficient feeding. If the child does not have independent control, the seating used during feeding will have to be addressed to determine if it gives the necessary support or if modifications are necessary. The help of the physical therapist will be very useful for this task. It is important to assess whether primitive reflexes are present. These may be seen in children with significant neuromuscular difficulties and may require adjustment of the way in which food is presented. The assessment should also determine whether the reflexes for swallowing, coughing, and gagging are present. It is important for the examiner and for all members of the team to remember that the absence of a gag reflex does not preclude safe oral feeding (Leder, 1997).

Observation of Eating

The observation of eating is the next area of assessment. In observing the child, notation should be made of effectiveness of independent eating. Is this easy for the child? Is the rate too slow or too fast? Does the child overfill the spoon? The OT on the team can contribute to this part of the assessment. If the child is fed, is the caregiver putting too much on the spoon or feeding the child too rapidly? Is there a problem with neatness, that is, does the food fall from the spoon? In many cases the caregiver may report that the child eats a certain amount but upon observation it may be noted that the child has lost much of the food and that it is collected on clothing. The clinician will want to look at management of liquids, nonchewable solids (such as applesauce), and chewable solids. Chewable solids vary from easy to eat (crunchy foods such as cookies) and foods that are more difficult to chew (meat or bread). In observing each of these foods, the clinician is first looking to see oral management. Does the child remove the food from the spoon by closing lips around it or is the caregiver dispensing food by wiping it off the top lip? Is there loss of food or liquids at the lips (dribbling), prolonged oral transit time, residual in the mouth after the swallow, delayed initiation of swallowing, and any indications of pharyngeal phase difficulties such as gagging, coughing, or choking?

The child's behaviors during eating should be observed. Is the child comfortable during the meal? Does the child tire as the meal progresses and have increased difficulty managing the food? Is the child cooperative?

The assessment also should include a trial of new food or liquid as appropriate to age and level of function. If the child is exclusively fed purees, tolerance of a mashed consistency should be explored. Mashed banana or mashed carrots are good foods to try. The child may be resistant to any texture changes or taste changes. If it is a taste issue, the cooked carrots can be mixed with the jarred carrots and the quantity of jarred food gradually decreased as acceptance of the home-prepared food increases. If texture is the issue, banana or carrots can be mixed with some milk to soften it further. A crunchy food that easily dissolves in the mouth can be offered by putting a very small piece on the molar table or the gums where the molars will come in. This should initiate some chewing movements. Children initially use a munching pattern with only up and down movements. The typically developing child usually has a rotary pattern by three years of age. This indicates that the child is moving the food from side to side in a more efficient pattern. Some children with oral motor deficits will mash chewables with their tongue against the palate and then swallow the items whole. If coughing is associated with liquids or if the child is not able to drink from a cup, thickened liquids can be offered to determine whether this is helpful. There are several thickeners on the market but thickening of liquid can be achieved with natural ingredients such as using pureed fruit or applesauce thinned slightly with juice or water. Milk can be mixed with yogurt to achieve a consistency that may be tolerated better. Recommendations made as the result of the clinical evaluation may include changes in positioning, modifications in diet or changes in the way the food is presented. Clinical intervention may be suggested, including speech therapy, physical therapy, and/or occupational therapy, as well as ongoing management by the dietician.

Instrumental Assessment

The clinical assessment may indicate the need for instrumental evaluation. A modified barium swallow is a fluoroscopic procedure that further investigates the management of food or liquid. It is usually conducted by an SLP/SLT and a radiologist. The examination is recorded and can be reviewed after the exam is completed. The goal of the examination is not to document aspiration but to assess the safest consistencies and the best manner in which to present the food. Barium is mixed into familiar food to highlight it. The child is placed in an upright position in appropriate seating and given liquids, purees, and solids as appropriate. If difficulties are seen, modifications may be trialed. It is important to remember that the modified barium swallow is only a moment in time. If the child continues to demonstrate difficulties at mealtime, it is important for the clinician to trust clinical judgment and to make needed modifications. The child's skills may deteriorate as the meal progresses and the child tires.

The recommendation is to scan the esophagus as part of the modified barium swallow examination to look for indications of reflux or decreased motility. As the esophageal portion of the examination is just a screening, it does not rule out reflux or candida esophagitis. If these are suspected based on history, the pediatric gastroenterologist on the team should be consulted. Further testing may include an upper GI series, pH probe monitoring, or endoscopic evaluation. Sometimes the pediatric gastroenterologist will give the child a trial of medication before undertaking these more invasive procedures.

Flexible endoscopic evaluation of swallowing (FEES) (Langmore, 2001) is a method of assessing swallowing that does not involve radiation and may be a choice for assessment at some centers. For this assessment, a thin tube is passed through the nose down to the pharynx just above the airway. Once the child accommodates to the tube a variety of food and drinks can be given. The child can be fed a full meal to assess function because there is no radiation involved. This allows for a determination as to whether skills decline as the child tires. The assessment is recorded for later review.

INTERVENTION

Nutrition must be the primary issue. The caregiver, dietician, and pediatric gastroenterologist will be critical in helping the child meet nutritional needs. Intervention for dysphagia falls into two broad categories: compensatory strategies and therapeutic treatment programs. The compensatory strategies are changes that are made to the posture, type of utensil (bottle, cup, spoon), bolus characteristics (puree vs. mashed vs. chewable), method of presentation of the bolus, and the environment in which the child is fed (Rosenthal et al., 1995). The SLP/SLT, PT, and OT will work together in assessing and determining the best strategies. The caregiver must be part of this discussion in order to achieve carryover to home and/or school. These strategies often are able to make significant change in a very short time and allow the child to be safely maintained on oral feeding and to meet their nutritional needs. It is important to remember that children may decompensate during periods of acute illness and require additional compensatory interventions before they return to their baseline. Rabie, Marais, van Toorn, Nourse, et al. (2007) note that manipulating the consistency and modifying feeding techniques frequently control the symptoms. Children should be offered high-calorie foods allowing them to meet their nutritional needs in a low volume meal (Table 12–4).

Therapeutic Intervention

The therapeutic treatment program has longer term goals of improving management and advancing skills. The oral sensorimotor approach to therapy in treating children with dysphagia (Arvedson, 2002; Clark, 2005; Sheppard, 2005, 2008) is one which has an evidence base to demonstrate its effectiveness. Feeding and swallowing are motor behaviors that depend on sensory input. When these behaviors are immature or disrupted, function is affected. The oral sensorimotor technique involves structured sensory and movement experiences which facilitate improved feeding and swallowing and improved acquisition of new feeding and swallowing skills. Oral feeding is the major goal. This approach is multimodal and encourages coordinated timing and sufficient muscle strength for food and liquid to be swallowed safely. It also elicits new movement components. The therapy may include some direct exercises but these are always preparatory to swallowing a bolus of food or saliva. The SLP/SLT will be the professional to take the lead in this treatment. It is important that all members of the intervention team, including the caregiver, be in agreement regarding techniques used.

In general, training for tolerance of a new food or for a new task should take place during a snack time or during a therapy time

Table 12–4. High Calorie Foods Recommended for Snack Time or Meals in Certain Cases

Food	Calories
Sweet potato	155 calories in 4 oz./113.4 grams
Cheese	Approximately 100 calories per oz./ 1162.3 grams
Avocado	194 calories per ½ cup/0.12 liters
Scrambled egg	75 calories per egg
Tuna fish packed in oil	268 calories per 3.5 oz./99.2 grams
Red kidney beans	110 calories per ½ cup/0.12 liters
Applesauce	110 calories per ½ cup/0.12 liters
Butter or margarine	45 calories/tsp.
Cream cheese	100 calories per oz./28.35 grams
Jelly or jam	50 calories per tablespoon
Olive oil	40 calories per teaspoon
Grated parmesan cheese	143 calories per oz./28.35 grams
Peanut butter	95 calories per tablespoon
Ground sesame seeds	159 calories per ¼ cup/0.06 liters
Ground raisins	190 calories per ¼ cup/0.06 liters

so as not to disturb the child's intake during meals. Meals are the time when the child should be attempting to meet nutritional needs in a positive manner, and should usually last for 30 minutes as the child generally eats the majority of what is going to be eaten in the first 30 minutes. The added time creates stress and burns calories so that the child may not benefit from the increased intake. It is better to provide high-calorie snacks between meals.

The goals of therapy are to help the child understand what is expected, develop sensory tolerances for the tasks, improve neuromuscular and praxic competency, and train the caregiver to work on carryover to home. The use of simple language and nonverbal cues are important for the child who has a language delay. It is critical that the SLP/SLT respond to the child's communication whether it be verbal or nonverbal. Nonverbal responses include eye gaze for the child who does not point. Verbalizing what the child has communicated helps the child to know that the need has been understood and to maintain the communication interaction. The recognition of the child's request should be done even if the response is negative, that is, cookies can be eaten after therapy.

The initial task may be a nonfeeding task such as putting pegs in a board in order to earn a reinforcer. This allows the child to understand what is expected. Once this is accomplished, food can be introduced as the work of therapy (McKirdy et al., 2008). The SLP/SLT orients the child to the task with verbal and signing cues, provides verbal support, and responds to the child's signals. The SLP/SLT then shapes the child's compliance to the adult's request. This often is done with a positive reinforcer, such as access to a book or toy for several minutes between bites or a song. This is paired with verbal praise. It is critical that the reinforcer be something that the child wants.

The SLP/SLT structures the management in such a way as to facilitate skill acquisition. Skills should be advanced in the developmental pattern that is seen in typically developing children. Once 2 to 3 oz. (56.7–85.05 grams) of a new food is being accepted, this food can be added to mealtime and a new food introduced at feeding therapy time. The difficulty and duration of the task should be graded in order for the child to achieve success, which may be as little as 3 trials of one-quarter of a spoon to start. The quantity is gradually increased both for the amount on the spoon and the number of bites taken. A new food may be alternated or mixed with a preferred food. Gradually, the amount of the new food is increased. Acquisition is defined as the learning of the new behavior. In developing fluency, the child practices so that the task can be completed accurately and quickly. Generalization allows the child to complete the learned behavior with various feeders, similar foods, and/or in various settings

In the study by Pressman and Morrison (1988), 19 of the 25 children (76%) treated for dysphagia demonstrated some degree of improvement in one or more areas. In 11 children, the dysphagia improved with position changes. Sixteen had diet adaptation to provide foods managed best at mealtimes. Seven children improved with the introduction of new foods that were different in taste and/or consistency. These foods were introduced at feeding therapy time and then introduced into the regular diet once they were being accepted. Changes in position and modification of the diet produced some degree of improvement in the first week. In 10 cases, oral feedings were concurrent with tube feedings or parenteral hyperalimentation. The goal for these children was to preserve skills and avoid tactile defensiveness that could interfere with returning to oral feeding in the future. Oral feedings were also encouraged to allow the intestinal enzymes to be induced and promote absorption. Ongoing nutritional monitoring is essential due to the fluctuations in health, secondary to infection and decompensation during periods of illness.

Special Medical Considerations

Children with tachypnea, tachycardia, or bradycardia may require 6 small meals per day as the effort of eating tires them out. They also burn significant calories with the effort of eating. Feeding should be limited to 20 to 30 minutes. If they are using oxygen, increasing the liters used during the meal and for 30 minutes after is sometimes helpful. This should be cleared with the pediatric pulmonologist or pediatric cardiologist. For children with oral and/or esophageal *Candida* the recommendation is smooth-textured, nonspicy foods, including purees and puddings. Crunchy foods which could have rough edges such as potato chips should be avoided. Foods with ascorbic acid, that is, orange juice and tomatoes also should be avoided. Cold foods are often best accepted. Mild sauces and gravies help to keep the food moist. In some instances, especially in young babies being nursed or bottle fed, there may be complete refusal of oral feeding. Children who have pain from *Candida* or from other sources may do better if a mild analgesic is given 30 minutes prior to the meal.

Failure to Thrive

For children with failure to thrive the pediatric gastroenterologist takes the lead. Medications such as proton-pump inhibitors (PPI) are often prescribed to treat symptoms of reflux. Often a trial of medication will be given before deciding to undertake invasive evaluation procedures. A motility agent may be given if there are indications of delayed stomach emptying. Caregivers are advised to feed children six small meals per day. Children should remain upright for 30 to 60 minutes after the meal. Proper positioning is critical here as a child who has poor trunk control may actually increase the reflux when seated in an infant or car seat as they slump down, putting extra pressure on the stomach. For young children holding them upright on the adult's shoulder is helpful. Some children do well when lying down with head elevated. Both of these positions allow the trunk to be extended. Children with reflux usually will not tolerate prone positioning. Side lying is sometimes helpful. For decreased appetite, medications such as Periactin® have been used as appetite stimulants with significant success for some children. When nausea and vomiting are present, small frequent meals are recommended. Cold foods and beverages are usually preferred as well as low-fat foods and bland foods. Spicy foods should be avoided.

Developmental Delay

Children with developmental delay will need to be positioned so that their head, neck, and trunk are in a stable position. If the child has to concentrate on remaining upright, the task of eating will be more difficult. If at all possible, children should not be fed in the feeder's lap, with the exception of breast or bottle feeding. The lap is an unstable base and each time that the feeder reaches to refill the spoon, the child's positioning is changed. Adaptive seating is available but costly. The PT and OT on the team can assist in achieving adequate positioning with the use of cushions or cardboard boxes. Some children who have been fed in the feeder's lap may be very resistant to alternative positioning. For these children, preferred foods such as pudding should be offered at a snack time in the seat. As the child improves their tolerance for the seat all feedings should be transferred. Children should be fed a consistency with which they are comfortable. If the child is unable to move beyond purees, the feeder should move from jarred purees to home prepared purees if possible. This will allow the child to become used to the taste of the family's food and will provide increased nutrition and calories. Once this is handled well, the food can begin to be mashed. Foods such as banana or cooked carrots mash well and are good transitional foods. In transitioning to table foods, the children will first do well with crunchy foods. Small pieces can be placed on the lateral tooth surfaces. This sensory input will usually elicit a chewing motion. Crunchy foods that easily melt in the mouth are the safest. Soft to chew foods would be offered next; foods such as rice or pasta are often handled well. Initially, they may need to be finely chopped. There should be some liquid or sauce on these foods to hold them as a cohesive bolus. This process of advancing food types will occur over a prolonged period of time. It is important to remember that there will be periods of regression when the child does not feel well. Some children with severe developmental disabilities may never move beyond pureed or mashed foods. It is important for the foods to have the highest caloric intake possible (see Table 12-4).

Liquids can be introduced by cup. Sippy cups have a valve that reduces leakage but requires the child to suck the same way that they suck from a bottle. The caregiver should remove the valve and assist the child in taking single sips. Gradually the child will advance to sequential sips. Drinking from an open cup can best be taught with thickened liquid. Yogurt can be mixed with milk. Applesauce or other pureed fruit can be mixed with water. The cup should have a wide mouth and be brought into the corners of the child's mouth. A small sip should then be dispensed. The cup is then withdrawn. As they acquire this skill, the children will begin to take sips. Initially they take single sips and eventually sequential sips. Gradually the liquid can be thinned and will be better managed.

Progressive Encephalopathy

Children with progressive encephalopathy usually will need to move backward from table food to soft to chew foods to possibly mashed and pureed foods. As they lose skills, eating becomes increasingly effortful. Some of the children are no longer able to be independent feeders and may require adaptive seating. This regression often is very difficult for families to accept. Children may begin to have difficulty taking thin liquids, indicated by coughing or distress. For these children liquids should be thickened as needed. Many children have been found to prefer drinking as skills further deteriorate.

The caregiver can use a prepared food supplement or can create interesting and high-calorie drinks to give the child. Some children will accept their pureed food in a cup, slightly thinned with liquid, and will drink their meal. For these children treatment may be palliative. It would be inappropriate to work on advancing skills and one should not expect that the child will eat enough to meet their nutritional needs. Instead, the goal is to help the child and caregiver manage intake of food and liquid in as easy a manner as possible. If the child does not wish to eat and/or is unable to meet nutritional needs, then the caregiver and the physician will need to decide on end of life treatment, which may or may not involve tube feeding. When the decision is not to use tube feeding the child should just be allowed to eat or drink as they wish.

Tube Feeding

Some children may require tube feeding for all or part of their nutrition. Tubes are placed either because the child is not able to meet their nutrition orally or because they are not able to swallow safely. A nasogastric tube (NGT) is very uncomfortable for the child both while it is in place and especially when the tube has to be changed. The adhesive used to keep it in place is placed on the face and is an added negative sensory experience. NG tubes are usually only recommended for the short term, up to 3 months. If the child is going to require longer term assistance, a gastrostomy tube (GT) or jejunostomy tube (JT) may be placed. The JT is often used to reduce reflux but may preclude bolus feedings. A fundoplication may also be considered if reflux is a significant problem. Many children continue to get some oral feeding while they are also tube fed. For these children, the tube may be used only to supplement oral feeding. For others, the tube is the primary means of nutrition and the oral feeding may be used to maintain skills, to teach acceptance of food by mouth, or for pleasure. It is best if the tube feeding can be bolus rather than continuous feeding, as this is similar to the way that we eat and may allow for some sense of hunger and satiation. The transition to tube feeding is always very difficult for the family. Nourishing our children by feeding them is the most basic instinct of mothers. Often the child is relieved to not have to work so hard to eat. It is helpful for the family and child if some amount of food or liquid can continue to be offered by mouth. Tube feeding may prolong life but limit the interaction that the child has with others. If the child does not have a reasonable quality of life, the family may choose to not have a tube placed. It is an important ethical question for the family to consider in consultation with members of the team, earlier in the illness. Tube feeding does not fully protect against aspiration. Reflux often is increased in tube-fed individuals, and if the refluxate reaches the oropharynx it can be aspirated.

Oral Hygiene

Oral hygiene is a critical issue for all children and the SLP/SLT, OT, dentist, and dental hygienist should be involved in this. Dentition and condition of the gums are a significant factor. If a child aspirates thin liquids then they are likely aspirating their saliva on a regular basis. All people aspirate saliva while sleeping. The saliva carries bacteria from the mouth. The dysphagia literature as well as the general medical literature demonstrate that bacteria from the mouth, if aspirated, can have a significant affect on respiratory status (Langmore, Terpenning, & Schork, 1998). The bacteria begins to regrow shortly after completing tooth brushing. Meticulous oral hygiene, three times per day, is critical in decreasing respiratory complications. Tooth brushing kills/reduces the bacteria in the mouth, so that the aspirated saliva does not bring bacteria along with it. Those who are tube fed still require meticulous oral hygiene as they continue to aspirate their saliva and the bacteria forms even if the child is not eating by mouth. The child can be positioned with head down while having the teeth brushed, if necessary. Any liquid will roll out of the mouth. The most important factor in tooth brushing is the friction that occurs from the toothbrush on the teeth. Dentifrice is less important and the dentist should be consulted regarding this. Young children and those with developmental disabilities need to have their teeth brushed by an adult in addition to any tooth brushing that they may do independently. Access to a dental member of the pediatric HIV/AIDS team may be indicated.

Broder, Russel, Catapano, and Reisine (2002), however, reported many barriers to obtaining dental care. These included poor interpersonal communication between dental staff and caregiver or child, shame and anger in mothers who were HIV+, family illness that interfered with keeping appointments, and the fact that oral health was a low priority for families. The study indicted that children often demonstrated pain secondary to *Candida albicans*, cytomegalovirus, herpes simplex virus, or oral ulcers. The team members should explore the barriers that the family may be encountering and assist them in helping the child to meet good oral hygiene goals. If there is pain secondary to *Candida* or viruses, medication needs to be used to improve the condition. The type of foods given should be considered if the child is experiencing pain. All foods with acid such as orange juice and tomatoes should be avoided. Cold, soft, and smooth foods such as ice cream and pudding will be tolerated best.

SUMMARY

For many children in developed countries, HIV/AIDS may be a chronic illness. For these children, as well as those who are acutely ill and those in developing countries who are unable to access the multiple medications needed, the ability to meet nutritional needs will have a significant affect on achieving and maintaining health. SLP/SLTs are specially trained to work with children with feeding and swallowing problems. They, along with their colleagues on the feeding team including medicine, nutrition, physical therapy, and occupational therapy can best serve the child in a team approach. It is critical to include the parent or caregiver as a member of the team so that they can provide information and have input as to the types of recommendations that are feasible in their lives.

Acknowledgments. The author wishes to thank James Oleske, M.D., Mary Boland, R.N., and the other members of the pediatric HIV/AIDS program in Newark, NJ that she was privileged to participate in.

REFERENCES

Angami, K., Reddy, S. V., Singh, K. I., Singh, N. B., & Singh, P. I. (2004). Prevalence of HIV infection and AIDS symptomatology in malnourished children—a hospital based study. *Journal of Communication Disorders, 36*(1), 45–52.

Arvedson, J. C., & Brodsky, L. (2002). *Pediatric swallowing and feeding.* Albany, NY: Singular Thomson Publishing Group.

Behardien, N. (2006). *Oral mucosal and facial manifestations of HIV/AIDS in children.* Thesis submitted to the Faculty of Dentistry University of the Western Cape, Cape Peninsula, South Africa. Februrary, 2006.

Broder, H. L., Russel, S., Catapano, P., & Reisine, S. (2002). Perceived barriers and facilitators to dental treatment among female caregivers of children with and without HIV and their health care providers. *Pediatric Dentistry, 24*(4), 301–308.

Butensky, E. A. (2001). The role of nutrition in pediatric HIV/AIDS: A review of micronutrient research. *Journal of Pediatric Nursing, 16*(6), 402–411.

Centers for Disease Control and Prevention. (2006). Reduction in perinatal transmission of HIV infection—United States, 1985–2005. *MMWR Weekly, 55*(21), 592–597.

Clark, H. M. (2005). Clinical decision making and oral motor treatments. *ASHA Leader, 10*(8), 34–38.

Davis-McFarland, E. (2002). Pediatric HIV/AIDS-Issues and strategies for intervention. *ASHA Leader, 7*(4), 10–14.

de Lange, J. (2003). *Feeding of infants with paediatric HIV/AIDS at care centers in Gauteng.* Masters dissertation, Department of Communication Pathology, Faculty of Humanities, University of Pretoria.

Dugger, C. W. (2008, March 9). Rift over AIDS treatment lingers in South Africa. *The New York Times.* Retrieved August 18, 2009, from http://www.nytimes.com

Fowler, M. G., & Newell, M. L. (2002). Breast-feeding and HIV-1 transmission in resource limited settings. *Journal of Acquired Immune Deficiency Syndromes, 30*(2), 230–239.

Gaur, A. H., Dominguez, K. L., Kalish, M. L., Rivera-Hernandez, D., Donohoe, M., Brooks, J. T., et al. (2009). Practice of feeding premasticated food to infants: A potential risk factor for HIV transmission. *Pediatrics, 124*(2), 658–666.

Lal, S., & Chussid, S. (2005). Oral candidiasis in pediatric HIV patients. *NY State Dental Journal, 71*(2), 28–31.

Langmore, S. E. (2001). *Endoscopic evaluation and treatment of swallowing disorders.* New York: Thieme.

Langmore, S. E., Terpenning, M. S., Schork, A., Chen, Y., Murray, J. T., Lopatin, D., et al. (1998). Predictors of aspiration pneumonia: How important is dysphagia? *Dysphagia, 13*, 69–81.

Leder, S. B. (1997). Videofluoroscopic evaluation of aspiration with visual examination of the gag reflex and velar movement. *Dysphagia, 12*, 21–23.

McKirdy, L. S., Sheppard, J. J., Osborne, M. L., & Payne, P. (2008). Transition from tube to oral Feeding in the school setting. *Language, Speech, and Hearing Services in Schools, 39*, 249–260.

McMeans, A. R. (2005). *Nutrition and HIV/AIDS.* HIV curriculum for the health professional. Retrieved February 19, 2008, from www.Baylor aids.org

McNeilly, L. G. (2005). HIV and communication. *Journal of Communication Disorders, 38,* 303–310.

Miller, T. L. (2003). Nutritional aspects of HIV-infected children receiving highly active antiretroviral therapy. *AIDS, 17*(Suppl. 1), S130–S140.

Oleske, J. M., Rothpletz-Puglia, P. M., & Winter, H. (1996). Historical perspectives on the evolution in understanding the importance of nutritional care in pediatric HIV infection. *Journal of Nutrition, 10*(Suppl.), 2616S–2619S.

Pressman, H. (1992). Communication disorders and dysphagia in pediatric AIDS. *ASHA, 34*(1), 45–47.

Pressman, H. (1995). Dysphagia in children with AIDS. In S. Rosenthal, J. J. Sheppard, & M. Lotze (Eds.), *Dysphagia and the child with developmental disabilities* (pp. 133–141). San Diego, CA: Singular Publishing Group.

Pressman, H., & Morrison, S. (1988). Dysphagia in the pediatric AIDS population. *Dysphagia, 2,* 166–169.

Rabie H., Marais, B. J., & Cotton, M. D. (2006). updAIDS in SA Family Practice—Preventing and diagnosing HIV infection in infants and children. *South Africa Family Practice, 48*(6), 35–41.

Rabie, H., Marais, B. J., van Toorn, R., Nel, E. D., & Cotton, M. D. (2007). Common opportunistic infections in HIV infected infants and children. Part 2: Non-respiratory infections. *South Africa Family Practice, 49*(2), 40–45.

Rabie, H., Marais, B. J., van Toorn, R., Nourse, P., New, E. D., Goussard, P. (2007). Important HIV-associated conditions in HIV-infected infants and children. *South Africa Family Practice, 49*(4), 19–23.

Rosenthal, S. R., Sheppard, J. J., & Lotze, M. (Eds.) (1995). *Dysphagia and the child with developmental disabilities.* San Diego, CA: Singular Publishing Group.

Shankar, A. V., Sastry, J., Erande, A., Joshi, A., Suryawanshi, N., Phadke, M. A., & Bollinger, R. C. (2005). Making the choice: The translation of global HIV and infant feeding policy to local practice among mothers in Pune, India. *Journal of Nutrition, 135,* 960–965.

Sheppard, J. (1995). Clinical evaluation and treatment. In S. Rosenthal, J. J. Sheppard, & M. Lotze (Eds.), *Dysphagia and the child with developmental disabilities* (pp. 133–141). San Diego, CA: Singular Publishing Group.

Sheppard, J. J. (2005). The role of oral sensorimotor therapy in the treatment of pediatric dysphagia. *Perspectives on Swallowing and Swallowing Disorders, 14*(2), 6–10.

Sheppard, J. (2008). Using motor learning approaches for treating swallowing and feeding Disorders: A review. *Language, Speech, and Hearing Services in Schools, 39*(2), 227–236.

United Nations International Children's Emergency Fund (UNICEF). (2008). Retrieved February 6, 2008, from http://www.unicef.org/lac/ OMS_PAEDS_Programming_Frameworks_WEB.pdf

U.S. National Institute of Allergy and Infectious Disease. (2004). *HIV infection in infants and children.* Retrieved August 18, 2009, from www.niaid.nih.gov/factsheets/hivchildren.htm

Van Rie, A., Harrington, P. R., Dow, A. & Robertson, K. (2007). Neurologic and neurodevelopmental manifestations of pediatric HIV/AIDS: A global perspective. *European Journal of Paediatric Neurology, 11*(1), 1–9.

CHAPTER 13

Dysphagia and Related Assessment and Management in Adults With HIV/AIDS

Alexandra M. Stipinovich

INTRODUCTION

. . . most deaths from AIDS are deaths of starvation
(Lehmann, 1997, p. 5).

The process of swallowing is complex and depends on coordinated neuromuscular interactions between the central nervous system (CNS), the enteric nervous system, and the muscular components of the swallowing apparatus (Miller, Bieger, & Conklin, 1997). Dysphagia results from abnormalities in deglutition occurring anywhere along the path between the lips and the stomach (Logemann, 1998; Massey, & Shaker, 1997). Thus, any biomechanical or physiologic changes affecting the oral, pharyngeal, laryngeal, or esophageal musculature may influence the integrity of swallowing (Perlman & Christensen, 1997). Swallowing difficulties (dysphagia) and odyno-phagia (painful swallowing) are frequently reported in individuals with HIV/AIDS (e.g., Bladon & Ross, 2007; Halvorsen, Moelleken, &

Kearney, 2003; Mhango-Mkandawire, 1995; Tirwomwe, Rwenyonti, Muwazi, Besigye, & Mboli, 2007), placing them at risk for pneumonia (due to aspiration of food material), malnutrition, dehydration, and reduced quality of life (Logemann, 1998).

HIV/AIDS AND NUTRITIONAL STATUS

Nutritional status and immune status are interrelated and as a result, survival in human immunodeficiency virus (HIV)/acquired immunodeficiency syndrome (AIDS) is directly related to nutritional status. The association between HIV morbidity and malnutrition may be bidirectional. On the one hand, HIV infection affects nutritional status via increased nutrient loss associated with chronic vomiting or diarrhea; malabsorption due to, for example, enteric infections; increased nutrient requirements associated with fever and infections; or decreased oral intake due to anorexia, food aversion, barriers to food access or preparation, swallowing, or feeding difficulties (Chantry & Moye, 2005; Pressman, 1995). On the other hand, malnourishment appears to affect the progression of the disease, causing a wide array of immunodeficiencies (Chantry & Moye, 2005).

Individuals at risk for dysphagia are those who present with conditions (such as dementia, cerebrovascular accidents, toxic or inflammatory encephalopathies, or space-occupying intracranial lesions) that result in the destruction or dysfunction of neural pathways involved in the control of swallowing. Individuals with neoplasms, reflux, or conditions that affect striated or smooth muscle function within the swallowing axis also are at risk for swallowing difficulties (Massey & Shaker, 1997). Owing to the central nervous system and structural manifestations of HIV and AIDS, individuals with HIV/AIDS are at risk for dysphagia and odynophagia with all phases of swallowing potentially affected (Halvorsen et al., 2003).

HIV results in severe immunodeficiencies in both adults and children. However, there are distinct differences between the two populations (Mintz, 1994 in Davis-McFarland, 2000). For example, the disease has a shorter incubation period from the time of infection to the manifestation of symptoms in children. Second, children are less likely to be plagued by opportunistic infections than HIV-infected adults. Furthermore, HIV-infected children exhibit greater

CNS involvement and less peripheral nervous system involvement than adults (Davis-McFarland, 2000). An important implication of these differences is that the management of HIV-associated diseases should differ between children and adults (Layton & Davis-McFarland, 2000).

ADULT DYSPHAGIA ASSOCIATED WITH STRUCTURAL MANIFESTATIONS OF HIV/AIDS

Infection with HIV leads to profound immunosuppression, resulting in the development of a variety of opportunistic infections and neoplasms. The oral cavity is particularly susceptible to infection (Naidoo & Chikte, 2004). Oral lesions are among the first symptoms of HIV infection (Gennaro, Naidoo, & Berthold, 2008; Tirwomwe et al., 2007), and are experienced by 40 to 50% of all individuals with HIV and by approximately 80% of those with AIDS (Coogan, Greenspan, & Challacombe, 2005; Petersen, Bourgeois, Ogawa, Estupinan-Day, & Ndiaye, 2005). Infectious esophagitis is also commonly seen in immunocompromized patients secondary to a variety of infectious diseases (Halvorsen et al., 2003). Oropharyngeal and esophageal disease may be caused by fungal, viral, or bacterial infections (Petersen et al., 2005) and also may occur secondary to antiretroviral therapy (Bladon & Ross, 2007; Coogan et al., 2005). The common structural oropharyngeal and/or esophageal manifestations of HIV/AIDS, which may influence swallowing, are described in Table 13-1.

Oral candidiasis (thrush) is the most common oral opportunistic *fungal* infection in individuals with HIV/AIDS and may be observed in four forms, namely, pseudomembranous candidiasis, erythmatous candidiasis, angular chelitis, and candidiasis of the hyperplastic type (Gennaro et al., 2008). The most common form of oral candidiasis is pseudomembranous candidiasis (Davis-McFarland, 2000), although the four forms of candidiasis may occur concomitantly (Gennaro et al., 2008). Candidiasis may have varying effects on swallowing and oral intake ranging from vomiting, to altered taste sensation and weight loss due to severe pain and discomfort associated with eating (Davis-McFarland, 2000; Lehmann, 1997; Mhango-Mkandawire, 1995). Oral candidiasis is strongly associated with the progression of HIV/AIDS and therefore has prognostic significance (Coogan et al.,

Table 13–1. Common Structural Oropharyngeal and/or Esophageal Manifestations of HIV/AIDS

Lesion	Appearance and Symptomatology
Fungal:	
Candidiasis:	
• Pseudo-membranous candidiasis	• Creamy white patches on any mucosal surface of the oral cavity that are easily rubbed off, leaving bleeding or redness. Lesions may expand into the pharyngeal area and into the esophagus. Associated with complaints of pain, dysphagia, odynophagia, dysgeusia, nausea, decreased salivation.
• Erythematous candidiasis	• Multiple flat, red patches on the palate, dorsum of the tongue, and occasionally on other intraoral mucosal surfaces.
• Angular chelitis	• Red fissures at the corners of the mouth that may bleed upon lip activity
• Hyperplastic	• Deep-rooted lesions. Cannot be rubbed off.
Viral:	
Oral hairy leukoplakia	• White, hyperkeratotic, vertical stripes on lateral border of tongue. Not removable when rubbed. Usually asymptomatic.
Cytomegalovirus	• Discrete ulcers with well demarcated borders. May be associated with gastrointestinal bleeding.
Herpes simplex	• Single or multiple vesicles that rupture and cause painful crusting ulcers. Burning and tingling may precede vesicle formation. Extraoral lesions may be found on the lips and heal within 7–14 days without scarring. Associated with dysphagia and odynophagia.
Herpes zoster	• Presents as small, painful, ulcerated areas of keratinised intraoral tissue in a unilateral pattern that follows the distribution of the trigeminal nerve. Associated with unilateral pain.

Table 13–1. *continued*

Lesion	Appearance and Symptomatology
Neoplasms:	
Kaposi's sarcoma	• Highly vascular tumor. Lesions can be flat or nodular. Occur commonly on the hard palate as one or more reddish, bluish, or purplish lesions with or without ulcerations adjacent to the gingival ridge.
Non-Hodgkin Lymphoma	• Tumoral mass extending from the gingival to the buccal vestibule or palate. Fast-growing. May mimic other oral tumors or infections.
Periodontal disease:	
Linear gingival erythema	• Distinct red band of gingival that bleeds easily.
Necrotizing ulcerative gingivitis	• Destruction of one or more interdental papilla, tissue sloughing, halitosis, and pain.
Necrotizing ulcerative periodontitis	• Rapid destruction of periodontal tissues and supporting bone.
Parotid enlargement	• Parotid glands are diffusely swollen and firm without evidence of inflammation or tenderness. The swelling is chronic with unilateral or bilateral involvement and may be accompanied by xerostomia.

Summarized from: Atkinson & O'Connell, 2005; Davis-McFarland, 2000; Gennaro et al., 2008; Little, 2005; Madariaga & Kalil, 2007; Murray et al., 1997; Naidoo & Chikte, 2004; Navarro et al., 2008; Petersen et al., 2005.

2005). The most common symptom of candidiasis of the esophagus is dysphagia, which is worse for solids than for liquids. Occasionally, patients may complain of heartburn, nausea, or vomiting (Murray, Rao, & Schulze-Delrieu, 1997).

Viral infections manifesting in the oropharynx and/or esophagus include oral hairy leukoplakia, cytomegalovirus (CMV) infections, herpes simplex virus (HSV), and herpes zoster virus (HZV) infections. Oral hairy leukoplakia, characterized by asymptomatic, white, hyperkeratotic, vertical stripes on the lateral border of tongue, is strongly associated with HIV infection in adults (Coogan et al., 2005; Naidoo & Chikte, 2004), whereas esophagitis characterized by one or multiple ulcers and occasional gastrointestinal bleeding (Madariaga & Kalil, 2007) is a common gastrointestinal manifestation of CMV infection. Oropharyngeal and/or esophageal HSV invades the mucosa, resulting in vesicles, which may enlarge, coalesce, and ulcerate. These lesions may also bleed, perforate, or cause tracheo-esophageal fistula (Murray et al., 1997).

Tuberculosis, a common *bacterial* infection in individuals with HIV/AIDS may lead to nonspecific ulceration and narrowing of the esophagus (Perlman, Lu, & Jones, 1997). As with oropharyngeal or esophageal candidiasis, patients with viral or bacterial oropharyngeal and/or esophageal manifestations of HIV/AIDS may report severe dysphagia and/or odynophagia, preventing the ingestion of much needed nutrients.

In addition to the above lesions, individuals with HIV/AIDS may present with ideopathic esophageal ulcer. This large, sometimes penetrating ulcer in the middle to distal oesophagus can occur early in the course of the disease after seroconversion, resulting in complaints of odynophagia (Perlman et al., 1997).

Patients with HIV/AIDS are at an increased risk for the development of *neoplasms* (Aboulafia, 2007). Oral neoplasms are more common in adults than children (Atkinson & O'Connell, 2005) with Kaposi's sarcoma strongly associated with HIV infection in adults (Coogan et al., 2005; Naidoo & Chikte, 2004). HIV-infected persons also are at heightened risk for the development of non-Hodgkin lymphoma (NHL) (Aboulafia, 2007), although dissemination of NHL to the mouth and jaw is not common and occurs in only 0.6% of cases (Kolokotronis et al., 2005 in Navarro, Shibli, Ferrari, d'Avila, & Sposto, 2008). Depending on the size, location, and number of neoplasms, swallowing may be affected.

Linear gingival erythema is a form of *periodontal disease* unique to HIV infection and is characterized by a red band of gingiva that bleeds easily. Other forms of periodontal disease seen less frequently but which are also associated with odynophagia include necrotizing ulcerative gingivitis, and necrotizing ulcerative periodontitis (Atkinson & O'Connell, 2005).

Salivary gland pathology is also associated with HIV/AIDS, although it is more common in children than adults. Enlargement of the salivary glands may be secondary to lymphatic infiltration of the salivary glands, or due to bacterial infection (Atkinson & O'Connell, 2005), and may result in reduced salivary flow (xerostomia). Xerostomia also may be a side effect of medications used in the treatment of HIV/AIDS (Bladon & Ross, 2007; Coogan et al., 2005). Saliva is essential for the maintenance of oral health due to its lubricating, physical cleansing, and antibacterial and antiviral properties (Atkinson & O'Connell, 2005). Lack of moisture and lubrication may contribute to the retention and decomposition of food in the oral cavity, with inflammatory fissuring and fungal overgrowth (Schulze-Delrieu & Miller, 1997). Thus, xerostomia may be associated with *dental decay*, which may be further exacerbated by sweetened medications and immunodeficiency (Atkinson & O'Connell, 2005).

There is a strong relationship between the oropharyngeal and/ or esophageal lesions of HIV/AIDS and immune status (Chidzonga, 1996 in Moynihan, 2005), as discomfort caused by these lesions may have a negative impact on nutrition through difficulty in chewing and drinking (Tirwomwe et al., 2007). Poor nutritional status may compound the impaired immune status associated with HIV/AIDS and in turn, contribute to the more rapid development of oropharyngeal and/or esophageal symptoms (Moynihan, 2005). Furthermore, HIV-positive individuals are required to take medications several times per day, most of which need to be taken orally (Davis-McFarland, 2000). Pain and discomfort caused by oropharyngeal and/or esophageal lesions may prevent or limit the oral intake of such medication. Early diagnosis and treatment of oropharyngeal and/or esophageal lesions is thus essential in HIV-infected persons. As the link between oral health and systemic health is becoming increasingly well understood, the need for improved integration of oral health care, research, and education (Gennaro et al., 2008; Sheiham, 2005) is becoming clear.

ADULT DYSPHAGIA ASSOCIATED WITH NEUROLOGICAL MANIFESTATIONS OF HIV/AIDS

Involvement of the nervous system is recognized as a major cause of disability and death in individuals with HIV/AIDS (Snider et al., 1983 in Scaravilli, Bazille, & Gray, 2007), and may also be associated with neurogenic dysphagia. The CNS manifestations of HIV/AIDS can be subdivided into 2 main groups, namely, those directly attributable to HIV brain infection, and those indirectly related to the effects of HIV disease on the brain, namely, CNS opportunistic infections, malignancies, and cerebrovascular disease (Civitello, 2005). These CNS manifestations may occur in isolation or in combination and may result in a range of swallowing difficulties.

Opportunistic infections of the CNS occur more frequently in adults than in children (Civitello, 2005), and include CMV, progressive multifocal leukoencephalopathy, cryptococcosis, and toxoplasmosis (Scaravilli et al., 2007). Prior to the advent of HAART, as many as 30% of individuals with HIV/AIDS presented with clinical or pathologic evidence of CMV-associated encephalitis. The majority of patients with CMV-associated encephalitis present with disorientation, confusion, seizures, fever, apathy, and focal deficits including cranial nerve dysfunction (Madariaga & Kalil, 2007). Progressive multifocal leukoencephalopathy (PML), a previously rare, viral encephalitis due to a papovavirus (Gray, Scaravilli, & Miller, 2007) is another of the neurologic complications of immune suppression resulting from HIV/AIDS. Clinical symptoms of PML include multifocal neurological signs, cognitive impairment, abnormal mental status, visual loss, and lack of coordination (Giancola et al., 2008). Magnetic resonance images characteristic of PML show multiple lesions, diffuse involvement and atrophy occurring anywhere in the brain, but most commonly in the frontal lobes and parieto-occiptal regions (Post et al., 1999 in Giancola et al. 2008).

CNS cryptococcosis is a further cause of mortality among individuals with HIV/AIDS. Clinical presentation of CNS cryptococcosis varies, with the common symptoms being headache, fever, altered sensorium, and neck stiffness (Lakshmi, Sudah, Teja, & Umabala, 2007). Toxoplasmosis is another common opportunistic infection associated with HIV/AIDS (Signorini et al., 2007). Toxoplasmosis encephalitis (TE) specifically occurs mainly in untreated patients presenting with advanced HIV infection. Although the introduction of HAART has markedly improved the prognosis of individuals presenting with TE, neurological manifestations remain common and include hemiparesis, seizure, and cognitive deficits (Hoffmann et al., 2007). Individuals with HIV/AIDS also are at higher risk of developing CNS herpes virus infection owing to decreased cellular immunity due to HIV infection (Kennedy, 2005 in Martínez et al., 2007). Clinical manifestations of CNS herpes virus infection include fever, headache, vomiting, focal abnormalities, photophobia, coma, seizures, and meningeal symptoms (Martínez et al., 2007).

In addition to the above CNS opportunistic infections, *lymphomas* of the CNS, either primary or secondary, also are common in individuals with HIV/AIDS. These lymphomas are usually high grade, non-Hodgkin and appear as partly necrotic multiple masses in the deep grey nuclei (Scaravilli et al., 2007). Primary CNS lymphoma presents insidiously over weeks to several months with the most common complaints being headache in association with focal neurologic deficits and personality changes (Aboulafia, 2007).

Young adults with advanced HIV infection appear to be at increased risk for *stroke*, either cerebral infarction or intracranial haemorrhage (Modi, Modi, & Mochan, 2006), with prevalence rates ranging between 6 and 34% (e.g., Rabinstein, 2003 in Ortiz, Koch, Romano, Forteza, & Rabinstein, 2007). Mechanisms of ischaemia in the HIV-infected population are variable and appear to include vasculitis and hypercoagulability (unusual in the general stroke population) (Ortiz et al., 2007), as well as opportunistic infections, intracranial neoplasms, and marantic and infective endocarditis. Furthermore, the introduction of antiretroviral medication may increase the risk of stroke in individuals living with HIV/AIDS (Modi et al., 2006; Ortiz et al., 2007; Tipping et al., 2007).

Initially, it was thought that opportunistic diseases such as those described above were the cause of all neurologic complications in HIV/AIDS (Gray et al., 2007; Scaravilli et al., 2007). However, the existence of a specific infection of the CNS has become apparent and is confirmed by viral detection within the nervous system (Shaw et al., 1985 in Scaravilli et al., 2007), together with the finding of multinucleated giant cells (Sharer, Cho, & Epstein, 1985 in Scaravilli et al., 2007). Three types of HIV-induced neuropathologic changes are observed in patients infected by the virus in the absence of any other cause. These changes, which may be variably associated, include HIV encephalitis, HIV leukoencephalopathy, and involvement of the gray matter (Scaravilli et al., 2007).

The above neurologic manifestations of HIV/AIDS place individuals with the disease at risk for neurogenic dysphagia, in which all phases of swallowing are potentially affected. These dysphagic symptoms may occur in combination or in isolation and may co-occur with the structural oropharyngeal and/or esophageal manifestations described earlier. The symptoms and complications arising from neurogenic dysphagia are due primarily to sensorimotor dysfunction of the oral and pharyngeal phases of swallowing (Buchholz & Robbins, 1997). Dysphagia resulting from neurogenic causes may present with obvious symptoms such as difficulty achieving voluntary mouth opening; problems with chewing; reduced sensitivity to certain tastes, textures, and temperatures; difficulty initiating swallowing; nasal regurgitation; drooling; abnormal responses to oral and/or pharyngeal residue; abnormal oral reflexes (e.g., a hyperactive gag reflex, tongue thrusting, or tonic bite reflex); and coughing and choking during eating (Buchholz & Robbins, 1997; Logemann, 1998). However, not all forms of neurogenic dysphagia present with obvious symptoms. Individuals with neurologic disorders may present with reduced sensitivity to aspiration owing to impaired sensory feedback regarding the position of food in the vocal tract and entry of food into the airway (Johnson, 1997; Logemann, 1998), resulting in silent aspiration (Buchholz & Robbins, 1997). Patient characteristics, which should alert the clinician to the possible presence of neurogenic dysphagia and associated aspiration risk, are listed in Table 13-2.

Chronic HIV exposure, associated with sizable neuronal loss, may induce HIV-associated dementia (Navia, Jordan, & Price, 1986 in Bhaskaran et al., 2008; Scaravilli et al., 2007). This specific progressive cognitive/motor syndrome is observed in approximately 20% of patients with AIDS (Scaravilli et al., 2007). Individuals with dementia (including HIV-associated dementia) may not fully understand their swallowing difficulty, and may develop an agnosia for food (Buchholz & Robbins, 1997; Logemann, 1998). As the dementia progresses, an apraxia for swallowing and feeding may develop (Logemann, 1998). In addition, the cognitive deterioration resulting from dementia contributes to eventual disability in independent eating, posing an increased burden on caregivers (Buchholz & Robbins, 1997).

Although the coordination of pharyngeal and esophageal muscle activity in swallowing may continue normally in individuals with extensive neurological damage to the cortex (Miller et al., 1997), neurologic deficits may cause incoordination between breathing and swallowing (Curtis & Langmore, 1997). In addition, clearance of the lungs of fluids depends primarily on lymphatics. Deficiencies in

Table 13-2. Patient Indicators to the Possible Presence of Neurogenic Dysphagia and Aspiration Risk

- Coma
- Mechanical ventilation/tracheostomy tube/intubation
- Respiratory distress
- Recurrent chest infections
- Temperature spikes
- Chest pain
- Weight loss
- Cognitive impairment/disorientation/confusion/changed mental status
- Drowsiness/reduced attention
- Inability to follow commands/answer questions
- Primitive oral reflexes
- Drooling
- Food agnosia
- Avoidance of specific food consistencies
- Poor mouth opening
- Reduced sensitivity to tastes, textures and temperatures
- Leakage/spillage of fluid or food from the mouth
- Difficulty chewing
- Poor bolus formation
- Pooling of food in anterior/lateral sulcus
- Delayed initiation of swallow
- Nasal regurgitation
- Coughing before, during or after swallowing
- Wet, gurgly vocal quality
- Multiple swallowing/infrequent swallowing
- Increased time taken to complete a meal

Summarized from: Buchholz & Robbins, 1997; Goodrich & Walker, 1997; Logemann, 1998; Pressman, 1995; Schulze-Delrieu, 1997.

lymphocyte function, as typified by infection with HIV, lead to pulmonary infection with a variety of opportunistic pathogens (Murray et al., 1984 in Curtis & Langmore, 1997). Thus, the immune system plays an important role in preventing lung infection (Curtis & Langmore, 1997). Individuals with CNS involvement are also at risk for increased fatigue, which in turn, may affect swallowing function (Logemann, 1998) and nutritional intake.

MULTIDISCIPLINARY APPROACH

Dysphagia in adults with HIV/AIDS may have multiple etiologies and may be present in all phases of swallowing. Accurate diagnosis and management of the swallowing and feeding difficulties in adults with HIV/AIDS is vital to prevent further respiratory complications, malnutrition, and dehydration. Consequently, the evaluation and management of dysphagia requires a multidisciplinary approach, wherein a team of different specialists communicate and collaborate (Massey & Shaker, 1997). Such a team should include a speech-language pathologist/therapist (SLP/T), physician, nursing staff, dietician, dentist, otolaryngologist, gastroenterologist, neurologist, occupational therapist, physiotherapist, pharmacist, radiologist, as well as the patient and his or her family and caregivers (Baser, 2006; Carrau, 2006; Leonard, 1997; Padda & Young, 2006b).

The SLP/T should combine the findings of the different team members and prioritize their recommendations based on where the patient is going to be housed after discharge from the hospital, the need for additional assessments, the need for therapy techniques that will benefit the patient, and the need for medication and surgery (Leonard, 1997; Logemann, 1998). Once the treatment plan has been finalized, the team should communicate it (verbally and in writing) to the patient, the family, and to the relevant caregivers. The patient, family, and caregivers should meet with members of the team on a regular basis to discuss the treatment plan. Thus, treatment planning should be an ongoing process during which risks, benefits, patient wishes, and underlying physiology are weighed in the selection of appropriate treatment strategies (Huckabee & Pelletier, 1999).

ASSESSMENT OF ADULT SWALLOWING AND FEEDING DIFFICULTIES ASSOCIATED WITH HIV/AIDS

Optimal dysphagia assessment is described in numerous texts (e.g., Goodrich & Walker, 1997; Hardy, 1999; Logemann, 1998; McKenzie, 1997; Murray & Carrau, 2001; Schulze-Delrieu & Miller, 1997) in which various forms and guidelines for this purpose are provided. In this text, the specific considerations that need to be taken into account in the clinical and instrumental assessment of the swallowing and feeding abilities of adults with HIV/AIDS are addressed.

Clinical Assessment of Adult Swallowing and Feeding Disorders Associated With HIV/AIDS

A clinical swallow evaluation is indicated in any patient presenting with weight loss, nutrition failure, or a pulmonary history suggestive of aspiration (Goodrich & Walker, 1997). As with all clinical swallowing and feeding evaluations, the clinical assessment of the swallowing and feeding abilities of the adult with HIV/AIDS aims to obtain information pertaining to his or her medical, swallowing, and feeding history and status; social history; oropharyngeal anatomy and motor functioning; respiratory functioning; and cognitive functioning and awareness of his or her swallowing difficulty (Goodrich & Walker, 1997; Logemann, 1998). A summary of the areas to be included in the clinical assessment of the swallowing and feeding difficulties associated with HIV/AIDS is provided in Table 13–3.

Medical History

Information pertaining to the medical history of the adult with HIV/AIDS may be taken from the medical records as well as from reports from the caregiver where available. Should dysphagia occur against a background of multiple medical problems and complications, as is the case in individuals with HIV/AIDS, systematic enquiry into the possible contributing historical and physical factors is required (Schulze-Delrieu & Miller, 1997). The clinician should determine whether there is a history of pulmonary and respiratory complications, including repeated upper respiratory infections,

Table 13–3. Areas Included in the Clinical Assessment of the Swallowing and Feeding Difficulties Associated with HIV/AIDS

• Medical history and status:
  – medical diagnosis
  – pulmonary and respiratory history
  – medications taken
  – nutritional status (including daily food intake)
 	
• Feeding and swallowing history:
  – nature and onset of feeding difficulties
  – methods of nutrition
  – caregiver and patient reports of swallowing and feeding difficulties
  – compensatory behaviours
 	
• Social history:
  – primary caregiver (relationship between patient and caregiver)
  – access to support
  – access to food preparation facilities
  – knowledge of food hygiene and safety
  – home and feeding environment
  – cultural and ethnic background
	• General observations of patient, e.g.:
	  – posture
	  – alertness and cognitive ability
	  – cooperation
	  – ability to follow commands
	  – tracheostomy tube and status
	  – respiratory rate
	  – ability to handle secretions
	  – vocal quality
	
	• Examination of oral anatomy
	
	• Examination of oral-motor control, e.g.:
	  – rate, range and accuracy of movement
	  – presence of abnormal oral reflexes
	
	• Feeding and swallowing evaluation:
	  – reaction to food placed in oral cavity
	  – oral movements
	  – changes in breathing
	  – handling of secretions
	  – complaints of pain during swallowing
	  – observation of caregiver feeding patient
	  – duration of meal
	  – amount of oral intake

Summarized from: Buchholz & Robbins, 1997; Chantry & Moye, 2005; Gennaro et al., 2008; Goodrich & Walker, 1997; Logemann, 1998; Mhango-Mkandawire, 1995; Schulze-Delrieu & Miller, 1997; Sheppard, 1995; Swigert, 1998; White et al., 1995.

pneumonia, and congestion as these may be symptomatic of swallowing difficulties. Information pertaining to the medications taken by the adult with HIV/AIDS should be obtained as certain medications used in the treatment of HIV and related opportunistic infections, may result in dysgeusia (changes in the taste of food), xerostomia, and increased reflux (Mhango-Mkandawire, 1995). Furthermore, medications may result in decreased arousal and suppressed brainstem function, myopathy, compromised neuromuscular transmission, suppression of the laryngeal cough reflex, movement disorders, and decreased or increased salivation (Buchholz & Robbins, 1997), all of which may affect swallowing.

Of particular relevance to the medical status of the adult with HIV/AIDS is information pertaining to his or her nutritional status. This nutritional assessment requires a team approach and entails examination of medical records, physical examination of the adult with HIV/AIDS, and laboratory studies investigating protein status and blood count (Chantry & Moye, 2005; White, Mhango-Mkandawire, & Rosenthal, 1995). Lachenmeyer (1995) recommends that the primary caregiver be asked to keep a daily food intake diary in which information pertaining to the time of food intake, the behaviors associated with intake, and the quantity of intake be recorded. Reasons for decreased intake or feeding problems need to be explored (Chantry & Moye, 2005). Certain questions pertaining to the adult's nutrition must be addressed, including whether or not the oral intake meets the daily requirements, whether or not alternative means of providing adequate nutrition are required, whether or not the number of daily meals and snacks needs to be increased, whether or not the amount of food offered each time should be modified, and whether or not food supplements are required (McNeilly, 2000).

Feeding and Swallowing History

Information pertaining to the nature of the onset of feeding and swallowing difficulties in the individual with HIV/AIDS, as well as the temporal course of symptoms is significant. For example, dysphagic symptoms associated with stroke usually present abruptly, whereas those associated with dementia may have a gradual onset (Buchholz & Robbins, 1997). Information pertaining to the different methods of nutrition also should be obtained, as individuals infected with HIV are likely to undergo forms of nonoral feeding to ensure adequate nutritional intake and to prevent malnutrition. Numerous complaints and symptoms reported by adults with HIV/AIDS themselves and/or their caregivers should alert the professional to the presence of swallowing and feeding difficulties. These include reports of excessive drooling, coughing on solids or liquids, slow feeding, abnormal chewing and bolus formation, gagging on solid foods, and hypersensitivity and oral defensiveness, unexplained food refusal, and complaints of pain when eating (Logemann, 1998; Pressman, 1995).

In addition to the above, it is essential that the clinician enquire specifically about behaviors that the adult with HIV/AIDS may have adopted to compensate for possible neurogenic dysphagia. For example, those who experience a gradual onset of neurogenic dysphagia may adapt by eliminating difficult-to-swallow foods or by developing habits such as cutting food into smaller pieces, chewing more thoroughly, washing down solids with liquids, double swallowing, throat clearing, or taking longer to complete meals (Buchholz & Robbins, 1997; Goodrich and Walker, 1997; Schulze-Delrieu & Miller, 1997).

Social History

Individuals with HIV/AIDS (particularly those in the late stages of the disease) are often dependent on caregivers for assistance in daily activities such as food preparation and feeding. For this reason, information pertaining to who the primary caregiver is, the relationship between the individual with HIV/AIDS and caregiver, access to support and food preparation facilities, food safety (knowledge and facilities to provide safe food preparation and storage), and the home and feeding environment are required (Goodrich & Walker, 1997). Furthermore, caregivers are often trained to assist in the implementation of, for example, diet modifications or postural changes to facilitate safe oral feeding. Families or caregivers living in rural areas may need to travel some distance to access services and may not have the resources to attend training appointments as scheduled. Thus, information pertaining to the availability of caregivers for training must be obtained as part of the assessment procedure to facilitate the later compilation of an effective management plan. Knowledge of the cultural and ethnic background of the family also should be obtained as this may influence future decisions made regarding food choices to facilitate oral feeding.

General Observations of the Adult with HIV/AIDS

Several general observations of the individual with HIV/AIDS can provide the clinician with helpful cues regarding the nature of the swallowing difficulty. For example, postural abnormalities may be symptomatic of weakness or paralysis. The presence of drooling also may be indicative of facial weakness, or a sign of reduced oral awareness. The inability to answer questions or follow commands, reduced general levels of awareness, impaired cooperation, and increased potential for fatigue (Goodrich & Walker, 1997; Logemann, 1998) may be indicative of neurologic manifestations of HIV/AIDS.

In addition to the above, the clinician should observe the respiratory rate of the adult with HIV/AIDS at rest, the timing of saliva swallows in relation to the phases of the respiratory cycle, the timing of any coughing in relation to respiration, and his or her rest breathing pattern (oral or nasal) (Logemann, 1998), as swallowing and breathing are reciprocal functions. Vocal quality and duration of phonation should be examined as neurologic problems resulting in swallowing difficulties also may cause dysphonia and dysarthria (Schulze-Delrieu & Miller, 1997). In addition, control of the motor subsystems observed in voice is evidence of the underlying sensory-motor competency available for swallow (Sheppard, 1995). Laryngeal agility should be assessed by having the adult with HIV/AIDS slide up and down his or her pitch range as this provides information regarding laryngeal elevation (Goodrich & Walker, 1997).

Examination of Oral Anatomy

Routine examination of the oral anatomy is an essential part of the general care of individuals with HIV/AIDS. As oral lesions are pathognomic of HIV/AIDS related opportunistic infections, the oral examination assists in identifying disease, promoting health, and determining overall health status (Gennaro et al., 2008). The oral examination may be performed by numerous members of the multidisciplinary team, and need not be performed only as part of the swallowing evaluation. Furthermore, although certain oral lesions, for example, Kaposi's sarcoma, need to be identified medically, oral lesions usually can be identified easily by appearance during an oral screening (Gennaro et al., 2008).

Gennaro et al. (2008) provide a detailed description of how to perform a quick, inexpensive, noninvasive oral screening and advocate that an examination of the extra-oral structures be performed prior to the examination of the intra-oral structures. Any skin changes and swellings, including red or white discoloration, ulcers, and lumps should be noted. The neck and submental/submandibular area should be palpated to determine the condition of lymph nodes, and the presence of scars or tumors as enlargement of cervical lymph nodes may be a sign of malignant lesion in the pharynx or a manifestation of lymphoma. Furthermore, the clinician should be on the alert for symptoms of dehydration, which include temporal wasting, sunken eyeballs, decreased skin tugor, and elevated temperature (Schulze-Delrieu & Miller, 1997).

The intraoral examination should include examination of lip texture and color; the anterior upper and lower labial mucosa, sulcus, and alveolus; the commissure, buccal mucosa, and lower and upper sulcus; hard and soft palate; the lower right and left lingual alveolar mucosa; the floor of the mouth; the anterior lower lingual alveolar mucosa; and the dorsum of the tongue at rest (Gennaro et al., 2008) for the presence of any oral lesions. The clinician should again take note of symptoms of dehydration, which include dry mucous membranes and shriveling of the tongue (Schulze-Delrieu & Miller, 1997). In addition to the above, the status of dentition and oral secretions should be assessed (Logemann, 1998). When combined with gingivitis and poor oral hygiene, halitosis may become pronounced (Schulze-Delrieu & Miller, 1997).

Oral-Motor Control Examination

Individuals with neurologic involvement may show impaired oral-motor control. For this reason, the oral-motor control examination should include evaluation of the range, rate, and accuracy of movement of the structures of the oral cavity (Logemann, 1998). Neuromuscular features, including the presence of joint stiffness, muscle weakness, and involuntary movements should be examined as these are indicative of neurologic involvement. The individual's oral postural control (alignment of oral structures at rest), voluntary movement of oral structures, oral secretions, and control thereof also should be examined (Sheppard, 1995). The clinician should note the presence of abnormal oral reflexes, for example, hyperactive gag, tongue thrusting, or tonic bite reflex (Logemann, 1998), as these also may be suggestive of neurologic problems (Goodrich & Walker, 1997). Sensation of the oral cavity should also be assessed, as reduced sensitivity to tastes, textures, and temperature may be associated with neurogenic dysphagia (Goodrich & Walker, 1997; Logemann, 1998).

Feeding and Swallowing Evaluation

Once the above information has been obtained, the swallowing therapist (usually the SLP/T) should determine the risks associated with having the individual with HIV/AIDS attempt trial swallows. Individuals with HIV/AIDS who are at risk for aspiration and who should not be fed orally include those with a weak voluntary cough, who are not alert and who cannot follow directions, who are having seizures, whose respiratory rate is so high it does not allow for normal cessation of breathing during swallowing, and those who are suspected of having a pharyngeal swallowing disorder (Logemann, 1998; Schulze-Delrieu & Miller, 1997). Such individuals should be placed on nonoral feeding until such time that trial swallows are considered safe.

Individuals with HIV/AIDS who are feeding orally should be given the opportunity to practice dry swallows prior to commencement of trial swallows with food. Logemann (1998) advocates that the clinician use approximately one-third of a teaspoon for liquid and paste consistencies, as these small volumes are unlikely to block a patient's airway. As with any clinical evaluation of swallowing function, the clinician should observe the reaction of the adult with HIV/AIDS to food placed in the oral cavity. The clinician should take note of food rejection, hypersensitivity to certain food textures or tastes, or excessive gagging (Logemann, 1998) as these may indicate the presence of neurogenic dysphagia or discomfort with eating associated with odynophagia. Oral movements in food manipulation, including the presence of abnormal oral reflexes, for example, jaw thrusting, tongue thrusting, tonic bite reflex, lip retraction, tongue retraction, and nasal regurgitation (all possible indications of neurologic problems), should be noted. The clinician should be on the alert for any coughing or changes in breathing during a meal (Logemann, 1998), as well as changes in and handling of secretions during a meal. Excessive drooling, for example, may be an indication of poor labial seal, or an indication of poor pharyngeal clearance and associated pooling of secretions in the hypopharynx (Schulze-Delrieu & Miller, 1997).

If the adult is attached to any monitors, changes in heart rate, respiratory rate, or oxygen saturation during feeding should be observed. Furthermore, the adult should be asked to describe feelings and symptoms during the clinical swallowing evaluation (Schulze-Delrieu & Miller, 1997). Complaints of pain during swallowing generally indicate disruption of mucosal integrity due to an infectious or inflammatory condition in the esophageal or oral mucosa (Gennaro et al., 2008; Schulze-Delrieu & Miller, 1997). This disruption may be produced by infections (e.g., candidiasis, cytomegalovirus, or herpes infections of the oropharynx and esophagus) (Schulze-Delrieu & Miller, 1997), which are frequently associated with HIV infection and which result in reduced oral intake owing to pain and discomfort during feeding.

Sheppard (1995) and Swigert (1998) advocate that observations of the caregiver offering different food consistencies with utensils used in daily feeding should be made. The feeding position of the individual with HIV/AIDS should be noted, including whether or not he or she is able to sit unsupported. Furthermore, the dependent and self-feeding behaviors of the adult must be evaluated. In addition to the above, the duration of the meal and amount of intake should be assessed (Logemann, 1998). Owing to the influence of fatigue on the swallowing abilities of individuals with dysphagia of neurologic etiology, Logemann (1998) recommends that the swallowing abilities of adults with neurogenic dysphagia be observed throughout the day.

Once the clinical swallow and feeding evaluation has been performed, the clinician must decide whether further instrumental assessment is required. Instrumental assessment of swallowing is strongly advocated in individuals with HIV/AIDS as diffuse pulmonary disease, often seen in this population, may mask the presence of aspiration pneumonia (Halvorsen et al., 2003). Furthermore, errors in the identification of aspiration have been found to range from 30 to 40% of patients in rehabilitation centres who were evaluated for dysphagia by clinical examination only (Perlman et al., 1997). In addition, according to Logemann (1998), 50 to 60% of patients who aspirate do not cough. This is particularly true of neurologic patients, whose pharyngeal and/or laryngeal sensitivity may be reduced (Aviv et al., 1996 in Logemann, 1998). In general, any patient who is suspected of aspirating, and whose swallowing disorder is suspected to be of pharyngeal origin, should be referred for an instrumental assessment procedure to define the abnormalities causing the swallowing difficulty and to assist in the identification of treatment strategies to promote safe oral feeding (Logemann, 1998).

Instrumental Assessment of Adult Swallowing and Feeding Disorders Associated With HIV/AIDS

The diagnostic procedure that currently provides the most information in a single evaluation session is the videofluorographic study known as the modified barium swallow (Logemann, 1998). As a result, videofluoroscopic examination of oropharyngeal function has become the gold standard for assessing the integrity of the oral and pharyngeal stages of the swallow (Perlman et al., 1997). Video-fluoroscopic studies provide information on bolus transit times, motility problems, and amount and etiology of aspiration (Logemann, 1998) and guide members of the multidisciplinary team in management decisions pertaining to swallowing therapy and enteral tube feeding (Buchholz & Robbins, 1997).

The focus of videofluoroscopy is primarily on the oral cavity, pharynx, and larynx (McKenzie, 1997). However, because abnormalities in the esophagus (such as the esophageal lesions associated with HIV/AIDS) may cause dysphagia or odynophagia, this organ should be evaluated along with the pharynx (Rosenquist, 1997). In addition, videofluoroscopy is usually not sufficiently sensitive to identify oropharyngeal or esophageal lesions such as candidiasis (Winter & Moye, 2005). As a result, endoscopic tests may be more helpful in the evaluation of the oropharyngeal and esophageal anatomy for lesions associated with HIV/AIDS.

Videoendoscopy, also known as flexible fiberoptic examination of swallowing (FEES), entails the insertion of a flexible scope, usually by the otolaryngologist, into the nose to the level of the soft palate or below (Logemann, 1998) and provides anatomic information regarding the oral cavity, pharynx, and larynx (Murray & Carrau, 2006). Esophagoscopy, on the other hand, is performed as part of standard upper gastrointestinal (GI) endoscopy as a diagnostic procedure for many esophageal disorders (Padda & Young, 2006a). During this procedure the endoscope is advanced through the upper esophageal sphincter with the entire length of the esophagus in direct view of the endoscope (Padda & Young, 2006a). Video-endoscopy and esophagoscopy provide the SLP/T with valuable anatomic information which assists in the understanding of swallowing difficulties experienced by individuals with HIV/AIDS.

Videoendoscopy is not without its own set of disadvantages, however. First, the oral stage of swallowing cannot be visualized by means of endoscopy. Second, because treatment for oropharyngeal swallow disorders is directed largely at the motor activity during the swallow, videoendoscopy makes it difficult to define the exact nature of the patient's physiologic disorder and the effectiveness of treatment strategies (Logemann, 1998). Finally, adults with cognitive disorders (such as those with HIV-associated dementia) or those who are agitated, are poor candidates for the procedure (Logemann, 1998). Thus, no one single instrumental procedure is able to provide all the required information in the assessment of the complex swallowing difficulties associated with HIV/AIDS. The clinician therefore needs to be knowledgeable regarding the different instrumental procedures available for the evaluation of swallowing, and select, in consultation with the relevant members of the multidisciplinary team, the procedure (or combination of procedures) that will best answer the questions arising from the clinical evaluation of the individual with HIV/AIDS.

Upon completion of the clinical and instrumental assessments of the swallowing and feeding difficulties of the adult with HIV/AIDS, the clinician should have sufficient information regarding the interactions between the many possible medical problems contributing to the dysphagia to develop an appropriate management plan.

Management of Adults with Swallowing and Feeding Difficulties Associated With HIV/AIDS

The life-threatening nature of dysphagia (particularly in the HIV/AIDS population) necessitates a high quality of service provision and a team approach. Owing to the changing states of wellness associated with individuals with HIV/AIDS, regular assessments of the patient's current health status are required (McNeilly, 2000). The establishment and maintenance of adequate nutrition is the primary issue in the management of individuals with HIV/AIDS owing to the role of nutrition in immune function in HIV/AIDS (Gennora et al., 2008; Pressman, 1995; White et al., 1995). A medical approach, entailing the establishment of baselines and regular follow-up examinations of the patient's nutrition and weight gain is thus required initially (Layton & Scott, 2000).

Mhango-Mkandawire (1995) provides suggestions for the sequence of nutritional management in HIV/AIDS. First, all ways to improve nutritional intake and to use foods readily available in the home should be exhausted. Second, high calorie, high protein foods and nutritional supplements to boost total caloric intake should be used. Third, all feedings must be tailored to secondary disease manifestations (e.g., lactose intolerance, thrush, and malabsorption). Finally, nonoral feeding must be considered if oral intake is not maintained. Table 13-4 provides an overview of the management techniques used in the management of odynophagia and dysphagia associated with HIV/AIDS in adults.

Promoting Increased Oral Intake via the Relief of Odynophagia and Xerostomia

Medical management of the oropharyngeal and/or esophageal manifestations of HIV/AIDS is essential. The medical management of candidiasis may be systemic (including antifungal medications such as fluconazole or itraconazole), or topical, depending on patient preference and adherence to the treatment regimen (Atkinson & O'Connell, 2005; Gennaro et al., 2008). The healing time of viral manifestations (e.g., oral hairy leukoplakia, CMV, HSV, and HZV) may be shortened by antiviral drugs, including azidothymidine, ganciclovir, or foscamnet (Madriaga & Kalil, 2007). Chemotherapy and surgery, depending on the number, size, and location of the lesions, may be used in the medical management of neoplasms (Gennaro et al., 2008). Antibacterial mouth rinses and antibiotics may be utilized in the management of periodontal disease (Atkinson & O'Connell, 2005). Rapid symptomatic relief to the pain caused by oral and esophageal lesions also may be provided by topical anaesthetics, which are usually administered before meals (Atkinson & O'Connell, 2005; Chantry & Moye, 2005; Lehmann, 1997; Pressman, 1995).

In addition to the pharmacologic and medical management of the numerous oropharyngeal and esophageal manifestations of

Table 13–4. Management of Odynophagia and Dysphagia in Adults with HIV/AIDS

Odynophagia:
- Medical and pharmacological management
- Promotion of good oral hygiene
  - regular visits to the dentist
  - brushing of teeth, gums, and tongue after every meal
  - frequent intake of water
  - limited intake of dietary sugars and sweetened liquids
  - limited use of tobacco
- Diet modifications
  - food texture and consistency: soft foods
  - food tastes: avoid acidic/spicy food
  - food temperature: foods served at room temperature/chilled
- Modification in food administration
  - Utensils, e.g., straws
  - placement and chewing of food on one side of mouth

Dysphagia:
- Compensatory techniques
  - postural techniques
  - bolus control techniques
  - increasing oral sensory awareness
  - diet modifications
- Rehabilitative techniques
  - face, mouth, and tongue exercises

Summarized from: Atkinson & O'Connell, 2005; Bladon & Ross, 2007; Chantry & Moye, 2005; Gennaro et al., 2008; Lehmann, 1997; McNeilly, 2000; Mhango-Mkandawire, 1995; Petersen et al., 2005; Tirwomwe et al., 2007.

HIV/AIDS, professionals such as SLP/Ts, dentists and nurses play a fundamental role in optimizing oral care in individuals with HIV/AIDS by educating and training them and their caregivers regarding the importance of good oral hygiene (Atkinson & O'Connell, 2005; Gennora et al., 2008). Regular referral of individuals with oropharyngeal lesions to a dentist for examination of the soft tissues and teeth (Lehmann, 1997) and frequent dental cleanings in the management of periodontal disease, is recommended (Atkinson & O'Connell, 2005). The gums, teeth, and tongue should be brushed after every meal, particularly as xerostomia (associated with salivary gland pathology and/or antiretroviral medication) can lead to dental decay and caries (Atkinson & O'Connell, 2005). As tooth brushing may be associated with discomfort (Tirwomwe et al., 2007), sore gums should be brushed with a soft brush. Lehmann (1997) suggests soaking a toothbrush in hot water before use to assist in softening the bristles and recommends that commercial mouthwashes be avoided if they cause pain or discomfort.

Optimal oral hygiene may be further facilitated by replacing toothbrushes on a monthly basis and by keeping the toothbrush clean by storing it with its head submerged in alcohol (which should be rinsed off before use) (Lehmann, 1997). The frequent intake of water to facilitate clearance of the oral cavity and to provide symptomatic relief to xerostomia should be encouraged (Atkinson & O'Connell, 2005; Gennora et al., 2008). The symptomatic relief of xerostomia may also be provided by the use of sugar-free gums or mints (Tougher-Decker, 2005 in Gennora et al., 2008).

Good oral hygiene may further be ensured and dental decay limited by controlling the intake of dietary sugars, as well as the frequency of intake of viscous sugars and sweetened liquids (Atkinson & O'Connell, 2005), all of which may leave a sugar residue in the mouth upon which candidiasis may feed (Lehmann, 1997). Highly sweetened medications should be administered by syringe to bypass the teeth and minimize the time in the oral cavity. Rinsing with saline solution (one teaspoon of salt to a glass of water, followed by subsequent rinse with fresh, plain water) will help maintain mouth freshness (Lehmann, 1997). Furthermore, professionals need to caution adults with HIV/AIDS against the use of tobacco as this has been estimated to cause over 90% of cancers in the oral cavity, and also is associated with aggravated periodontal breakdown, poorer standards of oral hygiene and thus premature tooth loss (Petersen et al., 2005).

Modifications in diet to accommodate pain and discomfort and to assist in easier chewing and swallowing also will provide relief and facilitate greater nutritional intake. Each of the feeding alterations or alternatives, however, should be carefully planned and discussed with the family and caregivers, taking the cultural and ethnic background of the family into account when assisting with food choices (Chantry & Moye, 2005; McNeilly, 2000).

As far as food texture and consistency are concerned, Lehmann (1997) recommends that foods such as mashed potato, cream or egg-drop soups, yogurt, macaroni and cheese, scrambled eggs, oatmeal, cottage cheese, soft tuna, or chicken be used as these are examples of nutritious foods that do not require much mechanical chewing. Lehmann (1997) further recommends that vegetables be cooked until soft, that solids be softened with blenders, and that liquid be added to pureed foods so that they may be drunk from a cup or sipped through a straw.

In addition to the above modifications to food texture, foods that are acidic or spicy should be avoided as these may exacerbate and irritate oropharyngeal and/or esophageal lesions, causing discomfort (Chantry & Moye, 2005; McNeilly, 2000; Mhango-Mkandawire, 1995; Tirwomwe et al., 2007). Thus, acidic fruits such as citrus, pineapple, or tomato should be avoided and spices such as pepper and curry replaced with basil or thyme (Lehmann, 1997). As far as temperature is concerned, foods presented at room temperature or slightly chilled generally are more comfortable to eat than hot foods. In addition, cold food may assist in numbing the pain. Beverages such as milk or juices may be iced. Purees of savoury foods may be chilled or frozen into popsicles, or blended to the consistency of soft ice cream. In the case of xerostomia, gravy, broth, or cream sauces may be added to foods for moisture or frequent sips of a beverage may be taken while eating (Lehmann, 1997).

Modifications in the use of feeding utensils may also provide symptomatic relief. For example, liquids may be taken in by means of a straw to bypass lesions (Chantry & Moye, 2005). In addition, patients with odynophagia have been found to compensate by chewing food on one side of the mouth to avoid food coming into contact with oral lesions (Bladon & Ross, 2007).

Management of Adult Neurogenic Dysphagia Associated With HIV/AIDS

The management of neurogenic dysphagia associated with HIV/AIDS should follow the same management principles that guide the general management of dysphagia. First, the patient's nutrition and hydration must never be jeopardized. Patient safety is a further priority and aspiration must be avoided or kept to a minimum (Logemann, 1998). A team approach to the management of dysphagia should be followed, wherein different specialities communicate and collaborate (Massey & Shaker, 1997).

The management of neurogenic dysphagia in individuals with HIV/AIDS may involve progressively changing strategies as the swallowing difficulties associated with this population are varied and complex and may increase with the progression of the disease (Bladon & Ross, 2007). Decisions regarding the selection of the therapy regimen are based on the patient's anatomy and physiology in the context of his or her medical status, prognosis, and behavioral or cognitive abilities (Logemann, 1998; McNeilly, 2000), and need to be reviewed over time (Bladon & Ross, 2007).

Compensatory techniques, aimed at controlling the flow of food without necessarily changing the patient's physiology of swallow (Logemann, 1998), usually are most appropriate in the management of neurogenic dysphagia associated with HIV/AIDS. As compensatory techniques are largely under the control of the caregiver or clinician, they may be used with patients of all cognitive levels (Logemann, 1998), including patients with cognitive difficulties associated with the primary and secondary CNS manifestations of HIV/AIDS. Furthermore, compensatory techniques involve less muscle effort than swallow exercises and manoeuvres do (Logemann, 1998), and therefore are less likely to fatigue the individual with HIV/AIDS. However, compensatory techniques must be used with every swallow to maintain safety for oral feeding (Huckabee & Pelletier, 1999). Patient and caregiver education and training are thus essential. Caregivers also should be encouraged to keep ongoing records of the patient's nutritional intake.

Compensatory techniques considered appropriate in the management of dysphagia associated with HIV/AIDS involve postural changes, bolus control techniques, increasing oral sensory awareness, and diet modifications. Postural techniques include adequate body positioning (often difficult for frail, institutionalized patients), the chin-down posture, chin-up posture, head rotation, head tilt, neck extension, and side lying (Huckabee & Pelletier, 1999; Logemann, 1998). The clinician must select the postural technique that best fits the patient's physiologic or anatomic swallowing disorder.

Bolus control techniques are those in which the flow of the bolus is redirected by function and include cyclic ingestion, bolus placement, modification of bolus size and adaptations in the rate of intake (Huckabee & Pelletier, 1999). Successful implementation of these techniques is again dependent on the cognitive abilities of the patient and caregiver support.

Techniques to improve oral sensory awareness prior to the swallow usually are beneficial in individuals with swallow apraxia, tactile agnosia for food, delayed onset of the oral swallow, reduced oral sensation, or delayed triggering of the pharyngeal swallow (Logemann, 1993b in Logemann, 1998). Sensory enhancement techniques include increasing downward pressure of the spoon against the tongue, presenting a cold bolus, presenting a larger bolus, and thermal-tactile stimulation. Such sensory enhancement techniques have been found to speed both oral acceptance and initiation of the oral stage of swallow (Logemann, 1998). Although the presentation of sour boluses or boluses requiring chewing are commonly used sensory enhancement techniques, these techniques may not be appropriate in individuals with HIV/AIDS who present with odynophagia associated with oropharyngeal and/or esophageal lesions. Thermal tactile stimulation may be helpful in patients who exhibit significant delay in the triggering of the pharyngeal swallow.

Neurologic dysfunction may necessitate modification of food consistency and routines (Chantry & Moye, 2005). Liquids, for example, may require thickening for ease of swallowing and increased fluid intake. Although thickening agents are commercially available, instant pudding and applesauce also work well to increase viscosity (White et al., 1995). In many cases, weak muscles owing to neurologic dysfunction may be strengthened by face, mouth, and tongue exercises. However, clinicians need to caution against the increased potential for fatigue in the individual with HIV/AIDS, who may not be able to tolerate facial exercises. In recent years, neuromuscular electrical stimulation has been investigated as a technique to stimulate inactive or atrophied muscles involved in swallowing.

The primary aim of swallowing therapy aims to improve the patient's swallowing function and ability to eat orally (Logemann, 1998). However, certain patients, for example those with advanced dementia, may not benefit from swallowing therapy. In such cases, a shift from oral feeding to partial or total nonoral feeding may be required.

Nonoral Feeding

Nonoral feeding refers to the provision of nutrition, hydration, and medications through a route other than the mouth and is prescribed when an individual is unable to ingest enough orally without the risk of medical complications (Davis & Conti, 2003). Nonoral feeding may take place through enteral route (i.e., directly into the gastrointestinal tract via tube feeds) or parenteral route (via intravenous nutrition) (Huckabee & Pelletier, 1999; White et al., 1995). Enteral feeding may occur through the nose, esophagus, stomach, jejunum, or duodenum (Huckabee & Pelletier, 1999). Decisions surrounding the placement of the tube depend largely on the duration required for enteral feeding. For example, nasogastric feeding is indicated in patients who are expected to return to oral feeding within a short period of time, whereas gastrostomy feeding is indicated in patients who are not expected to return to oral feeding within less than 30 days (Huckabee & Pelletier, 1999). A major advantage associated with tube-feeding in patients with oropharyngeal dysphagia is improved nutritional status as the tube bypasses the obstacles associated with the dysphagia and, provided the gastrointestinal tract is functioning well, all administered food is ingested (Leibovitz et al., 2004). However, should a patient not be able to digest nutrients via the gastrointestinal tract, enteral feeding is not an option, and intravenous nutrition must be considered (Huckabee & Pelletier, 1999).

Numerous factors, including the time taken to complete a meal and the presence of aspiration, must be taken into account when deciding whether or not a patient should receive nonoral feeding and, in most instances, the decision belongs to the patient or family (Logemann, 1998). Much controversy surrounds the placement of feeding tubes and decisions are often emotionally charged. On one hand, families may interpret the withholding of nutritional support as a sign of giving up hope and placing the patient at risk of death by starvation and dehydration. On the other hand, nonoral feeding may simply prolong the process of dying, causing undue suffering. The benefits of nonoral feeding are particularly unclear when the underlying illness (as in the case of HIV/AIDS) is grave and its future course is unknown (Van Rosendaal, Verhoef, & Kinsella, 1999). Information regarding the purpose of nonoral feeding, the method used, the advantages thereof, and potential complications thereof must be provided to caregivers by members of the multidisciplinary team. Complications associated with enteral feeding, for example, include tube displacement, infection, diarrhea, peritonitis, increased gastroesophageal reflux with subsequent aspiration, and even death (e.g., Feinberg, Knebl, & Tully, 1996 in Davis & Conti, 2003). Ideally, a health professional well known to and trusted by the patient and family should assist in the decision-making process (Van Rosendaal et al., 1999).

SUMMARY

In summary, the structural and CNS manifestations of HIV/AIDS place individuals with the disease at risk for odynophagia and/or neurogenic dysphagia. The complex and potentially life-threatening nature of the feeding and swallowing difficulties associated with this population necessitate a team approach and a high quality of service delivery. Owing to the direct relationship between nutritional status and immune status, the primary goal in the management of the feeding and swallowing difficulties in the individual with HIV/AIDS remains the maintenance of adequate nutrition. While much can be done to facilitate safe oral feeding in the individual with HIV/AIDS, partial, or total nonoral feeding may need to be implemented at certain stages of the disease process to maintain adequate nutrition.

REFERENCES

Aboulafia, D. M. (2007). AIDS-related non-Hodgkin lymphoma: Evolving clinical issues in the HAART era (highly active antiretroviral therapy). *Infections in Medicine, 24*(10), 445–451.

Atkinson, J. C., & O'Connell, A. (2005). Oral health and dental problems. In S. L. Zeichner and J. S. Read (Eds.), *Textbook of pediatric HIV care* (pp. 455–459). New York: Cambridge University Press.

Baser, S. M. (2006). The neurologist's perspective. In R. L. Carrau and T. Murry (Eds.), *Comprehensive management of swallowing disorders* (pp. 51–56). San Diego, CA: Plural Publishing.

Bhaskaran, K., Mussini, C., Antinori, A., Walker, S. A., Dorrucci, M., Sabin, C., et al. Changes in the incidence and predictors of human immunodeficiency virus-associated dementia in the era of highly active antiretroviral therapy. *Annals of Neurology, 63*(2), 213–221.

Bladon, K. L., & Ross, E. (2007). Swallowing difficulties reported by adults infected with HIV/AIDS attending a hospital outpatient clinic in Gauteng, South Africa. *Folia Phoniatrica et Logopaedica, 59*(1) 39–52.

Buchholz, D. W., & Robbins, J. (1997). Neurologic diseases affecting oropharyngeal swallowing. In A. L. Perlman & K. Schulze-Delrieu (Eds.), *Deglutition and its disorders: Anatomy, physiology, clinical diagnosis and management* (pp. 319–342). San Diego, CA: Singular Publishing Group.

Carrau, R. L. (2006). The otolaryngologist's perspective. In R. L. Carrau & T. Murry (Eds.), *Comprehensive management of swallowing disorders* (pp. 33–38). San Diego, CA: Plural Publishing.

Chantry, C. J., & Moye, J. (2005). Growth, nutrition and metabolism. In S. L. Zeichner & J. S. Read (Eds.), *Textbook of pediatric HIV care* (pp. 244–268). New York: Cambridge University Press.

Civitello, L. (2005). Neurologic problems. In S. L. Zeichner & J. S. Read (Eds.), *Textbook of pediatric HIV care* (pp. 431–444). New York: Cambridge University Press.

Coogan, M. M., Greenspan, J., & Challacombe, S. J. (2005). Oral lesions in infection with human immunodeficiency virus. *Bulletin of the World Health Organization, 83*(9), 700–706.

Curtis, J. L., & Langmore, S. E. (1997). Respiratory functions and complications related to deglutition. In A. L. Perlman & K. Schulze-Delrieu (Eds.), *Deglutition and its disorders: Anatomy, physiology, clinical diagnosis and management* (pp. 99–124). San Diego, CA: Singular Publishing Group.

Davis-McFarland, E. (2000). Language and oral-motor development and disorders in infants and young toddlers with human immunodeficiency virus. *Seminars in Speech and Language, 21*(1), 19–35.

Davis, L. A., & Conti, G. J. (2003). Speech-language pathologist's roles and knowledge levels related to non-oral feeding. *Journal of Medical Speech-Language Pathology, 11*(1), 15–30.

Gennaro, S., Naidoo, S., & Berthold, P. (2008). Oral health and HIV/AIDS. *American Journal of Maternal/Child Nursing, 33*(1), 50–57.

Giancola, M. L., Rizzi, E. B., Lorenzini, P., Rovighi, L., Baldini, F., Shinina, V., et al. (2008). Progressive multifocal leukoencephalopathy in HIV-infected patients in the era of HAART: Radiological features at diagnosis and follow-up and correlation with clinical variables. *AIDS Research and Human Retroviruses, 24*(2), 155–162.

Goodrich, S., & Walker, A. I. (1997). Clinical swallow evaluation. In R. Leonard & K. Kendall (Eds.), *Dysphagia assessment and treatment planning: A team approach* (pp. 29–40). San Diego, CA: Singular Publishing Group.

Gray, F., Scaravilli, F., & Miller, R. (2007). Changing patterns of human immunodeficiency virus-associated neuropathology. *Annals of Indian Academy of Neurology, 10*(2), 69–80.

Halvorsen, R. A., Moelleken, S. M. C., & Kearney, A. T. (2003). Videofluoroscopic evaluation of HIV/AIDS patients with swallowing dysfunction. *Abdominal Imaging, 28*(2), 244–247.

Hardy, E. (1999). *Bedside evaluation of dysphagia.* Bisbee, AZ: Imaginart International.

Hoffmann, C., Ernst, M., Meyer, P., Wolf, E., Rosenkranz, T., Plettenberg, A., et al. (2007). Evolving characteristics of toxoplasmosis in patients infected with human immunodeficiency virus-1: Clinical course and Toxoplasma gondii-specific immune responses. *Clinical Microbiology and Infection, 13*(5), 510–515.

Huckabee, M. L., & Pelletier, C. A. (1999). Compensatory interventions for dysphagia. In M. L. Huckabee & C. A. Pelletier (Eds.), *Management of adult neurogenic dysphagia* (pp. 93–145). San Diego, CA: Singular Publishing Group.

Johnson, R. E. (1997). Evaluation for dysphagia in neurogenic disorders. In R. Leonard & K. Kendall (Eds.), *Dysphagia assessment and planning: A team approach* (pp. 29–39). San Diego, CA: Singular Publishing Group.

Lachenmeyer, J. R. (1995). Behavior aspects of feeding disorders. In S. R. Rosenthal, J. J. Sheppard, & M. Lotze (Eds.), *Dysphagia and the child with developmental disabilities: Medical, clinical and family interventions* (pp. 143–152). San Diego, CA: Singular Publishing Group.

Lakshmi, V., Sudha, T., Teja, V., & Umabala, P. (2007). Prevalence of central nervous system cryptococcosis in human immunodeficiency virus reactive hospitalized patients. *Indian Journal of Medical Microbiology, 25*(2), 146–149.

Layton, T. L., & Davis-McFarland, E. (2000). Pediatric human immunodeficiency virus and acquired immunodeficiency syndrome: An overview. *Seminars in Speech and Language, 21*(1), 7–17.

Layton, T. L., & Scott, G. S. (2000). Language development and assessment in children with human immunodeficiency virus: 3 to 6 years. *Seminars in Speech and Language, 21*(1), 37–47.

Lehmann, R. H. (1997). *Cooking for life: A guide to nutrition and food safety for the HIV-positive community.* New York: Dell.

Leibovitz, A., Sharon-Guidetti, A., Seal, R., Blavat, L., Peller, S., & Habot, B. (2004). CD4 lymphocyte count and CD4/CD8 ratio in elderly long-term care patients with oropharyngeal dysphagia: Comparison between oral and tube enteral feeding. *Dysphagia, 19*(2), 83–88.

Leonard, R. (1997). Introduction—The team approach. In R. Leonard & K. Kendall (Eds.), *Dysphagia assessment and planning: A team approach* (pp. 1–6). San Diego, CA: Singular Publishing Group.

Little, R. F. (2005). Neoplastic disease in pediatric HIV infection. In S. L. Zeichner & J. S. Read (Eds.), *Textbook of pediatric HIV care* (pp. 536–548). New York: Cambridge University Press.

Logemann, J. A. (1998). *Evaluation and treatment of swallowing disorders* (2nd ed.), Austin, TX: Pro-Ed.

Madariaga, M., & Kalil, A. C. (2007). CMV infection: Trends, clinical presentations, and treatment. *Infections in Medicine, 24*(12), 519-535.

Marquis, J., & Pressman, H. (1995). Radiologic assessment of pediatric swallowing. In S. R. Rosenthal, J. J. Sheppard, & M. Lotze (Eds.), *Dysphagia and the child with developmental disabilities: Medical, clinical and family interventions* (pp. 189-208). San Diego, CA: Singular Publishing Group.

Martínez, P. A., Díaz, R., González, D., Oropesa, L., González, R., Pérez, L., et al. (2007). The effect of highly active antiretroviral therapy on outcome of central nervous system herpesviruses infection in Cuban human immunodeficiency virus-infected individuals. *Journal of Neuro-Virology, 13*(5), 446-451.

Massey, B. T., & Shaker, R. (1997). Introduction to the filed of deglutition and deglutition disorders. In A. L. Perlman & K. Schulze-Delrieu (Eds.), *Deglutition and its disorders: Anatomy, physiology, clinical diagnosis and management* (pp. 1-14). San Diego: Singular Publishing Group.

McKenzie, S. W. (1997). Swallow evaluation with videofluoroscopy. In R. Leonard & K. Kendall (Eds.), *Dysphagia assessment and treatment planning: A team approach* (pp. 83-100). San Diego, CA: Singular Publishing Group.

McNeilly, L. G. (2000). Communication intervention and therapeutic issues in pediatric human immunodeficiency virus. *Seminars in Speech and Language, 21*(1), 63-77.

Mhango-Mkandawire, S. C. (1995). Nutritional support for the child with AIDS. In S. R. Rosenthal, J. J. Sheppard, & M. Lotze (Eds.), *Dysphagia and the child with developmental disabilities: Medical, clinical and family interventions* (pp. 99-132). San Diego, CA: Singular Publishing Group.

Miller, A., Bieger, D., & Conklin, J. L. (1997). Functional controls of deglutition. In A. L. Perlman & K. Schulze-Delrieu (Eds.), *Deglutition and its disorders: Anatomy, physiology, clinical diagnosis and management* (pp. 43-98). San Diego, CA: Singular Publishing Group.

Modi, G., Modi, M., & Mochan, A. (2006). Stroke and HIV—causal or coincidental co-occurrence? *South African Medical Journal, 96*(12), 1247-1248.

Moynihan, P. J. (2005). The role of diet and nutrition in the etiology and prevention of oral diseases. *Bulletin of the World Health Organization, 83*(9), 694-699.

Murray, J. A., Rao, S. S. C., & Schulze-Delrieu, K. (1997). Esophageal diseases. In A. L. Perlman & K. Schulze-Delrieu (Eds.), *Deglutition and its disorders: Anatomy, physiology, clinical diagnosis and management* (pp. 383-418). San Diego, CA: Singular Publishing Group.

Murray, T., & Carrau, R. L. (2001). *Clinical manual for swallowing disorders.* San Diego, CA: Singular Thomson Learning.

Murray, T., & Carrau, R. L. (2006). Functional tests of swallowing. In R. L. Carrau & T. Murray (Eds.), *Comprehensive management of swallowing disorders* (pp. 75–80). San Diego, CA: Plural Publishing.

Naidoo, S., & Chikte, U. (2004). Oral-facial manifestations in pediatric HIV: A comparative study of institutionalized and hospital outpatients. *Oral Diseases, 10*(1), 13–18.

Navarro, C. M., Shibli, J. A., Ferrari, R. B., d'Avila, S., & Sposto, M. R. (2008). Gingival primary extranodal non-Hodgkin's lymphoma as the first manifestation of acquired immunodeficiency syndrome. *Journal of Periodontology, 79*(3), 562–566.

Ortiz, G., Koch, S., Romano, S., Forteza, A. M., & Rabinstein, A. A. (2007). Mechanisms of stroke in HIV-infected patients. *Neurology, 68*(16), 1257–1261.

Padda, S., & Young, M. A. (2006a). Gastroenterologic evaluation of swallowing. In R. L. Carrau & T. Murray (Eds.), *Comprehensive management of swallowing disorders* (pp. 87–90). San Diego, CA: Plural Publishing.

Padda, S., & Young, M. A. (2006b). The gastroenterologist's perspective. In R. L. Carrau & T. Murray (Eds.), *Comprehensive management of swallowing disorders* (pp. 47–50). San Diego, CA: Plural Publishing.

Perlman, A. L., & Christensen, J. (1997). Topography and functional anatomy of the swallowing structures. In A. L. Perlman & K. Schulze-Delrieu (Eds.), *Deglutition and its disorders: Anatomy, physiology, clinical diagnosis and management* (pp. 15–42). San Diego, CA: Singular Publishing Group.

Perlman, A. L., Lu, C., & Jones, B. (1997). Radiographic contrast examination of the mouth, pharynx and esophagus. In A. L. Perlman & K. Schulze-Delrieu (Eds.), *Deglutition and its disorders: Anatomy, physiology, clinical diagnosis and management* (pp. 153–199). San Diego, CA: Singular Publishing Group.

Petersen, P. E., Bourgeois, D., Ogawa, H., Estupinan-Day, S., & Ndiaye, C. (2005). The global burden of oral diseases and risks to oral health. *Bulletin of the World Health Organization, 83*(9), 661–669.

Pressman, H. (1995). Dysphagia in children with AIDS. In S. R. Rosenthal, J. J. Sheppard, & M. Lotze (Eds.), *Dysphagia and the child with developmental disabilities: Medical, clinical and family interventions* (pp. 133–142). San Diego, CA: Singular Publishing Group.

Rosenquist, C. J. (1997). Radiographic evaluation of the pharynx and esophagus. In R. Leonard & K. Kendall (Eds.), *Dysphagia assessment and treatment planning: A team approach* (pp. 73–82). San Diego, CA: Singular Publishing Group.

Scaravilli, F., Bazille, C., & Gray, F. (2007). Neuropathologic contributions to understanding AIDS and the central nervous system. *Brain Pathology, 17*(2), 197–208.

Schulze-Delrieu, K. S., & Miller, R. M. (1997). Clinical assessment of dysphagia. In A. L. Perlman & K. Schulze-Delrieu (Eds.), *Deglutition and its disorders: Anatomy, physiology, clinical diagnosis and management* (pp. 125–152). San Diego, CA: Singular Publishing Group.

Sheiham, A. (2005). Oral health, general health and quality of life. *Bulletin of the World Health Organization, 83*(9), 644.

Sheppard, J. J. (1995). Clinical evaluation and treatment. In S. R. Rosenthal, J. J. Sheppard & M. Lotze (Eds.), *Dysphagia and the child with developmental disabilities: Medical, clinical and family interventions* (pp. 37–76). San Diego, CA: Singular Publishing Group.

Signorini, L., Gulletta, M., Coppini, D., Donzelli, C., Stellni, R., Manca, N., et al. (2007). Fatal dissemination of tozoplasmosis during primary HIV infection. *Current HIV Research, 5*(2), 273–274.

Swigert, N. B. (1998). *The source for pediatric dysphagia.* East Moline, IL: LinguiSystems.

Tipping, B., de Villiers, L., Wainwright, H., Candy, S., & Bryer, A. (2007). Stroke in patients with human immunodeficiency virus infection. *Journal of Neurology, Neurosurgery, and Psychiatry, 78*(12), 1320–1324.

Tirwomwe, J. F., Rwenyonti, C. M., Muwazi, L. M., Besigye, B., & Mboli, F. (2007). Oral manifestations of HIV/AIDS in clients attending TASO clinics in Uganda. *Clinical Oral Investigations, 11*(3), 289–292.

Van Rosendaal, G. M. A., Verhoef, M. J., & Kinsella, D. (1999). How are decisions made about the use of percutaneous endoscopic gastrostomy for long-term nutritional support? *American Journal of Gastroenterology, 94*(11), 3225–3228.

White, K. R., Mhango-Mkandawire, S. C., & Rosenthal, S. R. (1995). Nutritional support. In S. R. Rosenthal, J. J. Sheppard, & M. Lotze (Eds.), *Dysphagia and the child with developmental disabilities: Medical, clinical and family interventions* (pp. 77–98). San Diego, CA: Singular Publishing Group.

Winter, H. S. & Moye, J. (2005). Gastrointestinal disorders. In S. L. Zeichner & J. S. Read (Eds.). *Textbook of pediatric HIV care* (pp. 510–520). New York: Cambridge University Press.

Index

A

Acinetobacter lwoffi, 70
Agnosia, food, 395
Alexander's law, 317–318
Anatomy. *See also* Physiology
  brainstem, 244, 296–297
  external/outer ear, 244
  inner ear, 244
  vestibular nucleus, 296–297
  vestibular system, 294
  vision, 298
ARC (AIDS-related complex), 333
ART (antiretroviral therapy). *See*
  ARV (antiretroviral)
  therapies
ARV (antiretroviral) agents. *See*
  also ARV (antiretroviral)
  therapies; HAART (highly
  active antiretroviral
  therapy)
  abacavir (ABC), 56, 303, 306,
    339, 361
  amprenavir, 361
  atazanavir, 57
  azidothymidine (AZT), 140, 255,
    257
  classes, 339
  combination alternatives testing,
    268–269
  compliance, 184–185

didanosine (ddl), 56, 249, 255,
  258, 339
didanosine (ddl)-hydroxyurea,
  256
efavirenz, 55, 361
emtricitabine (FTC), 56
fosamprenavir, 57
indinavir, 56, 361
lamivudine (3TC), 56, 57, 249,
  255, 257, 361
lopinavir, 57, 257
lopinavir-ritonavir, 255
nelfinavir, 361
nevirapine, 55, 56, 57, 255, 352,
  361
NNRTIs (nonnucleoside reverse
  transcriptase inhibitors),
  55, 56, 57, 339
NRTIs (nucleoside reverse
  transcriptase inhibitors),
  55, 56, 257–258
overview, 58–59
pediatrics, 57–58
ritonavir, 55, 56, 57, 255, 257,
  361
saquinavir, 56, 361
stavudine (d4T), 56, 57, 249,
  306, 339, 361
stavudine (d4T)-lamivudine
  (3TC), 255, 256
tenofovir (TDF), 56

ARV (antiretroviral) agents
(continued)
  zalcitabine, 256
  zidovudine (AZT), 56, 127, 140,
    249, 255, 257–258, 258,
    352, 361
  zidovudine (AZT) didanosine,
    256
ARV (antiretroviral) therapies. *See
  also* ARV (antiretroviral)
  agents; HAART (highly
  active antiretroviral
  therapy)
  for adults, 55–57
  adverse effects, 55, 361
  and cardiovascular disease, 55
  and CD4 count, 41
  and child-bearing-aged women,
    55
  compliance aids, 54
  and depression, uncontrolled,
    55
  in developing world, 184
  and dietary anomalies, 175
  expense, 55
  feeding/children, 352–353
  and genotypic analysis, 43
  global perspective, 5–6
  guidelines, 54–55. *See also*
    WHO (World Health
    Organization)
  and HIV-1 life cycle, 21
  and incidence, 32
  integrase inhibitors, 13
  and liver disease, 55
  management, HIV
    initial patient preparation for,
    50
  Micobacterium tuberculosis
    resistance, 289
  and monitoring of disease, 44
  overview, 183–184
  patient responsibility, 54

  pediatrics, 45
  PIs (protease inhibitors), 55,
    56–57, 257
    ritonavir-boosted, 55
  poor access to, 289
  and pregnancy, 44–45
  and psychosis, uncontrolled, 55
  regimen changes, 54, 55
  and resistance, 42, 54, 289
  second-line regiment selection,
    55
  side effects. *See* adverse effects
    in this section
  and testing, 33
ASHA (American Speech-Language-
  Hearing Association)
  dynamic communication
    assessment, 156–157
  meeting with IAPAC
    (International Association
    of Physicians in AIDS Care),
    1998, 174
Aspergillus, 302
Aspergillus flavus, 70
Aspergillus fumigates, 202
Aspergillus niger, 206
Assessment. *See also* Diagnosis
  auditory disorders, 263–275
  breast feeding
    risk assessment, 353–354
  CAT/CLAMS (Clinical Adaptive
    Test/Clinical Linguistic and
    Auditory Milestone Scale),
    155
  children/communication
    disorders, 153–157
  children/hearing disorders
    adaptations, 272–273
  audiologic evaluation, 154
  cultural/national relevance,
    155–156
  ELMS-2 (Early Language
    Milestone Scale), 154–155

EOWPVT (Expressive One-Word
Picture Vocabulary Test),
155
GFTA-2 (Goldman-Fristoe Test of
Articulation), 155
health status impression, 50
history of symptoms, 49
immunization discussions, 50
KLPA-2 (Khan-Lewis
Phonological Analysis), 155
McCarthy Scales of Children's
Abilities, 144
opportunistic infection
prophylaxis, 50
overview, 48
pediatrics, 143–144
PPVT-4 (Peabody Picture
Vocabulary Test), 155
RDLS-R (Reynell Developmental
Language Scales-Revised),
155
and referral, 179–180
risk factors exploration, 49–50
SALT (Systematic Analysis of
Language Transcripts), 155
of speech, 180–181
stages of presentation, 48
swallowing disorders, 181–182,
356, 371, 405
testing, 50
VDRL (veneral disease research
laboratory tests), 48
Audiology. *See* Hearing disorders
overview
Auditory disorders. *See also*
Children/hearing disorders
ABR (auditory brainstem
response), 265, 269–270
acoustic reflex testing, 265,
267–268
and antibiotic allergies, 213
assessment
team approach, 274–275
assessment of functioning,
263–271
audiograms, screening, 262
audiologic test battery, 264–265
audiometry, pure-tone, 264, 266
audiometry, speech, 264, 267
and *Bacteroides,* 221
biofilms, 221
case history taking, 261
central auditory pathway
disorders, 246, 249, 265,
270–271
and cigarette smoking, 213, 214
cochlear microphonic response,
270
Cogan syndrome, 250–251
cortical-evoked responses, 265,
270–271
cortical recruitment, 265,
267–268
external ear problems, 196–209,
229–231, 312
FM systems, 278, 279, 282
hearing aids, 278, 279, 280–282
and herpes zoster, 254
inner ear disorders, 250–252,
262, 265, 268–289
intervention, 276–282
sensorineural disorders,
258–259
Kaposi sarcoma (KS), 229–231
management, 205–206, 207
and meningitis, 225
middle ear problems, 209–216,
221–231, 264, 267,
273–274, 312, 335
and Moraxella catarrhalis, 213
and mycobacteria, 210
nasopharyngeal lymphoid
hyperplasia co-occurence,
215, 221
opportunistic infections,
228–231, 251–254

Auditory disorders *(continued)*
otomycosis, 206–209
otoscopy, 211, 221–223, 261
overview, 195–196, 231, 243
prevalence, 245–248
prevention of, 276–278
Prevnar vaccine, 213–214
screening tests, 261–262
sensorineural
    assessment adaptations,
        272–274
    audiometry, speech, 264, 267
    FM systems, 282
    hearing aids, 278, 279,
        280–282
    neural management, 281–282
    overview, 282–283
    sensory deficit management,
        279–281
    team approach, 274–275
and *Serratia,* 197
and straphylococci, gram-
    positive, 197
surgical debridement, 205–206,
    209
tympanocentesis, 213

B

Bacteroides, 221
Balance disorders. *See also*
    Hearing disorders overview
abacavir (ABC), 339
ABRs (auditory brainstem
    responses), 335
acoustic neuroma, 335
and alcohol intoxication, 323
Alexander's law, 317–318
amnesia, 311
anatomy, 294–297
and ankle strategy, 300
ARV (antiretroviral)
    agents/therapy, 339

and *Aspergillus,* 302
ataxia, 311
audiometry, diagnostic, 335
autoimmune inner ear disorders,
    342
Bell palsy, 313
and *Blastomycosis,* 302
blood tests, 335
BPPV (benign paroxysmal
    positional vertigo), 314,
    323, 333, 344–345. *See also*
    vertigo *in this section*
caloric testing, 311, 312, 325–326,
    332, 333. *See also* ENG
    (electronystagmography)
    in this section; VNG
    (videonystagmography) *in
    this section*
Candida, 302, 313
carcinoma, squamous, 313
and cardiovascular etiologies,
    307
cerebellopontine angle
    pathology, 309
cerebral hypoperfusion, 307
cholesteatoma, 312
clumsiness, 311
and CMV (Cytomegalovirus),
    302, 313
and CNS adaptability, 343
and *Coccidioides immitis,* 302
and cochlea, 294–295, 296
cochlear dysfunction testing,
    335
and COG (center of gravity),
    300
and cognitive impairments, 309
components of system,
    essential, 293
consciousness level, 307, 309
cover-uncover test, 319–320
and *Cryptococcus neoformans,*
    302

CSF (cerebrospinal fluid)
analysis, 311, 335
CT, 311, 335
dermatitis, seborrheic, 313
didanosine (ddl), 339
Dix Hallpike test, 311, 314, 323,
324. *See also* ENG
(electrostagmography) *in
this section*
dizziness, 294, 304–311
DVA (dynamic visual acuity)
test, 325
dysdiadokinesia, 311
and ear pressure, 306
ECochG (electrocochleography),
335
and eighth cranial nerve,
296–297
and elderly clients, 308
endo-/perilymph, 295
ENG (electronystagmography),
311, 331–333
and epiglottitis, 313
epilepsy, 334, 342
examinations, 308–313
eye movements, 299
and eye/vision function, 307
foot numbness, 311
frontal signs, 311
Fukuda stepping test, 315, 316
fullness, 306
and fundoscopy, 309
gait, ataxic/magnetic, 311, 315
gingivitis, 313
glioma, 303
and hair cells, 296
and hairy leucoplakia, 313
head and neck manifestations,
313
head impulse test, 320–321, 322
head thrust positive, 311
and herpes simplex (HSV), 302,
313

and hip strategy, 300
and *Histoplasma capsulatum,*
302
and hypo-/hyperreflexia, 310
immittance testing, 335
incontinence, 311
infections, concomitant,
302–303
inner ear, 294–296
intention tremor, 311
and IRIS (immune reconstitution
inflammatory syndrome),
303
and JC virus, 302
Kaposi sarcoma (KS), 303, 313
labyrinthitis, 302
leukoencephalopathy,
progressive multifocal, 302
and *Listeria,* 302
lymphoid hyperplasia, 215
lymphoma, 303
malaria, 303
and Ménière disease, 323, 335,
342, 343
meningitis, 309, 311
and micobacteriosis (MAC), 302
microvascular compression, 342
MRI, 311, 335
*and Mycobacterium
tuberculosis* (MTB)
complex, 202
nasal manifestations, 313
nasopharyngeal pathology, 309
neurocysticercosis, 303
neurologic disorders, 302, 307
neurosyphilitic tabes dorsalis,
310
and *Nocardia,* 302
non-Hodgkin lymphoma, 313
nystagmus. 323, 333–334. *See
also* BPPV (benign
paroxysmal positional
vertigo) *in this section*

Balance disorders *(continued)*
nystagmus testing. 315, 317–318,
320–321, 333. *See also* ENG
(electronystagmography) *in
this section*
OAEs (otoacoustic emissions),
335
oculomotor signs, 311
opportunistic infections, 302–303
optokinetic eye movements, 299
oral manifestations, 313
oscillopsia, 293, 309, 311, 340
otalgia, 306
otitis media with effusion
(OME), 335
otorrhea, 306
ototoxicity, 303, 306, 309, 311,
335, 339, 340, 343
OVAR (off-vertical axis testing),
334
overview, 289, 292–293,
337–338, 345
and papilledema, 309
pathology spectrum, 301–303
pendular tests, rotatory, 333
peri-/endolymph, 294, 295
and perilymph fistula, 234
periodontitis, 313
peripheral vestibulopathy, 310
physiology, 295–301
and *Pneumocystis jiroveci,* 302
positional/positioning testing,
321, 323, 333
and postural hypotension, 307
posturography, 311, 328, 329
presyncope, 307
processes of system, essential,
293
proprioceptive loss, 311
proprioceptive/somatosensory
system, 300–301
and psychological/psychiatric
problems, 307

and Ramsay Hunt syndrome,
302
retrocochlear pathology, 335
and rhinitis, 313
Rinne test, 309, 312
Romberg sign, 311, 314–315
rotational testing, 309, 311,
333–334
rotation chair testing, 327
RPR (rapid plasma reagin) test,
311
saccade testing, 319, 321
saccadic eye movements,
298–299
salivary gland involvement, 313
semicircular canal dehiscence,
234
semicircular canals, inner ear,
294, 295, 296
sensory loss, 311
skull base pathology, 309
and smooth pursuit eye
movements, 299
smooth pursuit testing, 319, 333
somatosensory/proprioceptive
system, 300–301
stavudine (d4T), 339
and step strategy, 300
and strabismus, 309
strokes, 303, 311
and *Strongyloides,* 303
and syphilis, 302, 340
system essential components,
293
throat manifestations, 313
and *toxoplasma gondii,* 303
treatment, 339–345
trypanosomiasis, 303
and tuberculosis, 315
Tulio phenomenon, 306
tuning fork testing, 309, 312
tympanic membrane
perforation, 312

ulcers, recurrent aphthous, 313
and Valsalva maneuvers,
234–325. *See also* ENG
(electronystagmography)
in this section; VNG
(videonystagmography) *in
this section*
and vascular compression, 323
VCR (vestibulocollic reflex),
293, 297
VDRL (venereal disease research
laboratory test), 311
VEMP (vestibular-evoked
myogenic potentials),
328–331
vertigo, 226, 227, 250–251, 294,
308, 311, 323. *See also*
BPPV (benign paroxysmal
postanal vertigo) *in this
section*
vestibular dysfunction, 242, 311,
315, 323, 327, 334–335,
340, 342–343
vestibular nuclei, 297
vestibular testing, 67, 309,
313–334
vestibulitis, 302
visual acuity, 311
visual fixation suppression,
incomplete, 333
vitamin deficiencies, 310, 311
VOR (vestibuloocular reflex),
293, 297, 299, 320–321,
322, 325, 327
VSR (vestibulospinal reflex),
293, 297
weakness, 311
Weber test, 309, 312
xerostomia, 313
X-ray testing, 335
Belmont Report (National
Commission for the
Protection of Human
Subjects of Biomedical and
Behavioral Research), 116
Biofilms, 221
Blastomycosis, 302
Breast feeding
mother-to-child transmission,
44–45
risk assessment, 353–354
and seroconversion (antibody
development), 353

C

Cancer, 68
Candida, 206, 208, 302, 313, 357,
375
Candida parapsilosis, 70
Carcinoma, squamous, 313
CDC (Centers for Disease Control
and Prevention)
hand hygiene, 76, 77
Universal (Standard)
Precautions, 65–66
CD4 T-cell count monitoring, 34,
40–41, 44
Cerebral palsy, 358
Children/communication
disorders, 135
versus adult opportunistic
infection patterns, 140
anorexia, 140
assessment, 153–157. *See also*
Assessment *main entry*
bacterial infection, recurrent,
140
brain atrophy, 140
candida esophagitis, 140
candidiasis, 160
CMV (Cytomegalovirus), 140
developmental delays, 143
encephalopathy, 140
fever, recurrent, 140
herpes, 140, 141, 142, 144

Children/communication disorders
(continued)
  HIV/AIDS pediatric case growth,
    135
    in USA, 137–139
    worldwide distribution,
      136–137, 138–139
  Kaposi sarcoma (KS), 140
  language deterioration/global
    cognitive ability, 145–149
  language functions, 145–153,
    152–153
  LIP (lymphoid interstitial
    pheumonitis), 140
  lymphadenopathy, 140
  manifestations/associated
    conditions, 140–159
  MLU (mean length of
    utterance), 145
  neuropathy, peripheral, 140
  non-Hodgkin lymphoma, 140
  overview, 135–139, 165
  perinatal transmission, 139–140
  Pneumocystis jiroveci
    pneumonia (PCP), 140
  treatment, 157–164
  tuberculosis, 140
Children/hearing disorders. *See
  also* Auditory disorders
  ABR (auditory brainstem
    response) testing, 143
  adenoidectomy, 220, 225
  antibiotic allergies, 213
  antibiotic resistance, 212, 213
  and ARV (antiretroviral)
    therapies, 210
  assessment
    adaptations, 272–273
    audiologic evaluation, 154
  azidothymidine prenatal
    exposure, 257
  and bacteremia, 212
  biofilms, 221

central nervous system (CNS)
    involvement, 250
  cerumen management, 211
  and child care centers, 213
  cigarette smoke exposure, 213
  and ciprofloxacin, 205
  CMV (Cytomegalovirus),
    congenital, 252
  cochlear implants, 282
  and developmental difficulty
    risk, 217–218, 224
  encephalopathy, hypoxic, 250
  eustachian tube dysfunction,
    143
  external otitis (EO), acute,
    196–201
  external otitis (EO), fungal,
    206–209
  and facial nerve paralysis, 203,
    204, 225
  and HAART (highly active
    antiretroviral therapy), 210,
    218
  hearing aids, 282
  and hearing assessment, 219
  hearing loss, 143, 250
  Kaposi sarcoma (KS), 230
  lamivudine prenatal exposure,
    257
  and lifestyle, 213
  malignant external otitis (EO),
    203
  mastoiditis, 225
  and meningitis, 212
  middle ear effusion, 246. *See
    also* otitis media with
    effusion (OME) *in this
    section*
  nasopharyngeal lymphoid
    hyperplasia co-occurence,
    215, 221
  nasopharyngeal reflux through
    eustachian tube, 221

neuromaturational
delays/deficits, 274
ossicular chain disruption, 224
otalgia, severe, 203
otitis media, 142, 143, 154,
209-227, 252, 267, 335
otorrhea, 203
otoscopy, 211
pain, 203
prevalence, 245-246
prevention, 213
self-limited conditions, 218
tympanic membrane, 203, 211,
224, 312
tympanocentesis, 143, 213
tympanometry, 264, 267, 273-274
tympanostomy, 218-220
typanomastoidectomy, 225
vaccine, heptavalent
pneumococcal conjugate,
213-214
VRA (visual reinforcement
audiometry), 273-274
zidovudine (AZT) prenatal
exposure, 257
Children/swallowing disorders. *See
also* Feeding/children;
Swallowing disorders
aspiration, 356, 360
assessment, 154, 356, 367-371
and bradycardia, 375
and brain tumors, 357
Candida, 357, 360-361
candida esophagitis, 144, 357
candidiasis, pseudomembranous,
360, 361
CMV (Cytomegalovirus)
esophagitis, 142, 144, 357,
361
and cryptococcus infection, 360
details, 357-358
discoordination, oral
mechanism, 142

encephalopathy, 144, 358-360
epiglottitis, 360
esophagitis, 361
and failure to thrive, 375-376
fungal infection, 360
gastritis, 361
GERD (gastroesophageal reflux
disease), 356
GI (gastrointestinal) symptoms,
144-145
gingivostomatitis, herpes, 142,
144, 361-362
hepatabiliary symptoms, 144
herpes gingivastomatitis, 357
and histoplasma infection, 360
indications for referral, 366
and infectious diseases, 360-362
intervention, 371-379
Kaposi sarcoma (KS), 141
and length of mealtime, 360
LPR (laryngopharyngeal reflux),
356
lymphoepithelial cysts, oral, 142
meningitis, 359-360
and morbidity, 358
and muscle wasting, 357, 362
nasal regurgitation, 359
nasopharyngeal incoordination,
358
and neurologic disease, 358-360
neuromuscular discoordination,
144
odynophagia, 142, 144, 357, 375
and oral candidiasis, 360
oral hygiene, 379-380
oral manifestations, 142
overview, 144-145, 351, 354-355
parotid enlargement, 142
phases affected, 144-145
and phases of swallowing,
355-356
and reflux, 375-376
self-feeding coordination, 359

Children/swallowing disorders
(continued)
  swelling, oral, 142
  and tachycardia, 375
  and tachypnea, 375
  tongue action, 358
  toxoplasmosis, 359–360, 361
  xerostomia, 142, 361
CMV (Cytomegalovirus), 259
  balance disorders, 302, 313
  pediatrics, 142, 144
  swallowing disorders, 388
CNS (central nervous system)
    problems, 176
Coccidioides immitis, 302
Cognitive impairments, 176–177,
    395
  pediatrics, 145–149
Communication disorders.
    See also Children/
    communication disorders
  apraxia of speech, 175
  assessment
    language, 181
    speech, 180–181
  and culture, 189–190
  dysarthria, 175
  and ethics, 118, 119, 126, 129,
    130–131. *See also* Ethics
    main entry
  HIV test results, 122
  infection control. *See* Infection
    control *main entry*
  intubation, 175
  Kaposi sarcoma (KS), 175
  language disorders, 176
  late disease stages, 175, 176
  overview, 173–174
  psychosocial influences, 97–105
  psychosocial resources. *See also*
    psychosocial influences *in
    this section*
  educational material design
    sensitivity, 109

  overview, 105–107
  psychological strength
    acknowledgment, 107
  strength-based intervention
    development, 108–109
  respiratory functioning
    compromise, 175–176
  and stethoscope contamination,
    69
  treatment, 182–184. *See also*
    ARV (antiretroviral) agents;
    HAART (highly active
    antiretroviral therapy)
  vocal quality, 175
Council for International
    Organizations of Medical
    Science (CIOMS)
  *International Ethical
    Guidelines for Biomedical
    Research Involving
    Human Subjects,* 126, 129
Cryptococcus, 259
Cryptococcus neoformans, 302
Culture, 189–190
  and ethics, 127–128
  sociocultural barriers, 100–101
Cytotoxic therapy, 231

D

Dermatitis, seborrheic, 313
DHHS (U.S. Department of Health
    and Human Services)
  viral load measurement
    guidelines, 39–40
Diabetes, 68
Diabetes mellitus, 201, 202
Diagnosis. *See also* Assessment;
    Testing
  of AIDS, 46
  CD4 T-cell count monitoring, 34,
    40–41
  and donors of blood/organs
    (early infection window), 44

and early infection, 43
ELISA (enzyme-linked
immunosorbent assay)
antibody tests, 34, 35-36
and early infection, 43-44
noninvasive, 37
and HIV natural history, 36
overview, 32-33, 58-59
p24 antigen test, 38, 39
and early infection, 43, 44
PCR (polymerase chain
reaction) test, 34, 38-39
and early infection, 44
pediatrics, 44-46
T-cell count monitoring, CD4
(cluster differentiation 4),
34, 40-41
testing rationales, 32-33
and viral load monitoring, 39-40
Western blot test, 34, 37-38, 49
window of early infection, 43, 44
Disability and infection propensity,
2
Disease progression. *See also*
Pathogenesis, HIV infection
acute HIV infection, 15, 17
to AIDS, 18
clinical asymptomatic HIV
infection, 17
to HIV-specific related disease,
18
immune response destruction,
22-23
immunocollapse, 18-19
immunopathogenesis
implications, 24-25
immunosuppression, advancing,
18-19
initial HIV response, 47
lymphadenopathy, persistent
generalized, 17-18
overview, 11
primary HIV infection, 20-21
"sanctuary site" invasion, 14

seroconversion (antibody
development), 15, 20-21
staging, adolescents/adults,
15-18. *See also* Staging,
adolescents/adults *main
entry*
transmission routes/targets, 14
viral replication of HIV, 23-24
Donors of blood/organs (early
infection window), 44
Drooling, 395
Drug-resistance testing, 42
Dysphagia. *See* Swallowing
disorders

E

ELISA (enzyme-linked
immunosorbent assay)
antibody tests, 34, 35-36
and early infection, 43-44
and initial assessment with HIV
diagnosis, 49
noninvasive, 37
with p24 antigen tests (4th
generation), 44
Encephalitis, 253
Enterobacter, 70
Epidemiology, HIV/AIDS, 290
Epiglottitis, 313, 360
Epstein-Barr virus
and non-Hodgkin lymphoma,
229
Escherichia, 221
Ethics
and access to care, 126-127
autonomy rights, 121-122
Belmont Report (National
Commission for the
Protection of Human
Subjects of Biomedical and
Behavioral Research), 116
beneficence/nonmalfeasance,
123-125

Ethics *(continued)*
confidentiality, 120–121
consent, 118–120
and culture, 127–128
decision making, 129–131
duties of service, 123–124
Helsinki Declaration, 128–129
Hippocratic oath, 123
and HIV-infected health care
workers, 125
and HIV testing, 121–122
*International Ethical
Guidelines for Biomedical
Research Involving
Human Subjects* (Council
for International
Organizations of Medical
Science [CIOMS]), 126, 129
justice principle, 125–127
Nuremberg Code, 128
overview, 115–116, 131
and research, 118–120,
126–127, 128, 129
respect for persons, 117–122
Tuskegee Syphilis Study, 126, 127
and universal precautions,
124–125
WHO (World Health
Organization), 129
and zidovudine (AZT)
administration, 127

F

Families
communicating with, 189
coping with loss, death, dying,
105
counseling of, 184
and HAART (highly active
antiretroviral therapy), 54
Feeding/adult nutritional status,
386–387

Feeding/children. *See also*
Children/swallowing
disorders
abacavir (ABC), 361
and anorexia, 140, 357, 362
appetite loss, 140, 362
ARV (antiretroviral) therapies,
352–353
assessment, 367–370
breast feeding, 353–354
caloric needs, 363
candida esophagitis, 357
CMV (Cytomegalovirus)
esophagitis, 357, 361
colitis, 361
and encephalopathy,
progressive, 377–378
enteral feeding, 145
esophagitis, 361
global perspective, 7–8
herpes gingivastomatitis, 357
herpes simplex (HSV), 361
hygiene, oral, 379–380
hyperalimentation, 357
indications for referral, 366
kwashiorkor, 358
malabsorption, 362
meal timing, 360
nausea, 361, 362
nutritional compromise risk,
357
nutritional needs, 372, 373
odynophagia, 357
oral compromise, 357
overview, 380
phases, typical, 355–356
psychosocial issues, 363–364
refusal of food, 360
transmission reduction, 352–353
tube feeding, 357, 358, 378–379
vomiting, 361
Feeding difficulties. *See*
Swallowing disorders

Fever spikes, 395
Food agnosia, 395

G

Genotypic analysis, 42-43
Gingivitis, 313
Glioma, 303
Global perspective, HIV/AIDS
and hearing disorders, 6-7
living with HIV/AIDS, 5-8
vulnerability, 1-2
of women, 3-4

H

HAART (highly active antiretroviral
therapy), 5, 173, 176. *See
also* ARV (antiretroviral)
therapies
Haemophilus influenzae, 210,
213, 214
Hearing disorders overview. *See
also* Auditory disorders;
Children/hearing disorders
balance disorders examination,
312. *See also* Balance
disorders *main entry*
and cerebrovascular disease risk
factors, 307
cochlear implants, 278
and diplopia, 307
and dysphagia, 307
ear pressure, 306
and ethics, 118, 119, 122, 129.
See also Ethics *main entry*
HIV test results, 122
external ear conditions,
196-209, 230, 231
and facial weakness/pain, 307
FM systems, 278
fullness sensation, 306
and gait difficulty, 307

and halting speech, 307
hearing aids, 278
infection, opportunistic, 174
infection control. *See* Infection
control *main entry*
and memory loss, 307
middle ear conditions, 209-231.
See also Ear disorder *main
entry*
otalgia, 306
otorrhea, 306
ototoxicity, 174, 248, 303, 306,
309, 311, 314, 335, 339,
340
and photophobia, 307
psychosocial influences, 97-105
psychosocial resources.
105-109. *See also*
psychosocial influences *in
this section*
and scotomas, 307
and seizures, 307
and stethoscope contamination,
69
Helsinki Declaration, 128-129
Hepatitis B (HBV), 64
vaccination plans/records
requirements, 85
Herpes gingivostomatitis, 142, 144,
361
Herpes simplex (HSV), 302
balance disorders, 313
feeding/children, 361
swallowing disorders, 388, 390
Herpesvirus, human (HHV),
229-230
Herpes zoster, 302
balance disorders, 313
oticus, 254
swallowing disorders, 388
Histoplasma capsulatum, 302
HIV-1
features, 12

HIV-1 *(continued)*
  versus HIV-2, 12
  life cycle, 19
  and ARV (antiretroviral)
    therapies, 21-22
  and RNA in life cycle, 12-13
  transmission, 14
  viral load assays, commercial, 39
HIV-2, 11-14
  and Western blot test, 38
HIV opportunistic infections
  adult, 19
  auditory disorders, 20, 174,
    228-231, 251-254,
    258-259
  balance disorders, 302-303, 340
  childhood, 26, 140-141
  of mouth/esophagus regions, 20
  swallowing disorders, 392-394
HIV overview, 47-48

I

IAPAC (International Association of
    Physicians in AIDS Care)
  meeting with ASHA (American
    Speech-Language-Hearing
    Association), (1998), 174
Immune reconstitution
    inflammatory syndrome
    (IRIS), 53, 103
Immunizations, 50
Infection control
  Acinetobacter lwoffi, 70
  Aspergillus flavus, 70
  and body orifices/microorganism
    transmission, 67
  CDC (Centers for Disease
    Control and Prevention)
    hand hygiene, 77
    Universal Blood and Blood-
      Borne Pathogen
      Precautions, 71-72

Universal (Standard)
    Precautions, 65-66
  cerumen exposure, 69
  cleaning of surfaces, 81
  in clinical setting overview,
    66-67. *See also* infection
    control *under*
    communication disorders;
    infection control *under*
    hearing disorders; infection
    control *under* swallowing
    disorders
  communication disorders
    relevance, 64
  contact transmission, 66-67
  Corynebacterium, 69
  critical instrument sterilization,
    82-83
  cross-contamination, 64
  defined, 64
  disinfecting of surfaces, 81
  employee exposure
    classification, 84-85
  Enterobacter, 70
  and eye protection, 74-76
  gloves, 72-74
  and gowns, 74-76
  hand hygiene, 76
    alcohol-based, no-rinse hand
      degermers, 76
    technique, 78-80
  and headset ear piece
    contamination, 69
  hearing instrument
    bacterial/fungal growth,
      69-70
  hepatitis B, 64
  hepatitis B (HBV) vaccination
    plans/records, 85
  implementation
    control development, 88-91,
      88-99
    overview, 87-88

protocols, 70–87
of work practices, 87–94
infection control plans, 83–87
infectious waste disposal, 82
instrument microbial
contamination, 69–70
intraoperative monitoring, 67
Lactobacillus, 70
and masks, 74–76
microbial contamination/
instruments, 69–70
OSHA (Occupational Safety and
Health Administration),
65–70, 84–87
overview, 63, 94–95
and patients subject to
immunocompromise, 67
personal barriers, 72–76
principles, foundational, 64
Pseudomonas aeruginosa, 70
relevance to service provision,
64–70
and scope of clinical practice,
67–68
Standard (Universal)
Precautions, 65–66, 70–72
Staphylococcus, 64, 68–69
Staphylococcus aureus, 69
Staphylococcus epidermidis, 69
sterilization, 81–83
and stethoscope contamination,
69
Streptococcus, 69
Universal Blood and
Blood-Borne Pathogen
Precautions, CDC, 71–72
WHO (World Health
Organization), 70
hand hygiene, 76–77
hospital-acquired for infection
prevention manual, 84
nosocomial infection control
guidelines, 65, 66

six standard precautions, all
patients, 71–72
work practice control
implementation, 87–94
*International Ethical Guidelines
for Biomedical Research
Involving Human Subjects*
(Council for International
Organizations of Medical
Science [CIOMS]), 126, 129
IRIS (immune reconstitution
inflammatory syndrome),
53, 103, 303

J

JC virus, 302

K

Kaposi sarcoma (KS), 16, 303
balance disorders, 313
communication disorders, 175
ear disorders, 229–231
and HAART (highly active
antiretroviral therapy), 230
pediatrics, 140, 141
and swallowing disorders, 389
Klebsiella, 221
Klebsiella oxytoca, 202

L

Labyrinthitis, 302
Lactobacillus, 70
Language disorders. *See*
Communication disorders
Leukoencephalopathy, progressive
multifocal, 302
Leukoplakia, hairy
balance disorders, 313
swallowing disorders, 388,
389–390

Lymphoid hyperplasia, 215, 313
Lymphoma, 303
  CNS, 291
  versus vestibular schwannoma,
    291

M

Malaria, 303
Management. *See individual
    conditions*
Management, HIV
  ARV (antiretroviral)
    initial patient preparation for,
      50
  assessment, initial with HIV
    diagnosis, 48–54. *See also*
    Assessment *main entry*
  prophylaxis with initial HIV
    diagnosis, 50
Ménière disease, 323, 335, 342, 343
Meningitis, 359–360
  bacterial, 253–254
  and balance disorders, 309, 311
  chronic, 311
  cryptococcal, 253
  and neurologic involvement,
    212, 290–291
  pediatrics, 212
  tuberculosis, 253
Micobacteriosis (MAC), 302
Micobacterium tuberculosis
  (MTB) resistance, 289
Migraine, vestibular, 323, 342
Moraxella catarrhalis, 213
Mother-to-child transmission, 4, 6,
    14, 44–45, 58, 127, 130,
    136, 139–140, 152, 153,
    290, 352
Multidisciplinary approach,
    106–107, 110, 121, 179,
    187–188
  and intervention, 182
  pediatrics, 153–154, 157

Mycobacteria, 19, 210, 302, 313,
    340
Mycobacterium avium complex,
    141
*Mycobacterium avium-
    intercellulare,* 259
Mycobacterium tuberculosis
    (MTB), 202, 259, 289

N

Nasal regurgitation, 359, 395
Neurocysticercosis, 303
Neurologic involvement, 174, 212,
    227, 290–291, 358–360,
    392–396
Neuronitis, vestibular, 323
Neurosyphilitic tabes dorsalis, 310
NIH (National Institutes of Health)
  on auditory dysfunction, 174
NINDS (National Institute of
    Neurological Disorders and
    Stroke)
  neurologic complications, 174
NNRTIs (nonnucleoside reverse
    transcriptase inhibitors),
    339
Nocardia, 302
Non-Hodgkin lymphoma
  balance disorders, 313
  ear disorders, 229–230
  and Epstein-Barr virus, 229
  swallowing disorders, 389
NRTIs (nucleoside reverse
    transcriptase inhibitors),
    257–258, 261, 339
Nuremberg Code, 128

O

OSHA (Occupational Safety and
    Health Administration), 70
  accidents/exposure follow-up
    plans, 86

annual training plans, 85–86
hepatitis B (HBV) vaccination
plans/records requirements,
85
infection control protocol
implementation, 86–87
infection postexposure
plans/records, 87
Universal (Standard)
Precautions, 65–66
written infection control plan
requirements, 84–87
Otosyphilis, 249, 252–253, 261
Ototoxicity, 174, 248, 254–259,
343
and age, 257
balance disorders, 303, 306,
309, 311, 339, 340
and noise exposure,
occupational, 257–258
reversibility of effects, 259
sensorineural disorders, 249

P

Pandemic overview, 31–32
p24 antigen test, 38, 39
and early infection, 43, 44
with ELISA antibody tests (4th
generation), 44
and pediatrics, 45
Pathogenesis, HIV infection. *See
also* Disease progression
abbreviations, 13
adult opportunistic
infections/conditions,
common, 19, 20
and aging, premature, 13
childhood opportunistic
infections/clinical
conditions, 26, 140–141
DNA and life cycle, 12–13
features, important, 12
HIV-1, 12

HIV-2, 12
HIV-1 life cycle, 21
immunopathogenesis
implications, 24–25
overview, 27–28
RNA and life cycle, 12–13
staging, adolescents/adults,
15–18. *See also* Staging,
adolescents/adults *main
entry*
subtypes, 11, 12
terms, 13
PCR (polymerase chain reaction)
test, 34, 38–39, 44, 45
Pediatrics. *See also* Children/
communication disorders;
Children/hearing disorders;
Children/swallowing
disorders; Feeding/children
Periodontitis, 313
Physiology. *See also* Anatomy
brainstem, 244
external/outer ear, 244
inner ear, 244
middle ear, 244
Pneumocystis carinii, 210
Pneumocystis jiroveci, 259, 302
Pneumocystis jiroveci pneumonia
(PCP), 140, 141
Pregnancy. *See* Mother-to-child
transmission
Prevnar vaccine, 213–214
Progression. *See* Disease
progression
Proteus, 221
Proteus mirabilis, 202, 226
Pseudomonas, 207
Pseudomonas aeruginosa, 70,
197, 201, 202, 210, 221,
226
resistant, 206
Psychosocial influences. 97–105.
See also Psychosocial
resources

Psychosocial resources. 105–110.
See also Psychosocial
influences

R

Ramsay Hunt syndrome, 254, 302
Regurgitation, nasal, 359, 395
Respiratory distress, 395
Rhinitis, 313

S

SARS (severe acute respiratory
syndrome), 65
Seroconversion (antibody
development)
and breast feeding, 353
confirmation, 44
disease progression, 15, 20–21
and HAART (highly active
antiretroviral therapy)
initiation, 51
symptoms when accomplished,
290
timing, 44
Simian immunodeficiency virus
(SIV), 11
SLP (speech-language pathology/
pathologists). *See* Children/
communication disorders;
Children/swallowing
disorders; Communication
disorders; Swallowing
disorders
SLT (speech-language therapy/
therapists). *See* Children/
communication disorders;
Children/swallowing
disorders; Communication
disorders; Swallowing
disorders
Speech disorders. *See*
Communication disorders

Speech-language pathology. *See*
Communication disorders
Staging, adolescents/adults
U.S. Centers for Disease Control,
AIDS Surveillance Case
Definition for Adolescents
and Adults, 15, 17, 46, 49
WHO (World Health
Organization), 15, 16, 18,
46, 49
Standard (Universal) Precautions,
65–66, 70–72, 183
WHO (World Health
Organization)
six standard precautions, all
patients, 71–72
Staphylococcus, 64, 68–69
Staphylococcus aureus, 69, 202,
210, 221, 225, 226, 227
Staphylococcus coagulase-
negative, 210
Staphylococcus epidermidis, 69
Streptococcus pneumoniae, 210,
213, 214, 225, 226, 253
Streptococcus pyogenes, 225, 226
Strokes, 303
Strongyloides, 303
Swallowing disorders. *See also*
Children/swallowing
disorders
agnosia for food, tactile, 412
apraxia of swallow, 412
aspiration
neurogenic indicators, 395
assessment, 181–182, 356, 371,
397–406
candidiasis, 177
and candidiasis (thrush),
387–389
cheilitis, angular, 177, 388
CMV (Cytomegalovirus), 388,
390
CNS (central nervous system)
involvement

opportunistic infection,
392-394
and dementia, 394
and encephalitis, 393-394
erythema, pseudomembranous,
177
and esophagitis, 390
and ethics, 129. *See also* Ethics
main entry
families, communicating with,
189
and food choices, 410
fungal lesions, 388
and gingival erythema, linear,
389, 390
and gray matter involvement,
393-394
herpes simplex (HSV), 388, 390
herpes zoster, 388
infection control. *See also*
Infection control *main*
entry
cleaning of surfaces, 81
disinfecting of surfaces, 81
and EMG, 67
gloves needed, 73
hand washing/hygiene,
64-65, 77
infectious waste disposal, 82
and nasoendoscopy/
nasometry, 67
overview, 94-95
protocol implementation,
86-87
and scope of clinical practice,
67-68
sterilization, 81-82
and videostroboscopy, 67
and Kaposi sarcoma, 389, 390
and leukoencephalopathy,
393-394
and leukoplakia, oral hairy, 388,
389-390
management, 406-414

manifestations of disease,
177-178
and medication regimen, 391
multidisciplinary approach, 396
and neoplasms, 389, 390
neurogenic dysphagia
indicators, 395
and neurological conditions,
392-396
and non-Hodgkin lymphoma,
389, 390
nonoral feeding, 412-414
odynophagia, 178, 385, 386,
388, 390, 403, 405, 410,
412
management, 408
of oral swallow, 412
overview, 174-175, 385-386,
414
and parotid enlargement, 389
periodontal disease, 177-178,
389
and periodontitis, necrotizing
ulcerative, 389
pharyngeal swallow triggering
delay, 412
and progressive cognitive/motor
syndrome, 394
and pseudomembranous
candidiasis, 388
regurgitation, nasal, 395
salivary gland pathology,
390-391
and structural problems, 387-391
and thrush (candidiasis),
387-389
treatment
nonoral feeding, 187
and tuberculosis, 390
viral infections, 389-390
viral lesions, 388
WHO (World Health
Organization) oral criteria,
177

Syphilis, 302, 310, 340
   otosyphilis, 249, 252-253, 261

T

T-cell count monitoring, CD4
   (cluster differentiation 4),
   34, 40-41
Testing. *See also* Diagnosis
   amino acid letter code,
      genotype reports, 43
   and ARV (antiretroviral)
      therapies, 33, 44
   and CD4 T-cell count
      monitoring, 34, 40-41
   and cell cultures, 39
   and disease monitoring, 44
   for drug-resistance, 42
   and early HIV infection, 43-44
   ELISA (enzyme-linked
      immunosorbent assay), 34,
      35-36
   and early infection, 43-44
   initial assessment with HIV
      diagnosis, 49
   noninvasive, 37
   finger price, 34
   4th generation (p24/ELISA
      combined), 44
   genotypic analysis, 42-43
   and HIV natural history, 36
   initial assessment with HIV
      diagnosis, 49, 50
   noninvasive, 37
   overview, 58-59
   p24 antigen, 38, 39
      and early infection, 43, 44
   PCR (polymerase chain
      reaction), 34, 38-39
      and early infection, 44
   pediatrics, 45-46
   rapid-test techniques, 36-37, 49
   rationales for, 32-33

saliva, 37
and T-cell count monitoring, CD4
   (cluster differentiation 4),
   34, 40-41
and ARV (antiretroviral)
   therapy, 44
urine, 37
and viral load monitoring, 39-40
Western blot, 34, 37-38
   and initial assessment with
      HIV diagnosis, 49
Toxoplasma gondii, 253, 259, 303
Treatment. *See also individual
   conditions*
   children/communication
      disorders, 157-164. *See
      also* treatment *under*
      Children/communication
      disorders
   communication disorders,
      185-186. *See also*
      treatment *under*
      Communication disorders
      main entry
   and mental status, 186
   swallowing disorders, 186-187.
      See also treatment *under*
      Swallowing disorders *main
      entry*
Trypanosomiasis, 303
Tuberculosis
   and balance disorders, 315
   multidrug-resistant strains, 258
   neurologic involvement, 290, 291
   pediatrics, 141

U

Universal Blood and Blood-Borne
   Pathogen Precautions, CDC
   (Centers for Disease
   Control and Prevention),
   71-72

Universal (Standard) Precautions,
    65-66, 183
    WHO (World Health
        Organization)
        six standard precautions, **all**
        patients, 71-72
U.S. Centers for Disease Control,
    AIDS Surveillance Case
    Definition for Adolescents
    and Adults, 15, 46
U.S. Department of Health and
    Human Service (DHHS). *See*
    DHHS (U.S. Department of
    Health and Human
    Services)

V

Vaccines
    development, 14, 25-27
    HBV (hepatitis B), 85
    Prevnar, 213-214
VDRL (veneral disease research
    laboratory tests), 48
Ventilation, mechanical, 395
Vestibulitis, 302
Viral load monitoring, 39-40, 53
Vitamin B deficiency, 310

W

Weight loss, 395
Western blot test, 34, 37-38, 49
WHO (World Health
    Organization), 70
    early infant treatment
        recommendations, 45-46,
        57, 58
    and ethics guidelines, 129
    hand hygiene, 76-77
    hospital-acquired for infection
        prevention manual, 84
    infant diagnostic testing
        recommendations, 46
    nosocomial infection control
        guidelines, 65, 66
    oral manifestation criteria, 177
    six standard precautions, **all**
        patients, 71-72
    staging, adolescents/adults, 15,
        16, 18, 46, 49
World Medical Association, 128

X

Xerostomia
    balance disorders, 313